Clinical Reasoning in Spine Pain. Volume II

Primary Management of Cervical Disorders Using the CRISP Protocols

And

Case Studies in Primary Spine Care

Dr. Donald R. Murphy

With

Gary Jacob, DC, LAc, MPH, DipMDT
Steven L. Heffner, DC, Diplomate MDT

©2016 Donald R. Murphy
Published by: CRISP Education and Research, LLC

• DEDICATION •

This book is dedicated to all those who have committed themselves to the establishment of primary spine care services as a designated service line in the health care system, and to the primary spine practitioner as a unique and valuable role within that service line.

And to my loving, supportive family, Laura, Jessica, Alison and Melissa. They make it all worthwhile.

• AUTHOR •

Donald R. Murphy, DC, FRCC
Director of Primary Spine Care Services,
Care New England Health System

Clinical Assistant Professor, Dept. of Family Medicine,
Alpert Medical School of Brown University

Professor, Part-Time University Faculty,
Southern California University of Health Sciences

Adjunct Associate Professor, Dept. of Research,
New York Chiropractic College

• CONTRIBUTORS •

Gary Jacob, DC, LAc, MPH, DipMDT
Private Practice
Pacific Palisades, California

Steven L Heffner, DC, Diplomate MDT
McKenzie International/USA Faculty

Photography:
Alison C. Murphy
Jesse Karlin Jacob
Georges Dagher, DC

Models:
Jessica L. Murphy
Kattie Bachar
Melissa G. Murphy
Georges Dagher, DC
Donald R. Murphy, DC, FRCC

Cover design:
Jessica L. Murphy

Cover photo courtesy of Cynthia Peterson, RN, DC, M.Med.Ed.

• TABLE OF CONTENTS •

• ACKNOWLEDGEMENTS •

In Volume I of this series, I acknowledged a number of individuals who have been helpful and influential to me in my career as well as in the development of this book series. I would like to again thank all of them here, though I will not list them individually as in the previous volume. Instead I will focus on those who have been particularly helpful in the development of this volume, as well as in the advancement of the primary spine care movement.

First, I would like to that the people who contributed directly to this volume. This foremost includes the outstanding authors who contributed the disc derangement section of Chapter 2, Gary Jacob, DC, LAc, MPH, and Steven Heffner, DC, Diplomate MDT. Their expertise in describing the end range loading examination for the identification of derangement is superb. They have taken a concept that is often difficult for people to grasp and made it more easily understood.

In addition, I would like to thank Jacqueline Beres, DC for contributing the foundation for one of the cases presented in Chapter 9. Some details of this case were changed for the purpose of this book, but it was her exceptional clinical skills that helped make this case a wonderful teaching tool. I would also like to thank Georges Dagher, DC for introducing me to the thoracic rotation exercise presented in Chapter 8.

I have received valuable input from several trusted experts on the content of various chapters. These individuals include Michael J. Schneider, DC, PhD; Stephen M. Perle, DC, MS; John Ventura, DC; Brian Justice, DC; Clifford Everett, MD; Philip McClure, PT, PhD; Carol Greco, PhD; Lisa Uebelacker, PhD; Geoff Schneider, PT, PhD; Paul Dougherty, DC; Lisa Killinger, DC; Howard Vernon, DC, PhD; Barry Levin, MD; and Julia Treleaven, PhD, BPhty.

I would like to thank all those who have made key contributions to the primary spine care movement, specifically toward establishing the primary spine practitioner as a designated role in the health care system. These individuals include Scott Haldeman, DC, MD, PhD;

Michael J. Schneider, DC, PhD; John Ventura, DC; Brian Justice, DC; Thomas Neuner, DC, JD; Ian Paskowski, DC, MBA; Richard E. Vincent, DC; Gary Jacob, DC, LAc, MPH; Michael Timko PT, MS; Christopher Bise PT, MS, DPT; Kris Gongaware, DC; Brian Mock, PT, DPT; John Scaringe, DC, EdD; Robb Russell, DC; Jacqueline Beres, DC; Melissa Nagare Kimura, DC, LAc; James E. Fanale, MD; Stephen M. Perle, DC, MS; Jan Hartvigsen, DC, PhD; Kim Humphreys, DC, PhD; Geoff Outerbridge, DC, MSc; Michael Allgeier, DC; Cameron Brown, DC; Marcia Miller Spoto, PT, DC.

Finally, I would like to thank God for Being.

Donald R. Murphy, DC, FRCC

8 June 2016

• PREFACE TO VOLUME II •

Welcome to Volume II of Clinical Reasoning in Spine Pain. For those who have Volume I, I hope it has been of benefit to you and, by extension, your patients, students, colleagues and anyone else to whom you might have brought the message of high quality spine care. For those who have not yet read the first volume, I urge you to obtain a copy. While I am confident that you will still learn a great deal from Volume II, your learning will be substantially enhanced after you have read the first volume.

The first chapter of this volume revisits the concept of primary spine care and the CRISP® protocols but with a much expanded view. It discusses where the primary spine care service line and the primary spine practitioner (PSP) fit in the new emerging value-based model that is rapidly becoming the standard in health care. It also reviews the CRISP® protocols in order to prepare the reader for the chapters that follow.

The following six chapters of this book present Clinical Reasoning in Spine Pain® (the CRISP® protocols) as they apply to patients with cervical disorders. These chapters are formatted in much the same way as in Volume I, being organized around the Three Essential Questions of Diagnosis. Chapters 2, 3 and 4 each presents one of the three questions from the standpoint of diagnosis. Chapter 5 covers outcome assessment in patients with cervical disorders. Then Chapters 6 and 7 present management strategies for the factors identified with diagnostic questions 2 and 3, respectively.

Chapter 8 covers thoracic disorders, applying the CRISP® protocols for diagnosis and management in the same manner in which these protocols are applied to patients with low back and cervical disorders.

It should be noted that in these chapters that are certain topics for which there is great overlap between the diagnosis and management of patients with low back disorders and those with cervical and thoracic disorders. Therefore, in some places in this volume the reader is directed to relevant chapters in Volume I.

This particularly applies to the general principles of primary spine care (Chapter 1 in Volume I) and patient management (Chapter 8 in Volume I), history taking (Chapter 3 in Volume I), many conditions that fall under diagnostic question #1 (Chapter 4 in Volume I), anti-inflammatory nutrition (Chapter 9 in Volume I), graded exposure to address nociceptive system sensitization (Chapter 11 in Volume I), addressing psychological perpetuating factors (Chapter 11 in Volume I) and maximum medical improvement, aftercare and referral decisions (Chapter 12 in Volume I).

Many of these topics are discussed in this volume as they specifically apply to cervical patients, and some are expanded upon beyond that discussed in Volume I. However, rather than reproduce the material in Volume I that completely overlaps with the care of patients with cervical disorders, the reader is simply directed to the relevant chapters in the first volume.

Finally, Chapters 9 and 10 in this volume, which are among the most enjoyable (and, in my view, useful) things I have ever written, present case studies in primary spine care. These chapters each include nine cases, with each case presenting a different clinical scenario. These cases (except one that is adapted from a case given to me by a colleague) are an amalgam of the innumerable patients I have seen over my many years of practice as a PSP.

Each case starts with the first visit and the initial history and examination, then follows the patient all the way from diagnosis to clinical decision making to management across the full cycle (see Chapter 1 to learn what "managing across the full cycle" means). At various key points along the way the reader is asked to stop and consider a number questions about the case – impressions regarding diagnosis, management decisions, whether or not referral is indicated, why the PSP made certain decisions or communicated certain messages to the patient, etc. I think these chapters serve as a wonderful learning tool. They help the reader put together the knowledge and skills that have been gained in the previous 19 chapters between the two volumes into the context of the "real world" clinical environment. I hope you find these chapters as useful as I do.

So we are off on the next step in our adventure together toward excellence in primary spine care. I greatly appreciate the feedback I have received from many readers on Volume I of this series, as well as the positive reviews that have appeared in online forums such as the Amazon.com page where the book appears (**http://www.amazon.com/Clinical-Reasoning-Spine-Pain-Management/dp/0615888577 accessed 27 May 2016**).

Donald R. Murphy, DC, FRCC

27 May 2016

Section I:

Introduction

•Chapter 1 •

Primary Spine Care Services, the CRISP® Protocols and the Value Model

Introduction

The purpose of this chapter is to briefly revisit and build upon several concepts presented in Volume I of this series. In Chapter 1 of Volume I, the primary spine practitioner (PSP) was discussed as a new practitioner type playing a unique and defined role in the health care system. Here we will expand this discussion to include not only this new practitioner type but also primary spine care services as a new health care service line. We will then review Clinical Reasoning in Spine Pain® (the CRISP® protocols) specifically in light of the unique role of the PSP. Finally, we will discuss how the PSP and the primary spine care service line can contribute to the creation of greater *value* to the health care system and society and greater *quality of care* for patients with spine related disorders (SRDs).

Primary Spine Care and the Primary Spine Practitioner

Primary spine care is an emerging service line in the health care system, and the PSP is a new practitioner type that is the linchpin of this service line. Primary spine care services and the PSP were developed in response to the need for greater efficiency, effectiveness and cohesiveness to spine care (see Haldeman and Murphy, et al in Recommended Reading list). Back in 2008 Haldeman and Dagenais (see Recommended Reading list) wrote of the "supermarket approach" to understanding the predicament faced by patients with SRDs. They likened this predicament to someone walking through a foreign supermarket, having no understanding of the products that are on the shelves. In the case of patients with SRDs, the foreign supermarket analogy refers to patients attempting to navigate the vast number of products, services and practitioner types that claim to have something to offer for back and neck pain. Most patients lack the ability to discern what is best for them, and have no one to guide them on a path to recovery.

In no other area in health care is there such a predicament, at least not to the extent that exists in the spine world. With other medical problems, such as diabetes, heart disease or even oral health problems, there is a primary care practitioner (in the case of oral health, this is the general dentist) who serves as the point person in the management of the disorder. When needed, there are specialists who may play a role in the care of any particular patient, depending on the circumstances. But it is the primary-level practitioner who initially diagnoses the disorder, manages the majority without the need for referral, makes decisions regarding the recommendation of special tests or specialist services, and generally guides the patient along the process of managing the condition.

In the area of SRDs, traditional primary care practitioners (which include family medicine and general internal medicine physicians, nurse practitioners and physician's assistants) are not well trained, and generally do not have the time, to provide optimal primary care for patients with SRDs. These fine professionals do the best they can, but patients are still left to navigate the spine care "supermarket" largely on their own. Thus the need for a designated primary-level provider for these patients – the PSP.

Primary Spine Care Services

This book series has discussed at great length the role of the PSP in spine care, and the place of this practitioner type in the health care system. Primary spine care services is the service line within which the PSP functions as the "hub of the wheel". Primary spine care services include any practitioner who acts as "first touch", i.e., first contact, within a community, be it an integrated practice unit, hospital, group practice, private office or emergency setting.

The primary spine care service line can include all primary care personnel as well as anyone else who may be the first contact that the SRD patient has with the health care system. This may include emergency department personnel, occupational medicine physicians, community chiropractic physicians and community physical therapists – as well as, of course, the PSP.

The ideal situation is one in which each of these "first touch" providers is trained in an evidence-based approach to front-line management of patients with SRDs. This should be coupled with an evidence-based decision-making process regarding when a patient requires referral for additional diagnostic testing or invasive procedures (which applies to a small minority of patients) or to the PSP.

The PSP, as stated earlier, manages the majority of patients without the need for referral, and functions in a team environment that involves any other specialized practitioner who may play a role in certain circumstances that require services that are beyond the PSP's skill set or time constraints. This team environment may be a formal integrated practice unit, a hospital system or other similar system, or may involve a more informal collection of individual practitioners who are capable of working together using a team approach.

The Team Approach to Spine Care

There have been recent calls for a better coordinated approach to health care in general, and spine care in particular. This has proven to be challenging because health care practitioners have traditionally functioned in "silos", with each practitioner working on his- or her own, or perhaps grouped according to specialty, such as orthopedics or rheumatology, rather than according to a particular patient population. To use the imagery of Atul Gawande, MD (see Recommended Reading list), doctors typically function as "cowboys" – independent, self-sufficient (seemingly, at least) and capable of handling whatever comes along without the need for others.

Gawande has recommended that the health care system move from the imagery of the practitioner acting as a lone "cowboy" to practitioners working together as part of a "pit crew". Gawande's "pit crew" analogy refers to auto racing. In this sport the pit crew functions as an integrated unit, with each individual playing a key, and very specific, role within the crew. Each individual is excellent at performing a particular function, or at least he or she had better be, if the crew as a whole is to be successful. Races can be won or lost on the basis of how effective the pit crew is able to work together. Thus, the jackman has specific job to do, which is different from the rear tire changer or the gas man (of course, a woman can, and often does, perform these roles).

Each pit crew must have a "crew chief" - the point person who is responsible for coordinating the activities of all the members of the crew. This is one of the roles of the PSP within the primary spine care service line.

Where the primary spine care service line differs from the pit crew in auto racing is that, in the majority of patients, the PSP is capable of handling the situation without needing the remainder of the crew. However, in a small, but sizable and critically important, minority of patients, an efficient "pit crew", with the PSP as "crew chief", is essential in establishing a successful spine care system.

Managing the patient across the full cycle

Michael Porter, one of the leading voices in bringing the value model to health care (see recommended reading list), emphasizes the importance of health care systems *managing the patient across the full cycle*. The *full cycle* means the entire process of care from the patient's initial encounter with the health care system for a certain problem to a designated end point. Obviously, the "end point" will widely differ depending on the patient and depending on the disease state. Many patients with chronic illnesses, such as diabetes and hypertension, may require ongoing follow up within that cycle, with no clear "end point".

The principle of managing patients across the full cycle is particularly important in the field of SRDs. One of the most important roles of the PSP is to serve as the point person who guides the patient across the full cycle of care. This means that it is the PSP who manages the situation from point A to point Z, i.e., from the point at which the patient is having a pain, disability and suffering experience (point A) to the point of resolution (or sufficient management) of that experience (point Z).

With most SRD patients, point A to point Z occurs purely with the PSP. In other words, as has been discussed repeatedly in this book series, one of the hallmarks of effective primary spine care is that the PSP is able to *manage the patient without the need for referral* in the majority of cases. However, in the relative minority who require additional testing, specialist consult or intensive or invasive procedures, it is the PSP who coordinates these processes and, most important, guides the patient every step of the way on the path to resolution. There may be other practitioners who play important roles in this process, but it is the PSP who directs the patient along the process, making sure the patient remains engaged and on track toward the most rapid and beneficial resolution possible.

This often requires a team approach, with each team member clearly knowing and accepting his or her role, as well as where this role fits within the cycle. For this reason, a highly beneficial environment for primary spine care services is within an integrated practice unit or pathway-oriented system in which care coordination can be maximized.

As stated earlier, "resolution" will mean different things to different patients. In the majority of cases it will mean the patient being released from the active care plan, free of pain (and often pain-free*), having been provided with several important tools (see Chapter 12 in Volume I of this series):

- Tools of prevention designed to lessen the likelihood of recurrence of the problem;

- Tools of self-management in case recurrence does arise, and;

- Tools of decision making if self-management of recurrence does not resolve the problem, or if a new SRD arises.

Clinical Reasoning in Spine Pain®

Clinical Reasoning in Spine Pain® (the CRISP® protocols) was developed based on the vast literature on the mechanisms, etiology, diagnosis and management of patients with SRDs. This involved my spending over 20 years studying the spine literature and finding that, while a lot of great work was done in this field, no single treatment was found to be most valuable. I concluded that this was because, first, SRDs are multifactorial in etiology and mechanism and, second, each patient experiences a SRD in his or her own unique way. I therefore concluded that a multi-modal approach that can be individualized to address the unique diagnostic features in each patient and that focuses on *the practitioner getting to know the patient as an individual* is needed for this complex and often confusing group of disorders.

*There is a difference between being pain-free and being free of pain, and understanding this difference is critical to the PSP. Being pain-free at any moment means not feeling any pain at that moment. Many patients, when they complete a care process under the direction of a PSP, will end up being pain-free. But that does not necessarily mean they are free of pain. This is because pain is a part of life, and pain related to the spine is a particularly common type of pain. Therefore, being pain-free at any given moment is great, however, there is a strong likelihood that pain will be experienced at some time in the future. There are strategies that one can engage in that lessen the frequency of future pain. But even if one engages in these strategies, it is almost certain that spinal pain will be experienced at some time in the future.

Being free of pain is different. Being free of pain means being fully in charge of life *in spite of the presence or absence of pain at any given moment*. When one is free of pain, any pain that may arise does not dictate one's quality of life and one's ability to live an effective life according to one's most deeply held values.

After completion of care, a patient who is pain-free but has not been taught to understand pain and its relationship to function, and has not been taught to manage future pain appropriately, may still not be free of pain!

It is essential that the PSP strive to move every patient in the direction of being free of pain. Helping the patient become pain-free is also a worthy goal. However, freedom from pain is the ultimate goal.

No one can live an entire life pain-free, but nearly everyone can live life free of pain.

Through my study I came to realize that there are a number of individual diagnostic and treatment approaches that are beneficial in addressing specific aspects of the SRD experience. But the randomized, controlled trials in the field generally show that each approach, when randomly applied to groups of patients without regard for diagnosis or individualization, contributes relatively little to the overall picture. This has led to many researchers and clinicians to conclude that nearly every diagnostic and treatment approach was virtually, or completely, worthless!

I decided to see it differently. It seems that the fact that each individual approach contributes a small amount means that a combination of approaches might add up to "contributing a lot". More importantly, the key to effectiveness is figuring out *in each individual patient* what combination of approaches is most important for *that person's problem*.

Moreover, it became apparent that a focus on "treating pain" was misguided because what we are "treating" is *an individual human being* who is suffering due to *pain and its resulting distress that comes from disability, fear and uncertainty*.

The logical conclusion was that any diagnostic and management approach that is going to be helpful has to involve the following features:

1. The recognition of the multifactorial nature of SRDs.

2. The recognition that for most of the contributing factors there is no single diagnostic test that definitively and objectively demonstrates its presence. Therefore a comfort level with "gray areas" was necessary to effectively help patients with SRDs.

3. The recognition that it is not a spine that is seeking our help, it is an individual human being who is having a pain, disability and suffering experience.

4. The recognition that patients want to know what is causing their suffering. They want a reasonable explanation. Telling them they have "non-specific back pain" or that they can be "classified" is unsatisfactory.

5. The recognition that while there are several treatments that have been shown to be beneficial in the treatment of SRDs (and many others that have not), it is the *communication context* in which the treatment is applied that plays a large role in the benefit to the patient.

6. Therefore, an integrated approach that allows the clinician to consider all of the possible contributing factors in each individual patient is needed in order to arrive at a diagnosis that is relevant to each patient.

7. And an integrated approach to treatment decision making is needed that addresses the various factors that are relevant to each individual patient.

As I further studied the literature I realized that there was no single study or group of studies that provided a definitive approach to SRDs. However, I discovered that there was a great deal of information from high-quality scientists that allowed me to develop an integrated approach that included all of the features listed above. This resulted in the CRISP® protocols.

A Review of Clinical Reasoning in Spine Pain®

To understand and appropriately apply the CRISP® protocols, certain important things must be understood:

1. The purpose of CRISP® is to provide a means by which the spine practitioner can apply an evidence-based approach to the evaluation of the patient in order to arrive at a diagnosis.

2. This process considers not only the individual clinical entities that may be present but *the whole patient*. As stated earlier, it is a whole human being who is having a pain, disability and suffering experience that brings him or her to the practitioner. Effective application of the CRISP® protocols requires this whole-person context.

3. The establishment of a working diagnosis identifying the key factors contributing to the patient's pain, disability and suffering experience allows the practitioner to make clinical decisions about the best management strategy. That is, as with all areas of medicine, the treatment plan is based on the diagnosis.

4. Within the context of the CRISP® protocols there are certain treatment approaches that are recommended for each potential contributing factor. Specifics regarding this can be found in Chapters 9, 10 and 11 in Volume I of this series and in Chapters 6, 7 and 8 of this volume. However, it is not simply the application of therapeutic techniques that provides benefit to the patient. The communication context is also critically important to obtaining a good outcome.

5. Regardless of the diagnosis and the clinical decisions regarding management, it is essential to monitor the results of the approach, using formal outcome assessment tools as well as relationship-centered communication. Expertly applied diagnostic and therapeutic methodology is irrelevant if it does not result in an improved quality of life for the patient.

The CRISP® protocols involve the practitioner asking the Three Essential Questions of Diagnosis:

1. Do the presenting symptoms reflect a visceral disorder, or a serious or potentially life?

2. Where is the pain coming from?

3. What is happening with this person as a whole that would cause the pain experience to develop and persist?

The first question considers traditional "red flag" conditions such as cancer, infection, fracture and cauda equina syndrome as well as other medical conditions that can produce pain in the spine such as gastrointestinal, genitourinary and neurological disorders.

The second question considers the possible presence of four clinical entities that can produce pain:

- Disc derangement

- Joint dysfunction

- Radiculopathy

- Myofascial trigger points

The third question considers mechanical, neurophysiological and psychological perpetuating factors such as:

- Dynamic and passive instability

- Nociceptive system sensitization

- Oculomotor dysfunction

- Fear

- Catastrophizing

- Passive coping

- Low self-efficacy

- Depression

- Anxiety

- Hypervigilance for symptoms

- Cognitive fusion

- Perceived injustice

In any given patient, one or more (usually more) of these factors contributes to the overall clinical picture, and there is often great interaction between the factors. Therefore, in most patients a multimodal approach is required. There are a number of general approaches that are applicable to all patients, as well as specific approaches that are designed to address the individual elements that make up the diagnosis.

It is also important to reiterate that the various pain generating and perpetuating factors listed above are *inextricably linked*. In other words, while the biological, psychological and social factors are discussed individually in this book series for learning purposes, it is essential for the practitioner to think and act in terms of the patient and the SRD that he or she is experiencing being an *integrated whole*.

Asking and answering the three questions of diagnosis, and applying therapeutic approaches that address the relevant factors, is what makes up the mechanics of the CRISP® protocols.

However, it must be realized that the real value of CRISP® comes in the whole, rather than the sum of its parts.

Bringing Value to Spine Care

Before discussing bringing value to spine care, we must first look at what value means in the context of health care in general and spine care in particular. In a nutshell, value is calculated simply as:

Value = outcome ÷ costs

Therefore, the highest value care is that which provides the best possible outcome at the lowest possible price.

However, it is important for us to not only provide high value care, but *high quality* care. High quality care is that which is not only of high value, but also provides the patient with the most pleasant and satisfying experience possible as well as providing maximum safety to the patient. Thus, the formula for quality of care might look something like this:

High quality care = (clinical outcome + patient experience) ÷ (financial cost + risk of harm)

This formula might not exactly be workable from a mathematical standpoint, but it illustrates the point that high quality spine care goes beyond mere value.

Primary spine care services as discussed in this book series seeks to satisfy both the value equation and the quality equation by focusing on accurate diagnosis, following the principles of minimalism and patient empowerment, and applying the least invasive approaches as a first-line approach.

Porter and Lee (see Recommended Reading list), in discussing improved value in spine care, provide an example of one Integrated Practice Unit in which each patient entering the system is seen by a team that includes two professionals – a physical therapist and a physician trained care in physical medicine and rehabilitation. In this system it is determined up front which patients require additional evaluation and which patients require surgical intervention, with the majority of patients receiving "physical therapy". All patients are managed within a system that consists of a team of professionals working in the best interest of the patient. They discuss the increase in efficiency that has resulted from this approach.

The implementation of primary spine care serves takes this one step further. The presence of an appropriately trained PSP dramatically improves the efficiency of this approach by having *one* professional see the patient on the front end, rather than two professionals. Right from the start, this doubles efficiency. The one front-end professional, the PSP, is trained to manage the majority of patients without the need for referral *in addition to* being able to make differential diagnostic decisions regarding additional investigation, referral decisions regarding intensive and invasive procedures *and* to follow and guide the patient across the full cycle. Because of this, the system not only has effective, safe, minimalist care for the majority of patients, but also a care coordinator who can help the patient navigate through the system. All in a single professional.

The implementation of PSP services brings simplicity to the current massive complexity of spine care. This helps reduce downstream costs by maximizing first-line care for patients with SRDs and providing right-sizing with regard to specialty care. That is, patients see the professional who is best suited to their current needs. This means non-surgical patients do not see surgeons, patients who do not need imaging do not receive imaging and patients who can be well-managed non-medically do not receive unnecessary prescription or injected medications. The other side of this, of course, is that the implementation of PSP services helps ensure that surgical patients see surgeons, patients who need injections receive them in a timely fashion and diagnostic testing is pursued when it is most needed and useful. This benefits patients and the healthcare system, but also benefits specialists because they see an appropriate case mix; the vast majority of patients the specialist sees are patients who are best suited for their unique knowledge and skills.

Add to this an organized and integrated spine care pathway. This is a system in which front-end personnel (PSPs as well as family medicine, internal medicine, occupational medicine and emergency medicine physicians, nurse practitioners, physician assistants), are trained to identify SRD patients who can be managed at the primary care level, as well as those who require immediate investigation (i.e., "red flag" patients). In addition, the non-PSP front-end professionals are also trained to identify patients who require PSP services. The PSP, as discussed at length here, then applies evidence-based care as well as coordination of care, follow-up and guidance across the full cycle. With the proper implementation of a system

such as this (which is not an easy task, but can be done), efficiency and, as a result, value and quality, are taken to a whole new level.

This is not just a theoretical concept. Early data suggests that this approach works in the real world (see Paskowski, et al and Allgeier, et al in Recommended Reading list).

Dramatic improvement in the value and quality of care for patients with SRDs is within our reach. By applying an organized, systematic approach to both the care of individual patients and to the implementation of primary and specialty spine care services, we can revolutionize the spine world. The result will be greater efficiency, increased cost-effectiveness and, most important, improved well-being for the millions of patients who suffer from SRDs.

Recommended Reading

Allgeier M, Ventura JM, Murphy DR. Replication of a Multidisciplinary Hospital Based Clinical Pathway for the Management of Low Back Pain. Spine J. 2016;15(10S):117S-8S.

Gawande A. Cowboys and Pit Crews. Commencement Address, Harvard Medical School. 2011.

Haldeman S. Looking forward. In: Phillips RB. The Journey of Scott Haldeman. Spine Care Specialist and Researcher. National Chiropractic Mutual Holding Company, 2009: 447-462.

Haldeman S, Dagenais S. A supermarket approach to the evidence-informed management of chronic low back pain. Spine J. 2008 Jan-Feb;8(1):1-7.

Murphy DR, Justice BD, Paskowski IC, Perle SM, Schneider MJ. The Establishment of a Primary Spine Care Practitioner and its Benefits to Health Care Reform in the United States. Chiropr Man Therap. 2011 Jul 21;19(1):17.

Murphy DR. Primary spine care services: responding to runaway costs and disappointing outcomes in spine care. R I Med J (2013). 2014;97(10):47-9.

Murphy DR, Hurwitz EL, Gregory AA, Clary R. A nonsurgical approach to the management of patients with cervical radiculopathy: A prospective observational cohort study. J Manipulative Physiol Ther. 2006;29(4):279-87.

Murphy DR, Hurwitz EL, Gregory AA, Clary R. A non-surgical approach to the management of lumbar spinal stenosis: a prospective observational cohort study. BMC Musculoskelet Disord. 2006;7:16.

Murphy DR, Hurwitz EL. A theoretical model for the development of a diagnosis-based clinical decision rule for the management of patients with spinal pain. BMC Musculoskelet Disord. 2007;8:75.

Murphy DR, Hurwitz EL, Nelson CF. A diagnosis-based clinical decision rule for patients with spinal pain. Part 2: Review of the literature. Chiropr Osteop. 2008;16:8.

Murphy DR, Hurwitz EL, McGovern EE. Outcome of pregnancy-related lumbopelvic pain treated according to a diagnosis-based decision rule: a prospective observational cohort study. J Manipulative Physiol Ther. 2009 Oct;32(8):616-24.

Murphy DR, Hurwitz EL, McGovern EE. A nonsurgical approach to the management of patients with lumbar radiculopathy secondary to herniated disk: a prospective observational cohort study with follow-up. J Manipulative Physiol Ther. 2009 Nov-Dec;32(9):723-33.

Murphy DR, Hurwitz EL, Nelson CF. A diagnosis-based clinical decision rule for spinal pain part 2: review of the literature. Chiropr Osteopat. 2008;16:7.

Murphy DR, Hurwitz EL. Application of a Diagnosis-Based Clinical Decision Guide in Patients with Neck Pain. Chiropr Man Therap. 2011 Aug 27;19(1):19.

Murphy DR, Hurwitz EL. Application of a Diagnosis-Based Clinical Decision Guide in Patients with Low Back Pain. Chiropr Man Therap. 2011 Oct 21;19(1):26.

Paskowski I, Schneider M, Stevans J, Ventura JM, Justice BD. A hospital-based standardized spine care pathway: report of a multidisciplinary, evidence-based process. J Manipulative Physiol Ther. 2011 Feb;34(2):98-106.

Porter ME, Teisberg EO. Redefining Health Care: Creating Value-Based Competition on Results. Boston, MA: Harvard Business School Press; 2006.

Porter ME, Lee TH. The strategy that will fix health care. Harvard Bus Rev. 2013;Oct:1-19.

Section II:

Diagnosis Using the Clinical reasoning in Spine Pain® Protocols

• Chapter 2 •

Diagnostic Question #1. Do the presenting symptoms reflect a visceral disorder, or a serious or potentially life-threatening illness?

Introduction

In the application of Clinical Reasoning in Spine Pain® (the CRISP® protocols) the first diagnostic question allows the practitioner to, through history and examination, consider certain illnesses, some serious and/or life threatening, some less so, that can produce cervical related complaints or headache. Chapter 4 of Volume I of this series discusses visceral disorders or potentially serious illnesses for which low back pain may be one of the initial symptoms. Many of the conditions discussed in that chapter, and the historical and examination factors that would lead the spine practitioner to suspect them, apply to patients with cervical disorders (CDs) as well. In addition, discussion of the use of imaging and special tests is provided in that chapter, and will not be repeated here except as it specifically applies to the disorders presented in this chapter. The reader is directed to Chapter 4 in Volume I for details. A thorough understanding of both this chapter and Chapter 4 of Volume I of this series is necessary to appropriately seek the answer to diagnostic question #1 in both cervical and low back disorder patients.

Conditions considered under diagnostic question #1 that are common to both low back and cervical patients are listed in Table 1. However there are certain conditions that the spine practitioner must be particularly cognizant of when considering diagnostic question #1 in cervical patients.

Included in this chapter are conditions that are of particular importance for the neck pain and/or headache patient. The most important condition of concern for the neck and/or arm pain patient, besides those covered in Volume I in this series, is cervical myelopathy. For the headache patient, the conditions of greatest concern are tumor, infection, subarachnoid hemorrhage, cervical artery dissection, temporal arteritis and meningitis.

Table 2-1. Conditions that are considered under diagnostic question #1 and their detection.

Disorder	Suggested by
Cancer	History of cancer No position of relief Fever Constitutional symptoms Unexplained weight loss Blood in the stool Pain in multiple sites
Benign tumor	Local severe pain No position of relief Relief with NSAID Pain on percussion
Infection	History of fever or chills Febrile (but often afebrile) Point tenderness Immunocompromised individual History of diabetes
Fracture	History of trauma History of osteopenia or osteoporosis Pain on percussion
GI disease	GI complaints Pain with food Positive abdominal exam

See Chapters 3 and 4 in Volume I of this series for general information regarding history taking particularly as it relates to diagnostic question #1.

The Neurological Screening Examination

A careful neurologic exam should be carried out in all patients. In a patient with cervical related disorders, the neurologic exam should at a minimum include sensory, motor and reflex examination of the upper and lower extremities. In headache patients, the full neurologic screening examination should be routinely carried out.

However, it is advisable for the spine practitioner who is not accustomed to performing the full neurologic screening examination to do so in all patients. This will allow the practitioner to refine his or her skills in performing the examination expertly and efficiently. Once this level of mastery of the full neurologic screening examination is achieved, the practitioner can tailor the examination to each particular patient situation.

An approach to screening the entire peripheral and central nervous system within four minutes is presented in Chapter 4 in Volume I of this series. Table 2 presents the components of this examination.

Table 2-2. The neurologic screening examination

Standing	Seated
Heel walking	Cranial nerve examination ◦ Visual fields ◦ Pursuit EOM ◦ Sensory ◦ Motor ◦ Tongue ◦ Palate ◦ Fundoscopy

Toe walking	Sensory to pinprick in the upper and lower extremities
Tandem walking	Motor of the upper and lower extremities
Romberg's position	Muscle stretch reflexes of the upper and lower extremities
	Plantar response
	Rapid alternating movements
	Heel-to-shin movements
	Finger-to-nose movements
	Pronator drift

Cervical Spondylotic Myelopathy

As discussed in Chapter 2 of Volume I in this series, a common cause of radiculopathy is spinal stenosis. When degenerative changes in the cervical spine lead to the development of osteophytes, facet joint hypertrophy, hypertrophy of the ligamentum flavum, or any combination of these, encroachment on the lateral canal or lateral recess (lateral stenosis) can cause radiculopathy (Fig. 2-1).

However if this same process occurs centrally (central stenosis), it can lead to encroachment on the spinal cord and cause cervical spondylotic myelopathy (CSM) (Fig. 2-2). It should be noted that central stenosis can occur asymptomatically, so if this finding is detected on imaging, it does not necessarily indicate the presence of CSM. The diagnosis must be made based on clinical findings.

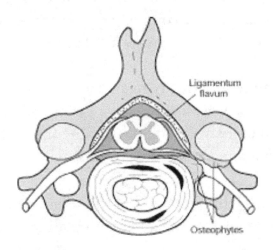

Figure 2-1. Lateral stenosis. Reprinted with permission from Murphy DR, ed. Conservative Management of Cervical Spine Syndromes. New York: McGraw-Hill, 2000.

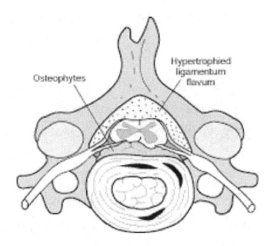

Figure 2-2. Central stenosis. This can, but does not always, lead to cervical spondylotic myelopathy. Reprinted with permission from Murphy DR, ed. Conservative Management of Cervical Spine Syndromes. New York: McGraw-Hill, 2000.

Historical Factors Associated with Cervical Spondylotic Myelopathy

Often the patient with CSM will present with neck and upper extremity pain, as the same stenotic process that leads to CSM can also cause radiculopathy. However the busy spine practitioner will encounter many patients who will only present with axial neck pain, without upper extremity pain who have CSM that may not have been previously detected.

- Age: Typically the patient with CSM will be over 50. In fact, CSM is the most common cause of myelopathy in older adults.

- Male predominance: CSM is more common in males by about a 2.4:1 ratio

- Pain: Particularly fleeting pains in the lower extremities

- Radicular sensory symptoms in the upper extremities with non-radicular sensory symptoms in the lower extremities: Often patients will complain of paresthesia or numbness in one or both upper extremities as well as in the lower extremities.

- Ataxia: This can either result from lower extremity spasticity related to anterolateral compression of the spinal cord (affecting the corticospinal tracts) or decreased proprioception related to posterior compression of the spinal cord (affecting the posterior columns). Or it can result from a combination of both these factors.

- Difficulty with fine motor movements of the hands: Examples of this are difficulty with buttoning a shirt, opening or closing a zipper, sewing and manipulating small items.

- Bladder difficulty: This is a late manifestation.

Examination Findings in Patients with Cervical Spondylotic Myelopathy

- Spasticity: This can often be seen on gait in the form of circumduction of one leg, stiff-legged walking, scissored gait, in which the knees are relatively close together while the patient walks, decreased arm swing or unsteadiness, with the patient falling toward the side of greater spasticity.

- Difficulty with heel walking: Often the earliest motor weakness in patients with CSM is manifested in the tibialis anterior. This weakness can be subtle and may not be detected on manual muscle strength testing. However, the patient may have difficulty walking on the heels on one or both sides. It is important to observe carefully because early in the disease the patient might be able to raise the forefoot, but not as fully as normal.

- Romberg's position: Particularly with involvement of the posterior columns, the patient may have difficulty standing in Romberg's position (standing still with the feet together) with eyes closed. For this reason it is important that the practitioner remain close to the patient in whom CSM is suspected while performing this test, in case the patient falls during the test.

- "Myelopathy hand": This is wasting of the intrinsic muscles of the hand that can be detected visually. Wasting of the shoulder musculature can also sometimes be found.

- Decreased joint position and vibration sense: As with Romberg's position, this particularly pertains to patients with posterior column involvement.

- Hyper-reflexia: Increased muscle stretch reflexes (often referred to as deep tendon reflexes) are found below the level of the lesion. Thus they are often found in both the upper and lower extremities but may be limited to only the lower extremities if the lesion is in the lower cervical spine. An "inverted radial reflex" is often found, i.e., when testing the brachioradialis reflex flexion of the fingers occurs. It should be noted that in a patient with CSM along with C6 radiculopathy, the brachioradialis reflex may be diminished or absent despite the presence of finger flexion upon reflex examination. In the lower extremity the practitioner may note a paradoxical ankle jerk, i.e., testing of the Achilles reflexes leads not only to plantar flexion of the ankle but also flexion of the knee.

- Upgoing toes: A true upgoing toe on plantar response testing (Babinski's sign) is a clear sign of an upper motor neuron lesion. However, interpretation of the plantar response is an art, as a true upgoing toe must be distinguished from a withdrawal response.

- Slowed movements: This can be tested in the upper extremities by having the patient perform rapid alternating movements, alternately tapping the hand on the thigh with the palmar and volar surface as rapidly as possible. It can also be tested by having the patient open and close the fist as rapidly as possible. Normally, patients should be able to do this 20 times in 10 seconds. It can be tested in the lower extremity by having the patient tap the toe against the floor or against the examiner's hand as rapidly as possible. Comparing one side to the other may help detect unilateral involvement.

- Lhermitte's sign: This can be identified by actively or passively flexing the patient's cervical spine. The sign is present if this causes an electric-like sensation down the spine and/or into the extremities.

Localizing the lesion

In a patient in whom examination findings create suspicion a central nervous system (CNS) process it is important to localize the lesion so a determination can be made as to what area of the CNS to investigate with imaging. A simple way to do this is as follows:

- Upgoing toes: In a patient who exhibits upgoing toes on testing the plantar response, a CNS lesion, specifically an upper motor neuron lesion, should be suspected. However, the presence of upgoing toes does not allow the practitioner to determine the level in the nervous system that is involved.

- Muscle stretch reflexes: A patient with an upper motor neuron lesion will typically have muscle stretch reflexes that when tested are graded 3+ (increased) or 4+ (clonus). In the CSM patient hyper-reflexia will usually be found in both the upper and lower extremities. However, this does not distinguish between a lesion in the cervical spine and a lesion in the brain.

  It is important to note that because CSM most commonly occurs in older people, comorbidities may affect the examination findings. This particularly applies to the patient with CSM who also has diabetes. Patients with diabetes in general often have diminished or absent muscle stretch reflexes. This especially applies to the ankle jerks. Thus, in a patient with diabetes who has +1 or +2 grade ankle jerks, hyper-reflexia should be suspected.

- Abdominal cutaneous reflexes (umbilical reflexes): These reflexes are examined by scraping the skin over the abdomen on either side of the umbilicus, both just below the umbilicus and just above the umbilicus. This is best done using the tail end of the reflex hammer. Absence of the reflex below the umbilicus suggests that the lesion is at least at the level of T10-12 or higher. Absence of the reflex above the umbilicus suggests that the lesion is at least at the level of T8-10 or higher. It is important to note that many people naturally have asymmetric abdominal reflexes. Thus, it is the *absence* of the reflex, bilaterally or unilaterally, that is of clinical significance.

- Hoffman's and Tromner's signs: There is some controversy over which of these signs is more sensitive in detecting a possible upper motor neuron lesion, but as both signs are elicited with the patient in the exact same position, it makes sense to examine for both signs. Hoffman's sign is elicited by flicking downward on the distal phalanx of the middle finger of the relaxed hand while Tromner's sign is elicited by flicking upward on the middle finger of the relaxed hand. The presence of flexion of the fingers and adduction of the thumb upon either of these maneuvers suggests that the lesion is at least at the C5 or C6 level or higher. It should be noted that some patients who are naturally hyper-reflexic, in the absence of an upper motor neuron lesion, may have the presence of Hoffman's or Tromner's signs. Thus, the false-positive rate of these signs is fairly high. However, in a patient with other signs and symptoms of an upper motor neuron lesion, these signs are still useful in the localization process.

- Scapulohumeral reflex: This is elicited by using the reflex hammer to tap on the acromion process and the spine of the scapula. The reflex is present if there is abduction of the shoulder with tapping of the acromion process and/or elevation of the shoulder with tapping of the spine of the scapula. The presence of this sign places the lesion at least at the level of the upper cervical spine or higher. As with Hoffman's and Tromner's signs, the scapulohumeral reflex is occasionally present in patients who are naturally hyper-reflexic even in the absence of an upper motor neuron lesion.

- Jaw jerk reflex: This is elicited by the practitioner placing his or her index finger on the patient's chin and having the patient slightly open the mouth and relax. The practitioner taps downward with the reflex hammer on the finger, looking for rapid closing of the mouth in response. Hyper-reflexia of the jaw jerk reflex suggests that the lesion is at the level of the brainstem or higher.

- Sensory level: In a patient who has sensory loss in the lower extremities and in whom cervical myelopathy is suspected, the practitioner gently touches the skin with a sharp object over the lower back to see if the patient can feel the sharp pinprick. If the patient cannot, the practitioner progressively moves up the spine, touching the skin at points at approximately one inch intervals, asking the patient to indicate whether there is a point at which he or she suddenly can feel the pinprick. The point at which sensibility becomes present is the sensory level. This helps localize the level of the spinal cord lesion.

Localizing the lesion on exam will help the practitioner make the decision as to what part of the nervous system to image. In a patient with CSM, the localization process will implicate the cervical spine as the location of the lesion. In other words, typically there will be upgoing toes, hyper-reflexia in the upper and lower extremities, absent umbilical reflexes and present Hoffman's and/or Tromner's signs. The scapulohumeral reflex may or may not be present, depending on how high the lesion is in the cervical spine. The jaw jerk will be normal. If the patient has sensory loss as a result of the CSM, there will typically be a sensory level at the level of the lesion.

Imaging

The imaging modality of choice in a patient in whom CSM is suspected is MRI of the cervical spine. This will demonstrate compression on the spinal cord and may or may not exhibit high signal in the cord on the T2-weighted images. High signal in the cord may represent edema, inflammation, ischemia, myelomalacia (softening of the cord), or gliosis (a collection of glial cells in response to neuronal damage). In some cases there may also be low signal in the cord on the T1-weighted images.

Measurement of severity of the myelopathy can be made using the modified Japanese Orthopedic Association scale (see Benzel, et al in Recommended Reading list):

Motor dysfunction score of the upper extremities

  0   Inability to move hands

  1   Inability to eat with a spoon, but able to move hands

  2   Inability to button shirt, but able to eat with a spoon

3 Able to button shirt with great difficulty

4 Able to button shirt with slight difficulty

5 No dysfunction

Motor dysfunction score of the lower extremities

0 Complete loss of motor and sensory function

1 Sensory preservation without ability to move legs

2 Able to move legs, but unable to walk

3 Able to walk on flat floor with a walking aid (i.e., cane or crutch)

4 Able to walk up and/or down stairs with hand rail

5 Moderate to significant lack of stability, but able to walk up and/or down stairs without hand rail

6 Mild lack of stability but walks with smooth reciprocation unaided

7 No dysfunction

Sensory dysfunction score of the upper extremities

0 Complete loss of hand sensation

1 Severe sensory loss or pain

2 Mild sensory loss

3 No sensory loss

Sphincter dysfunction score

0   Inability to micturate voluntarily

1   Marked difficulty with micturition

2   Mild to moderate difficulty with micturition

3   Normal micturition

This scale is scored by the practitioner, based on the clinical findings. A score $\geq$12 is considered mild. Any score <12 is considered moderate or severe.

A patient with moderate or severe CSM should be referred for spine surgical consult. The majority of patients with mild CSM do not progress (see Oshima, et al in Recommended Reading list), so immediate surgical referral is not necessary unless they have risk factors for progression. Risk factors for progression in patients with mild myelopathy, based on the study by Oshima, et al provided in the Recommended Reading list, include a large global cervical range of motion, kyphotic angle at the segment of maximal compression and spondylolisthesis at the point of maximum compression. Oshima, et al measured global range of motion radiographically and it is not clear how they went about this, but in the absence of flexion-extension radiographs it is reasonable to use physical examination to assess for global range of motion that is larger than would be expected based on the patient's age. In a patient with any signs or symptoms in whom clear evidence of passive instability is found (see Chapter 4), surgical consult is indicated.

In patients with mild myelopathy who do not have significant risk factors, a discussion should take place regarding the availability of surgical consult. However, a careful conservative approach can be taken in these patients. Cervical stabilization exercises (see Chapter 7) can be provided. It is important to monitor for increased symptoms as they are performing these exercises. Sometimes a cervical collar is advocated.

It is possible in a patient with mild CSM that minor trauma, such as a fall or a low-speed motor vehicle collision may lead to acute spinal cord injury, but the evidence is not entirely clear about this; the possible risk should be weighed against the risk of surgery.

In patients with mild CSM without risk factors who are managed conservatively, advice should be given to avoid high-risk activities. Examples of high-risk activities are heavy lifting and vigorous or prolonged flexion or extension of the head. The patient should particularly be advised against activities that involve risk of fall such as mountain climbing, rock climbing and walking on slippery surfaces. Further, these patients should be monitored at least every three to six months for signs of progression. Depending on comfort level, the primary spine practitioner may choose to provide this monitoring or may choose to refer the patient to a neurologist or neurosurgeon for this purpose.

There are times in which an acute centrally-located disc herniation can cause acute myelopathy. This is a neurologically unstable condition. Thus, these patients should be referred immediately for spine surgical consult, even if the myelopathy can be classified as mild.

Syringomyelia

Syringomyelia is a condition in which a cavity, called a syrinx, develops in the center of the spinal cord. This is essentially a focal dilatation of the central canal of the spinal cord, which can further expand as it becomes filled with cerebrospinal fluid. It can develop post-traumatically and there is often a delay in the development of symptoms by months or years (the average delay is nine years). Syringomyelia can also develop secondary to Arnold-Chiari malformation.

A spinal cord syrinx can develop asymptomatically, however when symptoms develop secondary to compression on neural structures, it can take on a characteristic pattern. Symptoms and signs can include:

- Pain: Either locally in the cervical spine or referred into the shoulders and/or upper extremities.

- Dissociated sensory loss: Patients will often have loss of pain and temperature sensation in a "shawl" distribution, i.e., in the shoulders and upper extremities (depending on the exact location of the lesion) with preservation of light touch, vibration and joint position sense. Often there is normal sensation below the lesion although if the syrinx is large it can disturb vibration and joint position sense in the lower extremities.

- Motor changes: These can be variable depending on the size of the syrinx. Patients may develop upper motor neuron findings below the level of the lesion and at times can develop lower motor neuron findings at the level of the lesion, if the anterior horn cells are affected.

Immediate surgical consult should be sought for a patient with symptomatic syringomyelia.

Diagnostic Question #1 in Acute Neck Pain and Headache

Cervical Artery Dissection

Cervical artery dissection (CAD) is a condition in which a tear forms in one of the cervical arteries. The cervical arteries include the internal carotid artery and the vertebral artery. CAD can lead to stroke related to one of these arteries. It is far more likely for the spine practitioner to encounter a patient with vertebral artery dissection (VAD) than internal carotid artery dissection*. While stroke from VAD is relatively rare, a busy spine practitioner may encounter this condition, as in more than 2/3 of cases the initial symptoms are neck pain with or without headache.

Historical Factors Associated with CAD

- Sudden onset of severe neck pain or headache: The pain is often occipital or suboccipital in location and is often described as sharp or throbbing. However it must be noted that the majority of patients who have this type of presentation do not have VAD.

- An association has been found between history of migraine headache and VAD. However, as migraine is a fairly common disorder and VAD is rare, the vast majority of migraineurs will never have VAD, thus limiting migraine history as a means to "rule in" the likelihood of VAD.

- Patients who have a history of migraine headache will often describe the headache related to VAD to be similar to their typical migraine. However there is a key difference that should be considered. This involves "the 3 S's". Migraine typically involves the gradual onset of pain that eventually becomes severe, then gradually subsides over the course of 24-48 hours. Headache from VAD is typically *sudden, severe and sustained* (i.e., the pain is severe from the initial onset and lasts greater than 72 hours - see Tarnutzer, et al in Recommended Reading list).

- Vertigo: This is the most common initial symptom and may accompany the neck pain and/or headache. As is the case with acute neck pain or headache, the vast majority of patients with vertigo do not have VAD. Thus the mere presence of vertigo does not, in and of itself, indicate that the patient has VAD.

- Symptoms suggestive of brainstem ischemia: This may include what have been referred to as the "5 D's And 3 N's" – diplopia, dizziness, drop attacks, dysarthria, dysphagia, ataxia, numbness, nausea and nystagmus. Nystagmus, of course, is an examination finding rather than a historical factor although some patients will report noticing a disturbing rapid eye movement.

---

*This is likely because patients with carotid artery dissection are more likely to experience neurologic symptoms at the onset of the disease, causing them to attend the hospital emergency department, whereas patients with VAD are more likely to experience neck pain and/or headache, causing them to seek the care of a spine practitioner.

- Horner's syndrome: Patients with internal carotid artery dissection may also present with partial Horner's syndrome (cormiosis and ptosis without anhidrosis) as well as amaurosis fugax (transient monocular blindness). Amaurosis fugax can have a number of different causes, including hypertension, arteriosclerosis, and drug or alcohol abuse. However when this symptom is accompanied by sudden onset of severe neck pain and headache with obvious Horner's syndrome along with other neurological symptoms (see above and below), internal carotid artery dissection should be suspected and immediate referral pursued.

- History of connective tissue disease: These include autosomal dominant polycystic kidney disease, Ehlers-Danlos Type IV, Marfan Syndrome or fibromuscular dystrophy. Patients with these disorders are at increased risk of developing VAD. Therefore the presence of one of these disorders should raise the spine practitioner's level of suspicion. However the majority of patients with VAD do not have any of these diseases, so their *absence* does not *rule out* the possibility of VAD.

Examination findings associated with CAD

In a patient with sudden onset of severe occipital or suboccipital pain, the possibility of CAD should be considered, however the majority of patients with this symptom will not have CAD. A full neurologic examination is warranted (see Table 2).

Examination findings related to brainstem or cerebellar involvement, such as cranial nerve dysfunction, nystagmus, difficulty with tandem walking, dysmetria, intention tremor or dysdiadochokinesia should be particularly watched for.

If history and neurologic examination are negative, and the remainder of the exam suggests a somatic cause of the pain, it is reasonable to carefully monitor the patient. There is no reason to suspect that treatment as discussed in Chapter 6 would be harmful. If neurologic deficit is noted on exam suggestive of brainstem and/or cerebellar dysfunction, CAD should be more strongly suspected and emergency medical attention considered.

Imaging and referral

In a patient whose history suggests the possible presence of CAD, but who do not have obvious examination findings suggestive of stroke, magnetic resonance angiography (MRA) is the imaging modality of choice. Doppler ultrasound is a second choice. While Doppler ultrasound is often more easily obtained and is less expensive, the advantage of MRA is that it can often detect the dissection itself, before there is a great deal of arterial occlusion.

In a patient who exhibits clear symptoms of stroke along with clear examination signs of brainstem and/or cerebellar dysfunction, the patient should be immediately transported by ambulance to the local emergency department. The patient should not try to self-transport or have a significant other transport to the hospital.

Spinal Meningitis

Meningitis is inflammation of the meninges. This can be caused by bacterial, viral or fungal infection. Meningitis can also be aseptic.

Historical factors associated with spinal meningitis

- The classic triad of symptoms are fever, headache and neck stiffness: It is important to ask about a history of fever and to ask if the patient has been exposed to someone with meningitis.

- History of compromised immune system: this can be a result of prolonged steroid use, HIV or recent organ transplant

- Recent history of spinal procedure such as epidural steroid injection

- Mental status changes and/ or lethargy

Examination findings in spinal meningitis

- Focal neurological deficits: These include motor loss in one or more extremities or cranial nerve dysfunction. In certain patients fundoscopy may reveal papilledema.

- Testing for nuchal rigidity: nuchal "rigidity" is actually not true rigidity, which is characteristic of an extrapyramidal disorder such as Parkinson's disease, but extreme resistance to passive flexion of the cervical spine due to protective muscle spasm.

- Testing for meningeal irritation: The most important test in patients with neck pain and headache in whom spinal meningitis is suspected is Brudzinski's Test. With this test, the patient lies supine and the practitioner flexes the cervical spine, looking for involuntary flexion of the hips and knees as a result of this movement.

A patient with suspected meningitis should be immediately transported to the local emergency department.

Other important considerations regarding diagnostic question #1 in headache patients

- Sudden, severe onset of headache should prompt consideration of subarachnoid hemorrhage. This typically involves the development of "thunderclap headache", i.e., headache that is more severe than any the patient has experienced. It may be accompanied by nausea, vomiting, confusion, irritability and visual disturbance. As such, these patients are not likely to present to an outpatient spine practitioner and are much more likely to attend the emergency department.

- Mental status changes should raise the suspicion of CNS infection.

- Bulbar symptoms: These are symptoms related to the brainstem (the "bulb") and include blurred vision, diplopia, dysarthria, dysphagia, vertigo, facial numbness or weakness and vertigo. These symptoms can suggest the possibility brainstem tumor, stroke or infection.

- Increased headache with coughing, sneezing or straining (DeJerine's triad) and/or with bending forward: This can occur in patients whose headache is caused by a brain tumor although, as with so many other isolated symptoms, many patients with benign headache, particularly migraine, will report DeJerine's triad during a headache episode, so this finding has to be considered in light of the remainder of the clinical picture.

- Headache accompanied by seizure: this can occur early in the process of a brain tumor.

- Pain in the temporal area in a patient over 50: This can be suggestive of temporal arteritis. Careful inspection of the temporal artery for swelling and strong pulsation as well as palpation of the artery for exquisite tenderness can be further evidence of this possibility. Some patients may report recent flu-like symptoms.

In headache patients a full neurologic screening examination should be routinely performed (see Table 2 in this chapter and Chapter 4 in Volume I of this series). It is particularly important to look for findings suggestive of cranial nerve dysfunction, papilledema, and cerebral or cerebellar dysfunction.

Significant factors related to diagnostic question #1 can be expected to be found in only about 1-3% of patients with CDs. Because visceral disorders or potentially serious or life-threatening illnesses are relatively uncommon, the spine practitioner must be particularly alert to the subtleties that often are found in these patients. As stated in the beginning of this chapter, presented here is information relevant to particular disorders that must be considered in CD patients with regard to diagnostic question #1. For a full understanding of the application of diagnostic question #1 in all spine patients, the reader must combine the information presented here with that presented in Chapter 4 of Volume I of this series.

Once the practitioner is comfortable with a "no" answer the diagnostic question #1, diagnostic questions #2 and #3 are considered. These questions are covered in the next two chapters.

Recommended Reading

Benzel EC, Lancon J, Kesterson L, Hadden T. Cervical laminectomy and dentate ligament section for cervical spondylotic myelopathy. J Spinal Disord. 1991 Sep;4(3):286-95.

Chang CW, Chang KY, Lin SM. Quantification of the Tromner signs: a sensitive marker for cervical spondylotic myelopathy. Eur Spine J 2011;20(6):923-7.

Blumenfeld H. Neuroanatomy Through Clinical Cases. 2nd ed. Sunderland, MA: Sinaouer Associates, 2010.

Goldberg S. The 4-Minute Neurologic Exam. Miami FL: MedMaster, Inc, 1999.

Gottesman RF, Charma P, Robinson KA, Arnan M, Tsui M, Ladha K, Newman-Toker DE. Clinical characteristics of symptomatic vertebral artery dissection. A systematic review. The Neurologist 2012; 18(5):245-254.

Murphy DR. Current understanding of the relationship between cervical manipulation and stroke: what does it mean for the chiropractic profession? Chiropr Osteopat. 2010;18:22.

Oshima Y, Seichi A, Takeshita K, Chikuda H, Ono T, Baba S, et al. Natural course and prognostic factors in patients with mild cervical spondylotic myelopathy with increased signal intensity on T2-weighted magnetic resonance imaging. Spine (Phila Pa 1976). 2012 Oct 15;37(22):1909-13.

Salvi FJ, Jones JC, Weigert BJ. The assessment of cervical myelopathy. Spine J 2006;6(6 Suppl):S182-9.

Shimizu T, Shimada H, Shirakura K. Scapulohumeral reflex (Shimizu). Its clinical significance and testing maneuver. Spine 1993;18(15):2182-90.

Tarnutzer AA, Berkowitz AL, Robinson KA, Hsieh YH, Newman-Toker DE. Does my dizzy patient have a stroke? A systematic review of bedside diagnosis in acute vestibular syndrome. CMAJ. 2011 Jun 14;183(9):E571-92.

Triano JJ, Kawchuk G, eds: Current Concepts: Spinal Manipulation and Cervical Arterial Incidents Clive, IA: NCMIC 2006.

• CHAPTER 3 •
Diagnostic Question #2: Where is the pain coming from?

Introduction

Another way of asking this question is "Are there characteristics of the pain generating tissue or tissues that can be identified and that allow treatment decisions to be made?" In the majority of patients with cervical disorders there is no way to identify the pain generating tissue objectively and with 100% certainty. But history and examination can increase the diagnostic probability of certain conditions. Treatment decisions can be made based on this increased probability and the practitioner can monitor the patient's response to treatment. It is not necessary to be absolutely certain of the pain generator to make treatment decisions.

Importantly, the patient can be provided with an evidence-based explanation as to the most likely cause of the pain - a critical aspect of a satisfying patient experience (see Laerum, et al and Verbeek, et al in Recommended Reading list).

In the context of Clinical Reasoning in Spine Pain® (the CRISP® protocols) there are four diagnostic entities that are investigated with diagnostic question #2:

1. Disc derangement: Diagnosed through historical factors and the end range loading examination.

2. Joint dysfunction: Diagnosed through historical factors and pain provocation maneuvers that are designed to identify pain from the cervical zygapophyseal joints (aka facet joints).

3. Radiculopathy: Diagnosed through historical factors, neurologic examination and pain provocation maneuvers designed to identify nerve root pain.

4. Myofascial pain: Diagnosed through historical factors and pain provocation maneuvers designed to identify myofascial trigger points.

Disc Derangement – the section on disc derangement was written by Gary Jacob, DC, LAc, MPH, DipMDT and Steven Heffner, DC, DipMDT

Cervical End Range Loading Examination and Treatment

This section concerns the use of end range loading strategies for the diagnosis and treatment of "derangement syndromes," first described by Robin A. McKenzie as part of the system he developed known as the McKenzie Method® or Mechanical Diagnosis & Therapy (MDT)®. The End Range Loading (ERL) exam and treatment strategies presented here for the management of derangement are but an introduction; the reader is encouraged to pursue training provided by the McKenzie Institute International® and to consult the texts authored by Robin McKenzie for providers and patients. See the Recommended Reading list for specifics.

Historical factors associated with cervical disc derangement include:

• Patients with disc derangement often report increased pain upon awakening in the morning, with gradual improvement as they get up and move for a period of time. As the day wears on they may worsen again, especially in response to movement or positioning in certain directions. This is ascribed to the imbibition of water into the disc at night due to lack of weight bearing, which increases intradiscal pressure. The nucleus, being hydrophilic, attracts water, thus water molecules attach themselves to the gel-like nucleus. This increases the nuclear volume within the disc, which being a closed container, causes intradiscal pressure to increase. The increased pressure that occurs as a result of non-weight bearing at night is relieved by weight bearing as the patient gets going in the morning (water is dispersed out of the nucleus). Sustained, sedentary postures during the day place asymmetrical loads on intradiscal material thus causing increase pressures in certain directions with increased symptoms. Pain that is worse upon awakening that lessens after a period of movement also indicates a lack of benefit from rest and benefit from movement. In addition, it suggests that anti-inflammatory interventions are not required.

- There can be maintained increase or decrease of pain with movement or positioning in certain directions. For most patients it is flexion and/or protrusion that are detrimental and for most patients retraction and/or extension that are beneficial. Other patterns of direction of benefit and direction of detriment are described below.

- The pain is often worse when the patient is sitting, particularly in "bad" posture, i.e., a posture in which the head is protruded: This position is common when a person is reading or working at a computer. Protruded head posture flexes the mid-to-lower cervical spine (increasing pressure on the anterior aspect of the lower cervical discs) and hyperextends the upper cervical spine (stressing joints and muscles of that area).

- The pain is often improved by standing and walking: The relative effects of sitting vs. standing/walking provide information regarding various ERL directions. As noted above, poor sitting posture extends the upper cervical spine and flexes the mid-to-lower cervical spine. Relative to the sitting posture, standing/walking reduces extension and promotes flexion in the upper cervical spine while reducing flexion and promoting extension in the lower cervical spine.

- Younger age: Patients with cervical disc derangements are typically between 22-55 years, the years in which the disc has most hydrostatic pressure. Certainly patients older than 55 can have disc derangement, but this is much less common. Also, in younger patients, especially children or adolescents, disc derangement is a common cause of "acute torticollis". Of course, it is essential to rule out other potential pernicious causes of this presentation, but in the majority of cases, this represents a "Torticollic Antalgia" (see below) and derangement is the causative factor.

- Antalgic posture: This will be discussed in detail later.

- Recurrent acute episodes: Patients will often report a history of acute episodes, many of which resolve spontaneously after a period of time, but then they will have one episode that does not spontaneously resolve, prompting the seeking of clinical care. In addition, episodic derangements usually begin centrally in the initial episodes and then peripheralize with progressive episodes.

Cervical End Range Loading: General Overview

For the cervical spine, diagnostic and therapeutic ERL strategies explore the movement plane directions of flexion, extension, rotation, lateral flexion as well as two-movements unique to the head/neck complex, those being protrusion and retraction. The protruded position loads the upper cervical spine at end range extension and loads the mid-to-lower cervical spine towards end range flexion. Retraction is the opposite of protrusion; the retracted position loads the upper cervical spine at end range flexion and loads the mid-to-lower cervical spine towards end range extension.

For most patients, cervical related complaints are created, aggravated or perpetuated with a slouched sitting posture wherein the head/neck is subjected to prolonged static protrusion. When the protruded head/neck position of sitting is provocative and the relatively retracted head/neck position of standing and walking is palliative, expectations are that upper cervical related complaints would respond to flexion achieved by retraction and that lower cervical related complaints would respond to extension from a retracted position.

In order to achieve the maximum degree of upper cervical flexion or lower cervical extension, the following tactics are employed. For the upper cervical spine, retraction achieves a greater degree of flexion than does the flexion of the usual cervical range of motion (ROM) exam. For this reason, retraction ERL often suffices for upper cervical-related complaints (e.g. headaches) without the need to perform chin-to-chest flexion. For the lower cervical spine, the maximum degree of extension is achieved if extension is initiated from a retracted head/neck position.

For cases that fail to respond to self-generated retraction or retraction-extension ERL, supine cervical retraction or supine cervical retraction-extension is performed under axial manual traction prior to concluding that extension ERL movements are of no therapeutic benefit and that movements outside the sagittal plane should be explored. When movements outside the sagittal plane are required, expectations are that upper cervical related complaints (e.g. headaches) would more likely to respond to rotation ERL *vs.* lateral flexion ERL, rotation being the "intrinsic" motion of the upper cervical spine. Expectations are that mid-to-lower cervical related complaints (e.g. non-radicular referral to the extremity) would likely to respond to lateral flexion ERL *vs.* rotation ERL, being the area where lateral flexion predominates over rotation.

Therapeutic movements outside the sagittal plane are typically performed ipsilateral toward the side of pain consistent with derangement theory about compressing intra-articular material in order to "relocate" it. It must be noted that although ERL "expectations" are noted above there are "atypical" patterns, the possibilities of which should be allowed for. Examples are when protrusion benefits headache, lateral flexion benefits upper cervical complaints or rotation benefits lower cervical complaints.

Another unique feature of the cervical spine is the lack of an intervertebral disc between occiput-atlas and atlas-axis. The McKenzie Method was originally developed for the lumbar spine for which the intervertebral nucleus was an important model to explain derangement related symptoms and mechanics. In spite of the lack of intervertebral discs, upper cervical derangement patterns are observed indicating derangement behaviors can exist for a variety of joint structures.

Mechanisms such as "intra-articular inclusions" or centrally mediated responses have been proposed to account for the derangement behaviors of such joints, thus expanding the possible explanation for all joints. While this chapter concentrates on the intervertebral disc model, the derangement patterns observed are more important than the proposed mechanism.

Cervical End Range Loading: Adopting a Strategy

For patients without antalgia, baseline ROM assessment is made. The usual cardinal planes are assessed (flexion, extension, lateral flexion, rotation) in addition to which protrusion and retraction are added. Following singular ROM assessments, repetitive and/or sustained retraction and/or retraction-extension motions are first explored. Expectations are that most patients will evidence an asymmetrical loss of extension and will improve symptomatically and mechanically with retraction-extension strategies. Repetitive protrusion is explored first (to demonstrate a possible adverse effect) followed by repetitive retraction and then repetitive retraction-extension. Before deciding that retraction-extension movements are without therapeutic benefit they are performed supine under manual traction. If supine manual traction strategies do not benefit, ipsilateral rotation ERL would be the next ERL to explore for upper cervical related complaints and ipsilateral lateral flexion ERL would be the next ERL to explore for lower cervical related complaints.

Exceptions to the above progressions include contraindications and antalgias. Contraindications are the same as for manipulation, another form of ERL. Of particular concern would be extension employed for a frank radiculopathy, especially in patients older than 50. For those patients, retraction, which produces slight extension in the lower cervical spine, may result in relief by "slacking" nerve roots, apparently a green light to exploring further extension. However, extension to end range in those patients may result in foraminal compression of nerve root structures with adverse consequences.

When patients present with antalgia, the ERL strategy is clear and does not require the exploration of repetitive motion in multiple directions to develop a treatment strategy, which is to load the spine in the direction opposite the antalgia. Antalgias represent the most extreme cases of derangements and afford the opportunity to study derangement properties and treatment protocols in the most difficult cases. In addition, the study of the "frank" antalgia derangements enhances the ability to classify derangements when antalgia is not present. Below, the cervical antalgias are employed as an educational tool to demonstrate the properties of and interventions for the 3 main types of derangements

Cervical Derangement: The Antalgia Based Criteria (ABC) Perspective

The most extreme cases of derangement are the three types of "acute" cervical antalgias (kyphotic, torticollic, lordotic). When a patient presents with an antalgia, the rules of treatment are clear – spinal loading is applied to reverse the antalgia. The majority of cervical derangements, however, do not present with antalgia. In cases where there is no presenting antalgia, it is important to investigate if there is a *recent history* of antalgia.

If there is no presenting or recent antalgia, an ERL history and exam allows the practitioner to identify whether derangement exists and, if so, which of the three antalgia pattern protocols are the best fit. If a patient presents with derangement without antalgia they are classified according to the type of antalgia their situation most represents and then the treatment for that antalgia is employed. In order to classify non-antalgic patients to the appropriate antalgic category, the mechanical and symptomatic properties of the various antalgias need to be fully appreciated.

Antalgia involves the spine being "fixed," "stuck," or "crooked" in one or more directions, with the patient unable to even achieve neutral posture in the opposite direction(s). Antalgic patients report the inability to achieve neutral posture due to pain and/or *the perception of a mechanical obstruction* to neutral positioning. The theory is that the antalgias occur as a result of displacement of intervertebral nuclear material. The derangements are named according to the direction of intervertebral nuclear material derangement that best explains the clinical presentation. The antalgias, corresponding derangement terminology and directions of lean (away or towards pain) are as follows:

- Kyphotic Antalgia: Posterior Derangement: Fixed in flexion; leans away from pain.

- Torticollic Antalgia: Posterolateral Derangement: Fixed in lateral flexion; lean away from the side of pain (contralateral); lean to side of pain is rare for the cervical spine.

- Lordotic Antalgia (Anterior Derangement): Fixed in extension; leans toward back pain.

Loading in Different Directions Has Different Effects

The pursuit and/or avoidance of ERL are of critical importance for diagnosing and treating derangements. The ERL exam involves dynamic (repetitive) loading *to* end range and/or static (sustained) loading *at* end range to determine the mechanical and symptomatic responses to particular movement plane directions. The ERL exam is conducted to identify the direction(s) that reduce derangement (the direction of benefit to be pursued) and the direction(s) that promote derangement (the direction of detriment to be avoided).

Direction of Benefit: Mechanical and Symptomatic Profile

The Direction of Benefit is commonly referred to as "Directional Preference." The Direction of Benefit is the ERL direction that results in positive mechanical and symptomatic responses. It is opposite the direction of the antalgia. ERL in the Direction of Benefit is typically restricted by the patient's perception of pain at an *obstructed* end range. Patients may report a sense of obstruction, as opposed to pain, as the reason for ROM limitation. Patients may say "it's not the pain that stops me, it just doesn't go any farther; that's the end; it's blocked". An important feature of the Direction of Benefit is that there are no symptoms during the arc of motion, i.e. during mid-range. *The Direction of Benefit exhibits no pain during the arc of motion, with pain at an obstructed end range only.*

Repetitive ERL in the Direction of Benefit results in beneficial mechanical and symptomatic responses, including reduction of the obstruction to movement in that direction and favorable changes in symptoms; the movements that previously provoked symptoms become less provocative.

Favorable changes *may* include a unique pattern of symptom changes, known as "centralization" involving the retreat of radiating symptoms that *may* be accompanied by increase of the more proximal symptoms.

Centralization: Retreat of Distal Symptoms

Centralization refers to patterns of symptomatic responses to ERL, wherein there is a *retreat of distal symptoms*, i.e. a reduction of the distance that symptoms radiate away from the spine. There are various changes that represent centralization.

Some examples are the following responses to ERL:

• Neck pain radiating to the hand changes to neck pain radiating to the elbow

• Neck pain radiating to the hand changes to neck pain radiating to the interscapular region

- Arm pain without neck pain changes to neck pain without arm pain

- A "circle" of central neck pain of 7cm in diameter reduces to 3cm in diameter

Centralization does not always occur as a result of loading in the Direction of Benefit. Centralization is sufficient, but not necessary, to identify the Direction of Benefit. A Direction of Benefit can be identified in the absence of centralization. Successful derangement reduction is often accomplished without Centralization.

Examples of this are when ERL in a certain direction results in the abolition of all symptoms (central and peripheral) simultaneously or when there is marked improvement in functional activities without change of symptom location.

One can speak of a Direction of Benefit with Centralization vs. a Direction of Benefit without Centralization. It has been our experience that the greater the obstruction to end range loading in the Direction of Benefit, the greater the likelihood that Centralization will occur and, as well, the greater the likelihood that Centralization will be associated with Proximal Increase of Symptoms.

Antalgias almost always centralize with Proximal Increase of Symptoms (see below).

Proximal Increase of Symptoms: A Centralization-Associated Response

Centralization involves the retreat of peripheral symptoms proximally, a favorable response to end range loading in the Direction of Benefit. In some cases, Centralization is associated with a significant increase in more proximal (central) symptoms. This increase of proximal symptoms is a "favorable response" as long as it is associated with centralization, i.e. the retreat of distal symptoms. The increase of proximal symptoms without centralization is not a favorable response. The Increase of Proximal Symptoms may be associated with Centralization but is not a necessary condition to determine that Centralization has occurred.

The more severe the obstruction to movement (i.e. the degree of ROM loss in the Direction of Benefit) the more likely there is to be Centralization and the more likely there is to be a Proximal Increase of Symptoms.

The Proximal Increase of Symptoms almost always accompanies Centralization when acute antalgias are corrected. *The antalgic position is assumed and perpetuated in order to avoid the Increase of Proximal Symptoms experienced when attempting to reverse the antalgia,* the very movement that is required for correction. The skilled practitioner must help the patient navigate through the counter-intuitive Increase of Proximal Symptoms.

In most cases, the Increase of Proximal Symptoms resolves or reduces to a tolerable level during the initial therapeutic intervention.

We noted above that the greater the obstruction to end range loading in the Direction of Benefit, the greater the likelihood that Centralization with Proximal Increase of Symptoms will occur. A proposed intradiscal mechanism explaining the proximal increase of symptoms is the proximal increase of intradiscal pressure as nuclear material is retuned to a more central location.

Direction of Detriment: Mechanical and Symptomatic Profile

The Direction of Detriment is the movement plane direction that results in negative mechanical and symptomatic responses. In patients with antalgia, the Direction of Detriment *is the direction of the antalgia*.

It was noted earlier that the Direction of Benefit has no pain during the arc of motion (i.e. mid-range), only pain at the painful obstructed end range. In the Direction of Detriment there can be *pain during the arc of motion as well as at end range*. ROM in the Direction of Detriment may

be excessive or aberrant (e.g. deviation from the intended movement plane direction).

When voluntary motion is limited in the Direction of Detriment, the reason offered by the patient is typically that it feels too painful or too unstable to go on vs. the perception of a mechanical obstruction prohibiting movement ("I *could* go further but it would hurt too much").

Negative mechanical and symptomatic responses within the Direction of Detriment include excessive or aberrant motions, increased symptom intensity or frequency, *peripheralization of symptoms* and a painfully obstructed end range in *another* (often opposite) movement plane direction.

Peripheralization phenomena are symptomatic responses to loading wherein there is an *advance* of symptoms in a more distal direction; it is the opposite of centralization - symptoms radiate further from the spine. There may be a decrease of proximal symptoms as distal symptoms increase, the opposite of the increase of proximal symptoms sometimes associated with the retreat of distal symptoms (centralization) that occurs in the Direction of Benefit.

ERL in the Direction of Benefit and Direction of Detriment Affect Each Other

Loading in the Direction of Detriment promotes peripheralization and/or aberrant mechanics (excessive motion including deviation from intended movement plane, etc.) in that same direction and results in a mechanical obstruction to movement (mechanically impeded end range) in the Direction of Benefit.

Loading in the Direction of Benefit promotes centralization, diminishes the mechanical obstruction in that direction and diminishes the detrimental effects of loading in the Direction of Detriment.

Mechanically, ERL in the Direction of Detriment promotes hypermobility in that direction and promotes a mechanically impeded end range in the Direction of Benefit. Loading at the mechanically impeded end range in the Direction of Benefit diminishes obstruction in that direction and diminishes the hypermobility in the Direction of Detriment.

Explanations of Direction of Detriment and Direction of Benefit behaviors and how they affect each other, based on intradiscal nuclear derangement theory, are as follows:

- Loading in the Direction of Detriment causes displacement of intradiscal material during the arc of motion that *may cause symptoms during the arc of motion*. The ROM in the Direction of Detriment may be excessive, as the displaced nuclear material no longer offers resistance to motion to compression within the part of the disc space that it has vacated. As the derangement increases, obstruction to ROM in the direction that the nuclear material displaced increases; in the most extreme cases antalgia develops, preventing neutral positioning. If the Direction of Detriment causes nuclear material to move laterally, so do symptoms, represented by peripheralization. As material moves from the center to the side, central symptoms may diminish as peripheral symptoms increase.

- The Direction of Benefit is the direction obstructed by displaced nuclear material. In the Direction of Benefit there is no pain during the arc of motion; pain is not experienced until end range, i.e. when the displaced nuclear material offers resistance to motion, experienced as a painfully obstructed end range.

Loading at the painfully obstructed end range in the Direction of Benefit returns displaced nuclear material to a more central location. This is reflected in Centralization that may be accompanied by Increase of Proximal Symptoms due to the "pressure pain" of returning the nuclear material to "a smaller container." Reduction of the derangement diminishes the effects of loading in the Direction of Detriment since nuclear displacement was reduced.

Phases of the Derangement Resolution

Antalgias demonstrate all the features of the derangement. Derangements that do not present as antalgias may not exhibit all of those features (starting with the antalgia itself) and may be considered to exhibit "partial patterns."

As antalgias resolve, antalgia-derangement "features" are increasingly subtracted from the clinical picture (conversely, as antalgia develops, antalgia-derangement features are added).

An idealized day-to-day scenario of the order in which derangement features are subtracted from the clinical picture as antalgias resolve is presented below (this is just an example and should not taken as standard). The opposite order would represent antalgia development.

In the treatment of disc derangement with antalgia, loading in the Direction of Benefit typically results in progressive improvement as follows:

Day 1: Increase of Proximal Symptoms associated with Centralization and recovery of movement in the obstructed direction permitting the ability to achieve neutral posture

Day 2: Increase of Proximal Symptoms no longer occurs as Centralization continues

Day 3: Symptoms and mechanical aberrations during the arc of motion in the Direction of Detriment resolve; improvement may or may not continue to involve Centralization.

Day 4: Symptoms at the end range of motion in the Direction of Detriment resolve; improvement may or may not continue to involve Centralization.

Day 5: The painful obstructed end range in the Direction of Benefit resolves; improvement continues typically without Centralization at this point.

Day 6: No complaints; no findings during motion or at end range in any direction

It should be noted that *the most basic and consistent mechanical and symptomatic pattern of derangement is the painfully obstructed end range in a movement plane direction that has no pain during the arc of motion, i.e. the Direction of Benefit*

Antalgia-Based-Criteria (ABC) Protocols:

ABC Criteria proceeds as follows. If one of the three antalgias is present, the corresponding protocols (described below) are employed. If there is no antalgia, the patient is treated according to the protocol for the antalgia that their mechanical and symptomatic responses to ERL most resemble.

Kyphotic Antalgia Treatment Protocols (Posterior Derangement Protocols)

- Direction of Benefit: Extension

- Direction of Detriment: Flexion

Kyphotic Antalgia Treatment Protocols: Extension Direction of Benefit

For patients with a frank kyphotic antalgia, symptoms may be central or may radiate into the upper extremity. The protocol is to employ retraction-extension and to avoid protrusion/flexion movements.

The majority of patients without antalgia, even those with symptoms radiating to the upper extremity respond to this protocol involving the pursuit of extension and the avoidance of protrusion/flexion. Non-radicular versus radicular extremity pain must be differentiated. True radiculopathy, especially in older patients who may have central or lateral stenosis, will generally be adversely affected by the extension component of the protocol. In younger individuals with non-radicular extremity pain, the intervertebral nucleus explanation for extension benefiting lateral complaints is that as extension reduces the posterior "component" of the nuclear displacement, the lateral component is "drawn along with it" to a more central location.

While patients presenting with kyphotic antalgia require retraction-extension, they cannot accomplish that by themselves due to the significant Increase of Proximal Symptoms associated with Centralization. Thus, manual traction is required in order to relieve the Proximal Symptoms associated with Centralization. Cases of Kyphotic Antalgia require the patient to be placed supine with the neck flexed with axial manual traction applied before initiating retraction and extension. The patient is asked to report on mid-range, end range, centralization and peripheralization phenomena with each repetition. In addition to judging the symptomatic responses, ROM or functional activities can be reevaluated subsequent to ERL. The progression is as follows:

Supine Retraction and Retraction-Extension during Manual Traction

- The supine patient is made comfortable, accommodating the antalgic position with the head resting on a pillow supporting the flexed position. Gentle retractions may be self-performed

- The supine patient's head is taken off the edge of the treatment table, with the edge of the table no higher than T1. Initially, the head is held in the least flexed position that is comfortable. The patient is asked to occlude (not clench) the teeth to avoid biting the tongue and/or moving the TMJ. The practitioner places the index and middle finger of one hand anterior and inferior to the chin, respectively (Fig. 3-1). The thumb and index finger of the other hand abuts the *inferior* border/ledge of the occiput. Axial traction is applied in the flexion antalgic position. While maintaining axial traction, cervical retraction mobilizations are performed in a slow, gentle, repetitive, ever increasing manner (Fig. 3-2). A momentary pause occurs at the end range of each retraction and after returning to the starting point of each cycle.

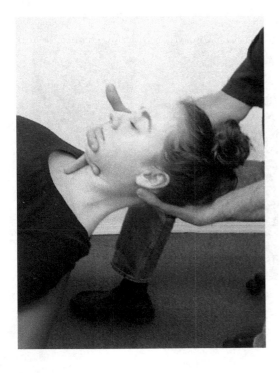

Figure 3-1. Starting position for supine retraction and retraction-extension. Note the slightly flexed positioning to accommodate the antalgia.

- Next, extension is introduced. This starts with the supine patient's head and neck in the retracted position under axial traction. As extension proceeds, the practitioner releases the retraction mobilization pressure but maintains the axial traction (Fig. 3-3). With each repetition further extension is attempted. At the end range of extension, very small and gentle rotations of the head are performed to facilitate further extension.

Sitting Retraction and Retraction-Extension

When the patient is deemed capable, a progression is made to self-generated ERL in the seated position. The patient is asked to perform these exercises periodically throughout the day. The maintenance of lumbar lordosis is essential (details of the body mechanics of sitting are discussed below) to reduce the degree of head and neck protrusion and to maximize the degree of extension. Sitting retraction to end range is first explored repetitively while symptomatic and mechanical responses are monitored (Fig. 3-4). The head must be level to avoid nodding or extending during the motion.

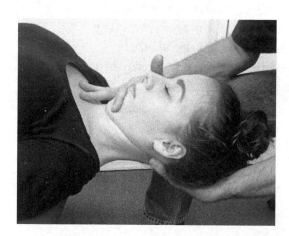

Figure 3-2. Supine retraction mobilization.

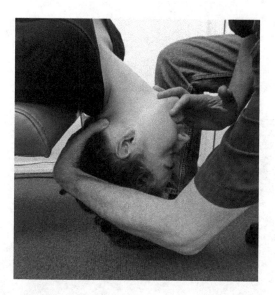

Figure 3-3. Supine extension.

Extension is then performed from the retracted position (Fig. 3-5). After initiating extension, there should be no attempt to maintain retraction. Gentle mini-rotations the width of one's eye are performed at end-range to permit further extension.

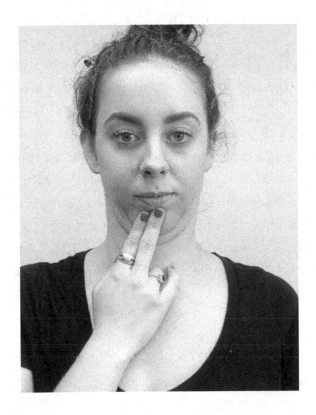

Figure 3-4. Self-generated retraction in the seated position.

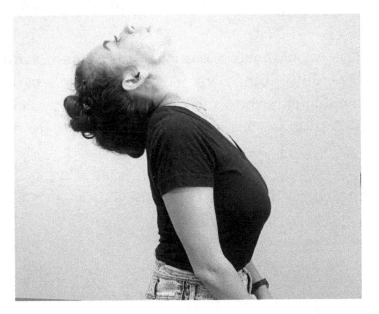

Figure 3-5. Self-generated extension in the seated position.

Kyphotic Antalgia Treatment Protocols: Avoiding Flexion Direction of Detriment

The kyphotic antalgia patient is advised to avoid any exercises, movements or positions that flex or protrude the cervical spine. Correction of sitting posture is essential for this.

If neutral sitting posture results in centralization and flexed, protruded head/neck positioning results in peripheralization, the reactions are used as educational and motivational tools.

In cases in which there is benefit from "sitting up", patients may not comply because they feel they "look weird" when doing so. The psychosocial obstacles to assuming better sitting posture can be overcome with simple educational techniques. Two effective approaches to teaching how to achieve neutral cervical positioning and how to help overcome the psychosocial barriers to lordotic sitting are McKenzie's "Slouch-Overcorrect-Relax 10%" and the senior author's (GJ) "Stand Alert-Sit Alert" and "Sit Slouched-Stand Slouched" exercises.

Slouch-Overcorrect-Relax 10%

Step 1: Slouched sitting posture - The patient is asked to assume a slouched, protruded head/neck sitting posture, which loads the mid-lower cervical spine at the end range of flexion (Fig. 3-6). Any adverse symptoms are noted.

Step 2: Over-corrected sitting posture - The patient simultaneously rolls the pelvis forward to increase lumbar lordosis, rotates the chest upward and retracts the head and neck backward, all to end-range. The shoulders should not be thrown back in a "military" posture but should relax "down." Essentially, body parts are moved to the end of range in the direction opposite the slouched positioning (Fig. 3-7).

Step 3: "Let go 10%" - From the overcorrected position, the patient is asked to let go ~10% to find correct lordotic sitting posture (Fig. 3-8).

For those who "feel weird" when "sitting up," the overcorrected posture feels even weirder. The result of this is that the normal lordotic sitting posture does not feel so weird after all.

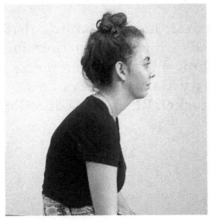

Figure 3-6.   Slouched sitting posture.

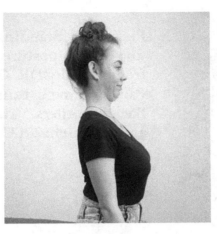

Figure 3-7. Over-corrected sitting posture.

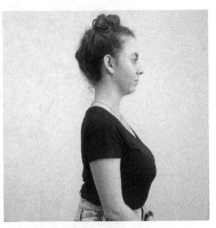

Figure 3-8. Correct sitting posture.

Stand Alert-Sit Alert

This trains lordotic sitting by maintaining the lordosis of standing.

Step 1: Stand alert - The patient is asked to stand with alert (not military) posture.

Step 2: Standing to sitting maintaining alert upper body posture - From alert standing, the patient is guided into a seated position while maintaining the lumbar lordosis of standing (Fig. 3-9). The practitioner's hands may be strategically placed on the sternum (to prevent flexion) and on the low back (to preserve lordosis) during the transition. The patient is asked to imagine having a glass on his or her head that is filled to the brim. Some patients may have to "stick the buttocks out backwards" a bit in order to ensure lordosis is maintained during the transition.

Step 3: Sitting to standing maintaining lumbar lordosis - From the lordotic sitting posture, the patient is transitioned from sitting to standing, maintaining lumbar lordosis. Again the practitioner's hands may be applied to ensure the maintenance of the lordosis.

With this exercise the patient realizes that sitting up does not look weird because, from the waist up, he or she looks the same as when standing.

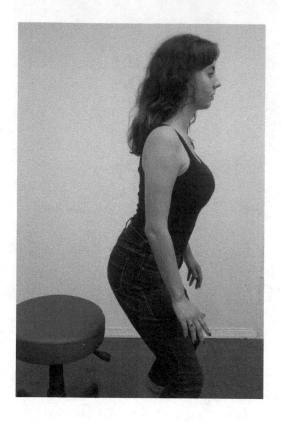

Figure 3-9. Standing to sitting maintaining alert upper body posture. Reprinted with permission from Murphy DR. Clinical Reasoning in Spine Pain Volume I: Primary Management of Low Back Disorders. Pawtucket, RI: CRISP Education and Research; 2013.

Sit Slouched-Stand Slouched

This exercise, employed subsequent to the Stand Alert-Sit Alert-Stand Alert Exercise, is merely a psychosocial ploy to help the patient better appreciate the how the slouched sitting posture that feels "normal" is not advantageous, whether the concern is about appearance or health.

Step 1: Sit slouched (Fig. 3-10) - The patient is asked to sit in a relaxed, slouched position.

Step 2: Sitting to standing maintaining upper body slouched posture (Fig. 3-11) - The slouched (flexed) position of the trunk is maintained as the patient is transitioned to standing.

The practitioner's hands may be strategically placed on the upper back and abdomen to maintain the slouched posture. Once standing, the practitioner removes the hands and the patient is left to contemplate the disadvantages of maintained flexion of the lumbar spine.

With this exercise the patient immediately understands that it looks strange and would be unduly stressful to stand and walk with the lumbar spine in the flexed, slouched position that is so often assumed when sitting. The patient can then easily generalize these principles to the sitting position. Neutral lordotic sitting becomes more attractive as the patient realizes it resembles the way he or she prefers to look and feel when standing and walking about.

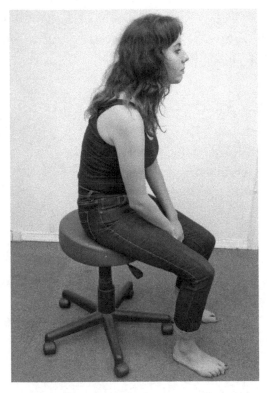 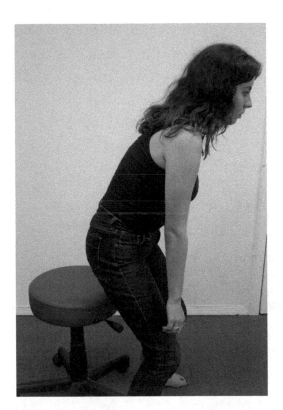

Figure 3-10. Slouched sitting posture. Reprinted with permission from Murphy DR. Clinical Reasoning in Spine Pain Volume I: Primary Management of Low Back Disorders. Pawtucket, RI: CRISP Education and Research; 2013.

Figure 3-11. Sitting to standing maintaining slouched posture. Reprinted with permission from Murphy DR. Clinical Reasoning in Spine Pain Volume I: Primary Management of Low Back Disorders. Pawtucket, RI: CRISP Education and Research; 2013.

Kyphotic Antalgia Treatment Protocols in the Absence of Kyphotic Antalgia

A majority of derangement patients without antalgia respond to extension end-range loading, independent of symptom location (including radiation to the upper extremity). The patient without antalgia who responds to extension typically has, at a minimum, a painfully obstructed extension end range with no pain during the arc of extension.

For the patient presenting with a Kyphotic Antalgia, the first intervention is supine axial traction and retraction (Fig. 3-2) followed by extension while under manual traction (Fig. 3-3). When deemed capable, the patient is instructed to perform cervical retraction-extension exercises in the sitting posture. For the patient presenting without a Kyphotic Antalgia for whom Kyphotic Antalgia Protocols are suspected to be of benefit, the progression is the opposite, starting in the sitting position (Figs. 3-12 and 3-13) and progressing to supine traction procedures only if sitting procedures fail to be of benefit.

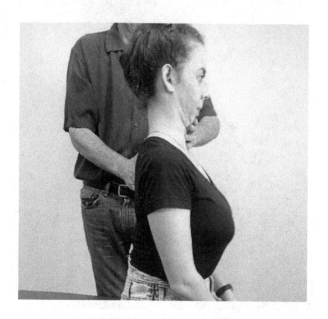

Figure 3-12. Practitioner-assisted retraction in the sitting position.

As stated earlier first step of Kyphotic Antalgia protocols is that of cervical retraction. In many cases of upper cervical related complaints, including cervicogenic headache, dynamic and/or static cervical retraction ERL exercises combined with the avoidance of protrusion suffice for resolution. In those cases, retraction followed by extension is of no benefit and may have adverse effects (by promoting upper cervical extension).

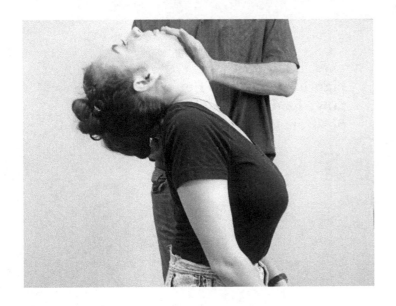

Figure 3-13. Practitioner-assisted extension in the sitting position.

When extension fails to benefit non-radicular radiating symptoms from the lower cervical spine to the shoulder girdle and/or upper extremity it is thought that the extension ERL is unable to "capture" the lateral component so as to "bring it along for the ride" centrally. In these cases extension may not only fail to provide benefit but may prove, initially, to be a Direction of Detriment. In some of these cases extension may actually promote the lateral derangement by "squeezing it out to the side". In those cases Lateral-Torticollis-Antalgia Protocols must be considered.

Torticollis (Coronal) Antalgia Protocols: Posterolateral Derangement
- Direction of Benefit:
  - o Initially: Lateral Flexion in direction opposite antalgia
  - o Subsequently: Extension
- Direction of Detriment:
  - o Initially: Lateral Flexion in direction of antalgia; Flexion; Extension
  - o Subsequently: Extension not detrimental after lateral flexion is recovered

Most cases of unilateral derangement complaints are amenable to Kyphotic Antalgia Protocols that manage to address the lateral component as well. For Torticollis, which is the most extreme version of posterolateral derangement, Kyphotic Antalgia Protocols would be detrimental as an initial intervention, as extension is insufficient to reduce the lateral component and may in fact promote it. In these cases, lateral ERL is required. After reduction of the lateral component, the extension ERL that initially would have been detrimental

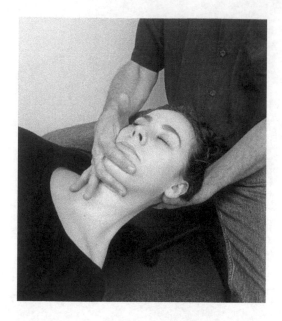

Figure 3-14. Lateral flexion end range loading in the supine position.

proves to be beneficial. Torticollis Protocols are employed for patients who present with torticollis antalgia and are the first protocols considered for lower cervical related symptoms that do not respond to ERL in the sagittal plane.

Cervical torticollis derangement presentation typically involves a combination of contralateral antalgia away from the side of pain as well as antalgia in the flexed position, the latter sometimes not noticed. The contralateral antalgia is considered to be in the direction opposite the "lateral component" of the posterolateral derangement while the flexion antalgia is considered to be due to the "posterior component" of the posterolateral derangement.

Treatment proceeds in two steps. The first step is to employ lateral ERL to reduce the lateral derangement; after that is accomplished, Kyphotic Antalgia Protocols are employed to reduce the posterior component. As with kyphotic antalgia, practitioner-induced manual axial traction is initially required. Shortly thereafter, the responsibility of treatment is transferred to the patient, employing techniques resembling those the practitioner employed.

The patient is supine. As with the Kyphotic Antalgia Treatment protocols, the head is held in slight flexion to accommodate the flexion component (Fig. 3-1). The practitioner's manual contacts are the same as were employed with the cervical kyphotic antalgia. Axial traction is applied, keeping the head and neck comfortably flexed (Fig. 3-1). While maintaining axial traction, lateral flexion ERL is conducted in the direction opposite the antalgia until the painful obstruction is met at which point there is a momentary pause (Fig. 3-14). The practitioner then backs off slightly to reduce the discomfort, pauses a moment (traction being maintained throughout) and repeats the procedure, moving further in the direction opposite the antalgia, gaining more lateral flexion with each repetition.

The Torticollis Protocol requires a degree of flexion to be maintained when recovering lateral movements. While it is important for the torticollis patient to avoid flexion, the degree of lordosis (extension) that is tolerated may be limited until after the lateral component is reduced. As the patient progresses, lateral ERL is performed with progressively less flexion, and more neutral lordotic positioning. After benefit has been attained from lateral ERL in a slightly flexed position, the next progression is lateral ERL from a neutral head/neck position and then lateral ERL from a retracted head and neck position. When the patient is deemed capable, lateral ERL can be self-performed in the supine position, and then progressed to sitting (Fig. 3-15). Subsequent to reduction of the lateral component (e.g. subsequent to centralization and recovery of lateral motion), the Kyphotic Protocol of sitting cervical retraction-extension is explored whether a Kyphotic Antalgic component is present or not.

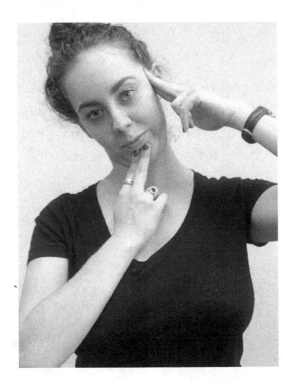

Figure 3-15. Lateral end range loading self-performed in the sitting position.

Torticollis treatment protocols for those with and those without torticollis

In the presence of Torticollis, a ROM exam is not needed. Torticollis Protocols are employed after ruling out a potentially serious underlying condition as cause of the torticollis. In addition, it must be determined whether the torticollis is a result of true radiculopathy (e.g. due to lateral stenosis), which would be very unlikely to benefit from compressing the side of pain.

For patients presenting with unilateral lower cervical complaints, in the absence of torticollis, who fail to respond to extension ERL in the sagittal plane (including supine manual traction tactics), lateral flexion in the direction of complaints is the first direction considered. Lateral flexion can first be explored sitting, from a retracted position (Fig. 3-15) and then, if there is a lack of response, the supine-traction maneuvers (Fig. 3-14) can be explored before assuming the approach has been exhausted.

Lordotic Antalgia Treatment Protocols (Anterior Derangement Protocols)

- Direction of Benefit: Flexion
- Direction of Detriment: Extension

The treatment protocols for Lordotic Antalgia are the opposite of those for the Kyphotic Antalgia. Flexion end range loading exercises are advised. Extension is avoided. Flexion may be performed from the supine, sitting or standing position (Fig. 3-16). Manual traction is not required nor is there need to correct sitting posture to promote lower cervical extension.

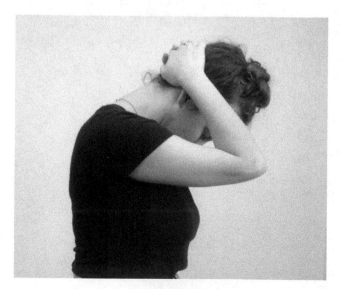

Figure 3-16. Flexion end range loading in the sitting position.

Considering the flexion stressors in everyday life (e.g. prolonged sitting, bending) one would predict that flexion as a treatment of mid-lower cervical complaints would be the exception rather than the rule. The reverse is true for the upper cervical spine, which is habitually held in an extreme extended position as a result of habitual protrusion of the head and neck.

The lordotic antalgia is uncommon and when present is difficult to visualize in the cervical spine. Flexion, however, is diminished with pain at the obstructed end range only, without pain during the arc of motion. Flexion ERL is the therapeutic exercise and extension is avoided. Postural vigilance is not required.

For the mid-lower cervical spine, the patient may report feeling better when sitting (flexion reducing the derangement) and worse when standing (extension increasing the derangement). Associated with anterior derangement of the lower cervical spine is the curious symptom of pain with swallowing that can be abolished with repetitive flexion ERL.

For the upper cervical spine, the greatest degree of flexion is accomplished with retraction ERL versus the flexion performed upon typical cervical ROM exams. For upper cervical complaints and cervicogenic headaches in which the patient reports that symptoms are worse with sitting and better with standing, dynamic or sustained retraction (Fig. 3-4) or rotation to end range from a retracted position (Fig. 3-17) often prove to be Directions of Benefit.

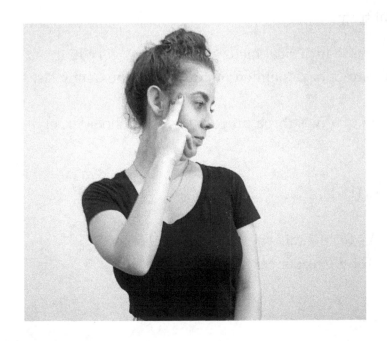

Figure 3-17. Rotation to end range from a retracted position.

For cervicogenic headaches, static (sustained) loading for a minute or two at end range retraction or at end range retraction-rotation may be required to obtain a positive response. For the upper cervical spine, the effects of poor sitting promote extension, the opposite of what happens to the mid-lower cervical spine. Upper cervical related symptoms that benefit from flexion require the correction of sitting posture as has been described above.

Joint Dysfunction

Historical factors associated with cervical zygapophyseal (facet) joint pain include:

- The pain is often well localized to the cervical spine with the exception of the lower cervical segments, which can cause referred pain into the upper thoracic, upper trapezius and scapula areas. However, the pain does not typically extend into the upper extremity (see Fig. 3-18)

- The pain is often unilateral

- The pain is often accompanied by headache

- The pain is often increased with rotation combined with extension

- There is often a history of cervical trauma

It should be noted that the specificity of these historical factors is likely not very high, so while they can be generally useful, they cannot be depended on to confirm the diagnosis.

Examination for cervical joint dysfunction involves three procedures (see Schneider, et al in Recommended Reading list):

- Palpation for segmental tenderness (PST)
- Manual joint palpation (MJP)
- The Extension-Rotation Test (ERT) – for the mid- to lower cervical spine
- The Flexion-Rotation Test (FRT) – for the upper cervical spine

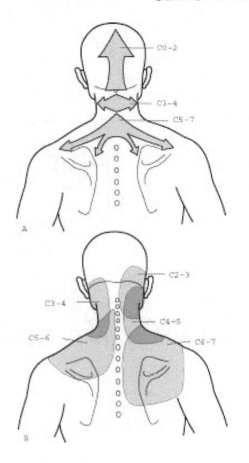

Figure 3-18. Referred pain patterns of the zygapo-physeal joints of the cervical spine. Reprinted with permission from Murphy DR, ed. Conservative Management of Cervical Spine Syndromes. New York: McGraw-Hill, 2000. Adapted from Aprill, et al, Dwyer, et al and Dreyfuss, et al (see Recommended Reading list).

Palpation for segmental tenderness

The purpose of this procedure is to detect tenderness of the muscles immediately overlying the joint, particularly the semispinalis cervicis and multifidus. The patient lies prone and the practitioner stands at the head of the table (Fig. 3-19). It is important to apply the palpation as close to the deep muscles as possible. Therefore, the overlying tissues must be moved out of the way first. To do this the practitioner starts by placing the thumbs on the lateral aspect of the cervical spine (Fig. 3-20) and moves the superficial tissues medially. The practitioner feels for the joint line and applies pressure with the tips of the thumbs gently but firmly on tissues overlying the joint (Fig. 3-21). The practitioner asks if this is painful and, if it is, whether this reproduces all or part of the patient's chief complaint.

Manual joint palpation

Manual joint palpation involves the assessment of both pain and resistance to motion. In this context "resistance to motion" refers to the amount of movement that occurs at the involved segment before the *barrier*, is reached. The barrier is the point at which the practitioner initially senses resistance to further movement (see Chapter 10 in Volume I and Chapter 6 in this volume for a more detailed discussion of the barrier). It is important to note that resistance to motion can be highly variable across different patients. However,

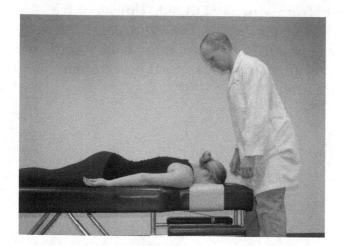

Figure 3-19. Starting position for palpation for segmental tenderness and manual joint palpation.

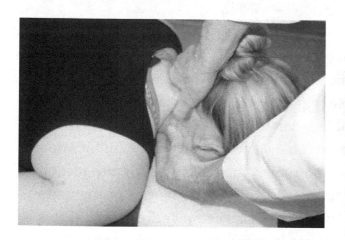

Figure 3-20. Moving the superficial tissues from lateral to medial for palpation for segmental tenderness and manual joint palpation.

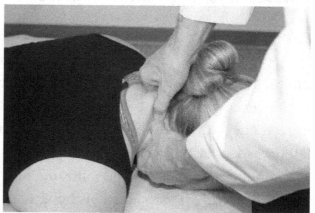

Figure 3-21. Palpation of the tissues overlying the joint during palpation for segmental tenderness.

resistance to motion should typically be symmetrical within the same patient. That is, a normal segment is likely to have similar resistance to motion on the left side as on the right. So asymmetry of resistance to motion is more important to consider than trying to assess for "normal" resistance to motion. It is also important to note that the patient's report of pain is more clinically relevant than the practitioner's sense of resistance to motion. So greater importance should be placed on what the patient reports than on what the practitioner perceives.

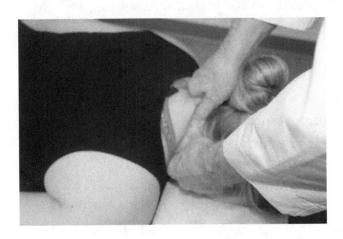

Figure 3-22. Manual joint palpation.

As with PST, the patient lies prone and the practitioner stands at the head of the table. In fact, these tests are best performed sequentially. It is important to apply the palpation as close to the joint surface as possible. Therefore, the overlying tissues must be moved out of the way first. To do this the practitioner starts by placing the thumbs on the lateral aspect of the cervical spine and then moves the superficial tissues medially (Fig. 3-20). The practitioner then uses the flat surface of both thumbs (as opposed to the tips of the thumbs that were used during PST) to palpate for the joint line. The practitioner then applies gentle but firm pressure into the segment at the joint line (Fig. 3-22). The practitioner feels for the amount of resistance to motion and asks whether the maneuver causes pain. If it does, the practitioner asks the patient whether this reproduces all or part of the patient's chief complaint.

With both PST and MJP, is important to compare the palpated segment with "control" segments, i.e., the segment on the opposite side of the cervical spine (if the pain is unilateral) or other levels of the cervical spine. If the amount of resistance to motion and the pain are substantially different at other segments, the practitioner can be confident that the segment at which familiar pain was reproduced is, in fact, the primary pain generating segment. If all segments are equally painful, the practitioner should repeat the procedures, but with less firm pressure. If after reducing the amount of applied pressure the patient continues to report equal amounts of pain at all segments, the practitioner should be less confident in the diagnosis of joint dysfunction (though this does not rule out this diagnosis) and should consider the possibility of the presence of nociceptive system sensitization (see Chapter 4).

Of course, before drawing any firm conclusions about the presence or absence of joint dysfunction, the practitioner must consider all three criteria for this diagnosis, i.e., PST, MJP and ERT.

Each segment of the cervical spine can be examined individually. Although in most cases it is likely not possible to be completely certain as to which numbered segment the practitioner is palpating at any given time, the most important task is to be as precise as possible and to identify the "painful segment", regardless of which numbered segment this is.

The Extension-Rotation Test

The patient is seated and the practitioner extends the patient's the head and neck to end range (Fig. 3-23). The practitioner then passively rotates the head to one side (Fig. 3-24) and asks the patient whether this is painful and, if so, if it reproduces the presenting neck pain. It is important to test rotation to both sides, even in patients with unilateral pain, as the pain can be provoked with rotation toward or away from the side of pain.

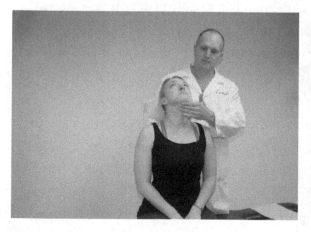
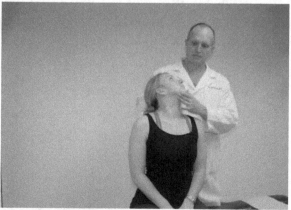

Figure 3-23. The first step in the Extension-Rotation Test – extension of the cervical spine.

Figure 3-24. Adding rotation to the Extension-Rotation Test.

The Flexion-Rotation Test

The patient is lying supine and the practitioner stands at the head of the table. The practi-tioner passively flexes the lower cervical spine to end-range, then passively flexes the upper cervical spine to end range (Fig. 3-25). The practitioner then rotates the head to one side (Fig. 3-26) and asks the patient whether this is painful and, if so, if it reproduces the presenting pain.

As with the Extension-Rotation Test, it is important to test rotation to both sides, even in patients with unilateral pain, as the pain can be provoked with rotation toward or away from the side of pain.

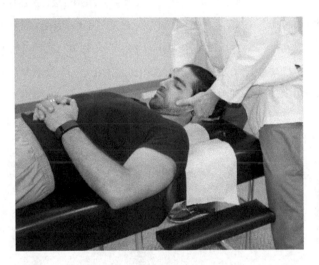

Figure 3-25. The first step in the Flex-ion-Rotation Test – flexion of the en-tire cervical spine.

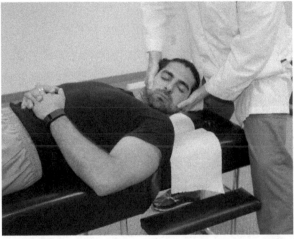

Figure 3-26. Adding rotation of the upper cervical spine to the Flexion-Rotation Test.

Protocol for applying these tests:

- Perform PST and MJP first. These tests in combination are very sensitive. So if they are negative, it is very unlikely the patient has joint dysfunction.
- If PST and MJP are positive, the patient likely has joint dysfunction but to increase the specificity of the diagnosis, perform ERT (for suspected mid- to lower cervical joint dysfunction) or the FRT (for suspected upper cervical joint dysfunction).
- If all three are positive, joint dysfunction is very likely the diagnosis

- If PST and MJP are positive but ERT or FRT is negative, joint dysfunction is still the likely diagnosis, but consider other possibilities, particularly disc derangement or myofascial pain.

See Schneider, et al and Hall, et al in the Recommended Reading list for further information regarding these tests.

Palpation of the first costotransverse joint

The first costotransverse joint can be a source of pain at the cervicothoracic junction and can sometimes cause referred pain into the upper extremity. Palpation of this joint is best performed with the patient sitting. The practitioner stands behind the patient and contacts as close the joint as possible (Fig. 3-27). The practitioner moves the patient's head and cervical spine into ipsilateral lateral flexion, slight contralateral rotation and slight extension. The practitioner then applies gentle but firm pressure into the joint (Fig. 3-28) feeling the amount of resistance to motion and asking whether the maneuver causes pain. If the maneuver causes pain, the practitioner asks the patient whether this reproduces all or part of the patient's chief complaint.

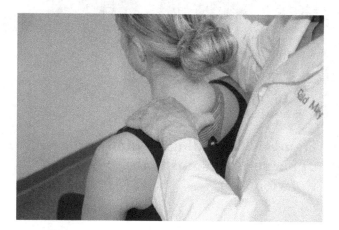

Figure 3-27. Contacting the first costotransverse joint.

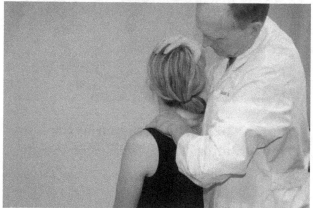

Figure 3-28. Examination of the first costotransverse joint.

Anesthetic joint injections (joint blocks) are occasionally used in an attempt to identify pain arising from the cervical facet joints. However, joint blocks are invasive and expensive and require a meticulous approach to blinding and confirmation in order to produce reasonably reliable findings. Most important, however, is that in most cases it is not necessary to know with *absolute certainly* the precise tissue origin of pain in order to make treatment decisions based on the historical and examination findings presented here. Therefore, injections for diagnostic purposes are uncommonly necessary, particularly at the primary spine care level.

Nevertheless, joint injections are an option in cases in which diagnostic clarity is lacking, and a more precise tissue diagnosis is considered to be clinically important. Substantial temporary improvement in pain intensity strongly suggests that the joint that was injected is the primary pain generator. Pain intensity should be measured prior to and after the injection using a numeric pain rating scale. "Substantial" pain improvement is defined as a minimum of 80% improvement in pain intensity following the injection compared to prior to the injection. The ideal approach is a double block methodology in which substantial short-duration pain relief occurs following injection of a short-acting anesthetic, such as lidocaine, and substantial longer-duration pain relief occurs following injection of a longer-acting anesthetic, such as bupivacaine. However, the double block methodology is not always practical. So in most clinical circumstances, the single block approach is adequate.

If 80% improvement in pain intensity occurs after joint injection, medial branch block (MBB) is used to confirm the presence of facet joint pain. The medial branch of the spinal nerve innervates the facet joints. MBB is an injection technique in which the medial branch is anesthetized temporarily. As with joint blocks, if 80% improvement in pain occurs shortly after the procedure, based on pre- and post-injection pain measures, the facet joint at that level is implicated. MBB is only recommended if radiofrequency neurotomy is being considered (see Chapter 6). Therefore, both joint injections and MBB are typically only indicated in patients who have not experienced substantial improvement with a reasonable trial of primary spine care.

Joint injections and MBBs should be performed under fluoroscopic guidance and are typically performed by an interventional physician, most commonly an anesthesiologist or a physiatrist.

It is recommended that the primary spine practitioner confer with local interventional physicians with regard to the utilization of these procedures.

Radiculopathy

For the purpose of this book, the diagnostic term radiculopathy is used for any disorder involving a nerve root. This can involve nerve root pain in isolation, neurologic dysfunction (such as paresthesia, sensory loss or motor loss) in isolation, or both pain and neurologic dysfunction. The most common causes of radiculopathy are spinal stenosis and disc herniation. Younger patients with radiculopathy are more likely to have disc herniation and older patients are more likely to have spinal stenosis. See Chapter 2 in Volume I of this series for a discussion of the pathophysiology of radiculopathy.

Historical factors associated with radiculopathy are:

- Upper extremity pain, usually with neck pain, though occasionally a patient with cervical radiculopathy will not have neck pain.

- The extremity pain is typically more intense than the neck pain.

- About half of patients also have ipsilateral scapular pain. This is particularly common in patients whose radiculopathy is secondary to disc herniation.

- Neurologic symptoms such as paresthesia, dysesthesia, sensory loss or motor loss.

- Certain arm positions dramatically relieve the pain. If the patient reports that the pain is relieved by holding the arm in adduction, there is a good likelihood of the presence of C5 radiculopathy. If the patient reports that the pain is relieved by raising the arm overhead (often referred to as "Bakody's sign"), there is a good likelihood that he or she has a C6 radiculopathy. Holding the arm against the side and pressing the hand against the chest for relief suggests C7 radiculopathy. However, holding the arm overhead ("Bakody's sign") may be a position of relief with radiculopathy at any level.

- Occasionally, symptoms of myelopathy, including lower extremity neurologic symptoms, ataxia and difficulty with fine motor movements of the hands (see Chapter 2).

Examination for radicular pain involves tests that are designed to apply pressure or tension on the nerve root, thus reproducing the pain, or reducing pressure or tension on the nerve root, thus relieving the pain. An important part of this process is the neurodynamic exam.

The most important cluster of tests in identifying cervical nerve root pain are (see Wainner, et al in Recommended Reading list):

1. The Brachial Plexus Tension Test (BPTT) (sometimes referred to as the Upper Limb Tension Test)

2. Cervical rotation toward the side of symptoms

3. The Cervical Distraction Test

4. The Foraminal Compression Test (sometimes referred to as the Maximum Cervical Compression Test or Spurling's Test)

The Brachial Plexus Tension Test

The BPTT is part of the neurodynamic exam. The neurodynamic exam is discussed in Volume I of this series as it applies to patients with lumbar radiculopathy. This discussion is reproduced here as it applies to patients with cervical radiculopathy. For a more complete exploration of neurodynamics in general the reader is directed to the work of Butler, Shacklock, Neurodynamic Solutions and the NOI Group, all listed under Recommended Reading.

During the neurodynamic exam, the practitioner utilizes maneuvers that apply tension to the nerve root, looking for reproduction of the patient's pain. Maneuvers are then applied that slacken the nerve root to see if this reduces or eliminates the pain. The neurodynamic exam actually applies tension and slackening not only to the nerve roots but to the entire neural tract that the nerve roots are a part of. So, strictly speaking, the neurodynamic exam is designed to identify pain that is arising from a neural source anywhere along the neural tract to which the movement is being applied. The history and the remainder of the examination can then provide clues as to the likelihood that the source of pain is the nerve root itself (although, as will be seen, there are aspects of the neurodynamic exam that can help in this localization).

Because patients with nerve root pain may have other manifestations of radiculopathy, namely neurologic deficit, a careful neurologic exam should be performed (see Chapter 4 in Volume I of this series and Chapter 2 in this volume).

There are three principles that are useful in maximizing the understanding and utilization of the neurodynamic exam:

1. All neural structures are part of an anatomical continuum: As mentioned earlier, the nerve root is anatomically just one aspect of a continuous neural tract that extends from the brain, along the spinal cord to the nerve root and plexus and ending at the distal end of the peripheral nerves. During the neurodynamic exam, tension is applied at several levels of the tract, which ultimately causes tension to be applied along the entire tract. This tension results from movement of the parts of the body through which that neural tract extends.

2. Tension is applied first and to a greatest extent at the point closest to which movement is initiated: For example, if a person were to sit upright and laterally flex the head and spine to one side, then extend the elbow, wrist and fingers, this would apply tension to the nerve roots, brachial plexus and peripheral nerves of the upper extremity, particularly the median nerve. The greatest tension is applied to the cervical nerve roots, as these are closest to the initiation of the movement. The movements that followed would then increase this tension even further. This is helpful in conducting the neurodynamic exam because starting the examination procedure close to the suspected pain source (i.e. the nerve root) may be helpful in maximizing tension on the nerve root, which increases the likelihood that nerve root pain will be reproduced. Clinical application of this group of movements will be discussed below.

3. Structural differentiation: The movements that produce tension on neural structures also produce tension on certain musculoskeletal structures. Therefore, pain with these movements does not necessarily implicate the neural structure as the pain source. Maneuvers that *slacken* the neural structure, without changing the tension on the musculoskeletal structures, will help to differentiate the pain source. If pain that is elicited on the initial maneuver is lessened or eliminated with a structural

differentiation (i.e., neural slackening) maneuver, it is likely that the pain is of neural origin. However if the structural differentiation maneuver fails to reduce or eliminate the pain (particularly if more than one structural differentiation maneuver fails to do this) it is unlikely that the pain is of neural origin.

The initial positioning in the application of the BPTT is very sensitive but is not very specific. That is, a patient with cervical radiculopathy is very likely to have pain with this positioning (high sensitivity). But there are a fairly large number of patients who do not have radiculopathy who will also report pain with this positioning (low specificity). This is the purpose of structural differentiation as discussed above – to increase the specificity of the BPTT in the identification of pain of neural origin.

There are three positions in which the BPTT can be carried out. Each of these positions "biases" the test toward a certain peripheral nerve, thus toward a particular nerve root or group of nerve roots. The nerve roots that are primarily affected by each position are:

- Median bias position: primarily C5-7

- Ulnar bias position: primarily C8-T1

- Radial bias position: primarily C7

The position that is most commonly positive in patients with cervical radiculopathy is the "median bias" position. In the examination of the patient with suspected radiculopathy, this position should be applied first. If no clear significant findings are identified with this position, the ulnar biased position should be explored next, followed by the radial bias position.

The BPTT in the Median Bias Position

The patient lies supine and the practitioner sits facing the superior. In preparation for the test, the patient's arm is placed in 90 degrees of shoulder abduction and 90 degrees of elbow flexion (Fig. 3-29). The practitioner depresses the shoulder girdle by pressing downward on the shoulder (Fig. 3-30). The practitioner then extends the wrist and fingers (Fig. 3-31), supinates the forearm (Fig. 3-32), externally rotates the shoulder (Fig. 3-33) and extends the elbow (Fig. 3-34) to the point at which the practitioner feels tension develop and/or the patient reports pain.

The tension is usually felt by the practitioner in the form of elevation of the patient's shoulder girdle.

It is important that the tension that was developed at each point in the maneuver is maintained as the maneuver is continued. If the maneuver is painful, the practitioner asks if this reproduces the patient's pain.

Structural differentiation during the application of the BPTT in the median bias position

When performing the BPTT in the median bias position, structural differentiation can be applied in several ways. The simplest and most useful method is for the practitioner to let up on the pressure that is maintaining shoulder girdle depression, allowing the shoulder girdle to rise (Fig. 3-35). This reduces tension on the neural tract without changing the stretch on the muscular and joint structures of the arm. If this maneuver reduces or eliminates the pain, this suggests that the pain is of neural origin.

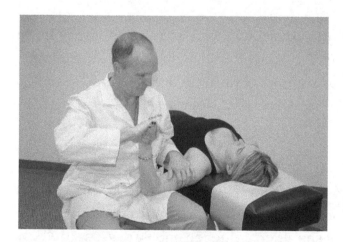

Figure 3-29. Starting position for the Brachial Plexus Tension Test in both the median bias position and the ulnar bias position.

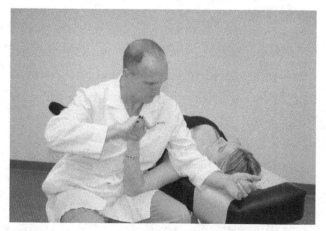

Figure 3-30. Depression of the shoulder girdle during performance of the Brachial Plexus Tension Test in the median bias position.

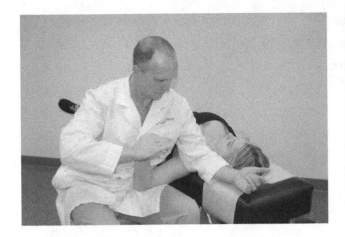

Figure 3-31. Extension of the wrist and fingers during performance of the Brachial Plexus Tension Test in the median bias position. Note that the thumb is extended as well as the remaining fingers.

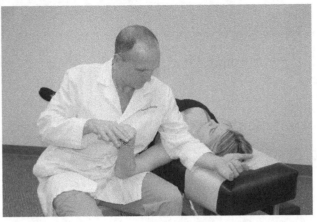

Figure 3-32. Supination of the forearm during performance of the Brachial Plexus Tension Test in the median bias position.

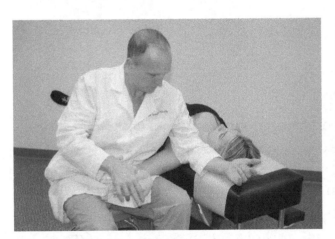

Figure 3-33. External rotation of the shoulder during performance of the Brachial Plexus Tension Test in the median bias position.

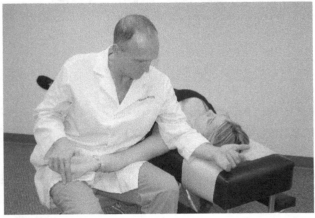

Figure 3-34. Extension of the elbow during performance of the Brachial Plexus Tension Test in the median bias position.

The structural differentiation can be confirmed by the practitioner re-applying downward pressure on the shoulder girdle so that the pain is again reproduced, then flexing the wrist and fingers, reducing tension on the distal end of the neural tract (Fig. 3-36). If this reduces the pain, the suspicion of a neural source of pain is supported.

There are some patients with suspected radiculopathy in whom the application of the BPTT in the median bias position does not clearly reproduce the patient's pain. One useful modification is to position the patient's head in lateral flexion away from the side that is being tested (recall that this places greater emphasis on the nerve roots) and to re-apply the test (Fig. 3-37). If this reproduces the patient's pain, structural differentiation can be applied by having the patient return the head to the neutral position. If this lessens or eliminates the pain, a neural source of the pain is suspected.

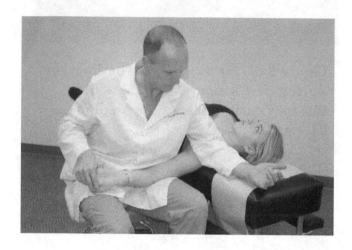

Figure 3-37. Application of the Brachial Plexus Tension Test in the median bias position with the head placed in lateral flexion away from the side being tested.

The BPTT in the Ulnar Bias Position

The patient again lies supine and the practitioner sits facing the superior. In preparation for the test, the patient's arm is placed in 90 degrees of shoulder abduction and 90 degrees of elbow flexion (Fig. 3-29). The practitioner depresses the shoulder girdle by pressing downward on the shoulder. For testing in the ulnar bias position, it is best for the practitioner to use his or her hand for this purpose. The practitioner extends the wrist and fingers, however, unlike the median bias procedure, only the 4th and 5th digits are included (Fig. 3-38). The practitioner then pronates the forearm (Fig. 3-39), externally rotates the shoulder (Fig. 3-40) and flexes the elbow and shoulder so that the patient's hand moves toward the ear (Fig. 3-41). If this maneuver is painful, the practitioner asks if this reproduces the patient's pain. Structural differentiation can be pursued by the practitioner letting up on the shoulder depression to determine whether this lessens or eliminates the pain. Further confirmation can be sought by re-applying shoulder depression to the point at which the pain is again reproduced, then flexing the wrist and fingers and/or moving the elbow away from the flexed position to determine whether this lessens or eliminates the pain.

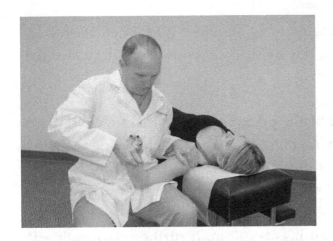

Figure 3-38. Extension of the 4th and 5th digits during performance of the Brachial Plexus Tension Test in the ulnar bias position.

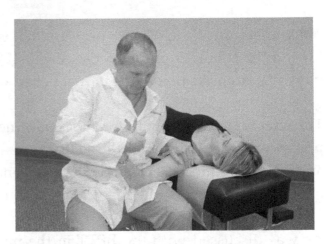

Figure 3-39. Pronation of the forearm during performance of the Brachial Plexus Tension Test in the ulnar bias position.

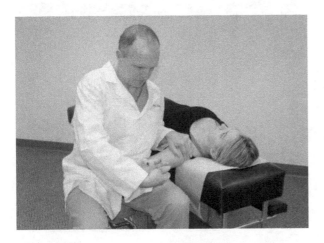

Figure 3-40. External rotation of the shoulder during performance of the Brachial Plexus Tension Test in the ulnar bias position.

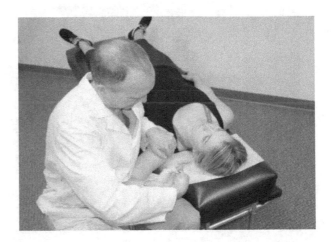

Figure 3-41. Flexion of the elbow and shoulder during performance of the Brachial Plexus Tension Test in the ulnar bias position.

Structural differentiation during the application of the BPTT in the ulnar bias position

When performing the BPTT in the ulnar bias position, structural differentiation can be applied in in a similar manner as when performing the BPTT in the median bias position. First, the practitioner can let up on the pressure that is maintaining shoulder girdle depression, allowing the shoulder girdle to rise (Fig. 3-42). If this maneuver reduces or eliminates the pain, this suggests that the pain is of neural origin.

The structural differentiation can be confirmed by the practitioner re-applying downward pressure on the shoulder girdle so that the pain is again reproduced, then flexing the wrist and fingers, reducing tension on the distal end of the neural tract (Fig. 3-43). If this reduces or eliminates the pain, the suspicion of a neural source of pain is supported.

As was discussed with the BPTT in the median bias position, if further clarification is needed the test can be performed with the head placed in lateral flexion prior to commencement of the procedure (Fig. 3-44). If reproduction of pain occurs during the test, structural differentiation can be pursued by having the patient return the head to the neutral position.

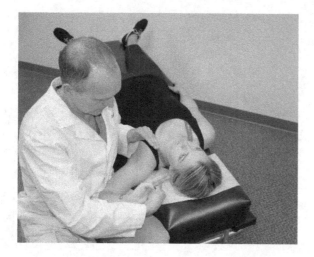

Figure 3-42. Letting up on the depression of the shoulder girdle for structural differentiation during performance of the Brachial Plexus Tension Test in the ulnar bias position.

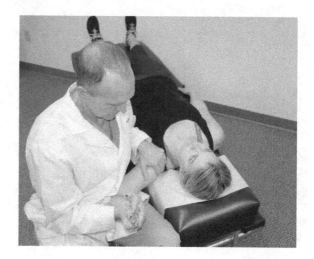

Figure 3-43. Flexion of the wrist and fingers for structural differentiation during performance of the Brachial Plexus Tension Test in the ulnar bias position.

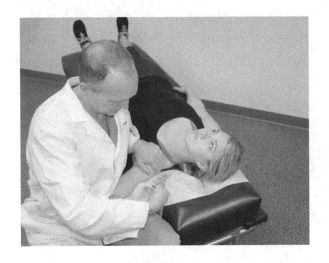

Figure 3-44. Application of the Brachial Plexus Tension Test in the ulnar bias position with the head placed in lateral flexion away from the side being tested.

The BPTT in the Radial Bias Position

The patient is again in the supine position but this time the practitioner is facing the inferior. As with the median and ulnar bias tests, the patient's arm is placed in 90 degrees of shoulder abduction and 90 degrees of elbow flexion. The practitioner depresses the shoulder girdle by pressing with the hand downward on the shoulder (Fig. 3-45). The practitioner then flexes the wrist and fingers (Fig. 3-46), pronates the forearm (Fig. 3-47), internally rotates the shoulder (Fig. 3-48) and extends the elbow (Fig. 3-49). As with the other tests, the practitioner asks if this is painful, and if it reproduces the patient's pain.

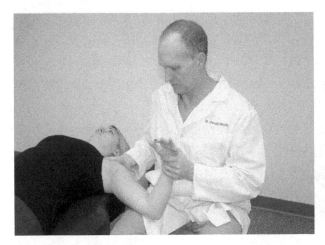

Figure 3-45. Depression of the shoulder girdle during performance of the Brachial Plexus Tension Test in the radial bias position.

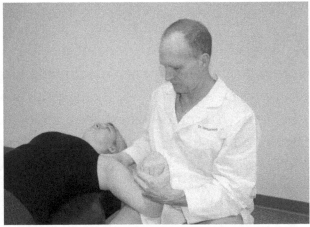

Figure 3-46. Flexion of the wrist and fingers during performance of the Brachial Plexus Tension Test in the radial bias position.

Structural differentiation can be pursued by the practitioner letting up on the shoulder depression to determine whether this lessens or eliminates the pain (Fig. 3-50). Confirmation can be sought by the practitioner re-applying shoulder depression to the point at which the pain is again reproduced, then reducing the wrist and finger flexion or reducing the elbow extension (Fig. 3-51). Also, as with the other tests, if further confirmation is required the test can begin with lateral flexion of the head away from the side being tested (Fig. 3-52).

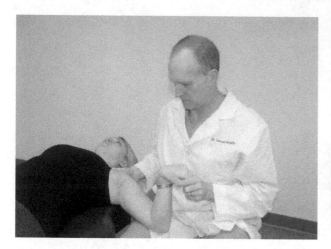

Figure 3-47. Pronation of the forearm during performance of the Brachial Plexus Tension Test in the radial bias position.

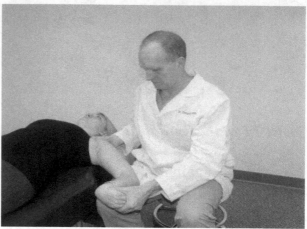

Figure 3-48. Internal rotation of the shoulder during performance of the Brachial Plexus Tension Test in the radial bias position.

Ideally, with the BPTT a "positive" test is exact reproduction of the patient's arm pain, with lessening or elimination of the pain with structural differentiation maneuvers. However there are a number of patients with radiculopathy in whom the BPTT will be painful, but will not precisely reproduce the patient's pain in the *exact* same location. In these cases, it is useful to perform the test on the uninvolved side. As mentioned earlier, patients without radiculopathy will often experience discomfort with the BPTT – stretching of neural structures is somewhat uncomfortable for most people. However, in normal circumstances the discomfort, as well as the range of movement of the upper extremity during the performance of the test, is symmetrical bilaterally.

So in cases in which the test does not clearly reproduce the patient's exact pain pattern, greater discomfort and/or reduced range of movement on the side of involvement compared to the non-painful side should be considered a "positive" test.

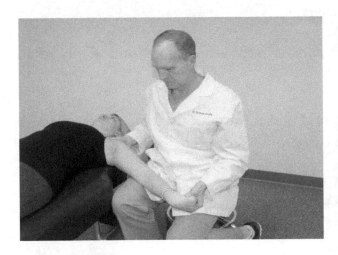

Figure 3-49. Extension of the elbow during performance of the Brachial Plexus Tension Test in the radial bias position.

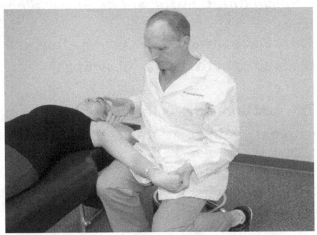

Figure 3-50. Letting up on the depression of the shoulder girdle for structural differentiation during performance of the Brachial Plexus Tension Test in the radial bias position.

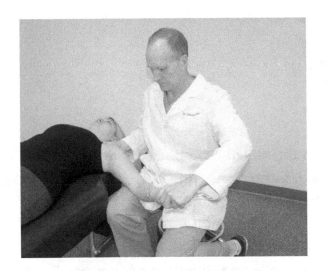

Figure 3-51. Extension of the wrist and fingers for structural differentiation during performance of the Brachial Plexus Tension Test in the radial bias position.

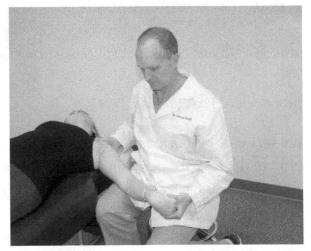

Figure 3-52. Application of the Brachial Plexus Tension Test in the radial bias position with the head placed in lateral flexion away from the side being tested.

Cervical Rotation Toward the Side of Symptoms

This can be carried out simply by having the patient in the seated position actively rotate the head toward the side of symptoms.

The practitioner asks the patient if this is painful and if it reproduces the patient's upper extremity pain. If it does not the practitioner can provide additional passive rotation (Fig. 3-53).

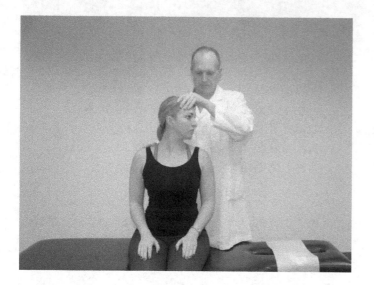

Figure 3-53. Practitioner-assisted cervical rotation in examining for cervical radiculopathy.

The Cervical Distraction Test

This test can be performed with the patient in the seated or supine position. It is best to perform the test in a position in which the patient's arm pain is provoked, since the purpose of the Cervical Distraction Test is to attempt to relieve the pain.

In the supine position, the practitioner places one hand under the occiput and the other beneath the chin. The practitioner flexes the cervical spine slightly, and then applies long axis traction (Fig. 3-54). The practitioner asks the patient if this relieves the arm pain. Alternate methods include the practitioner placing both hands under the occiput or one hand under the occiput and the other on the forehead.

In the seated position, the practitioner places both hands under the mastoid processes with the thumbs under the occiput. The practitioner lifts the head straight upward to distract the cervical spine (Fig. 3-55). The practitioner asks the patient if this relieves the arm pain. Relief of arm pain with this maneuver constitutes a positive test.

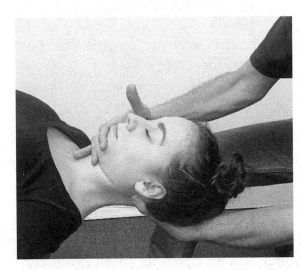

Figure 3-54. The Cervical Distraction Test in the supine position.

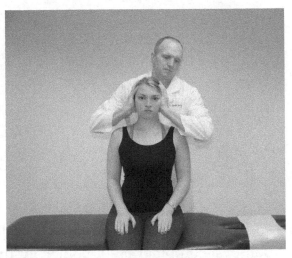

Figure 3-55. The Cervical Distraction Test in the seated position.

Foraminal Compression Test (Maximum Cervical Compression Test, Spurling's Test)

The patient is seated and the practitioner stands behind the patient. The practitioner laterally flexes the head toward the side of symptoms, rotates the head slightly toward the side of symptoms and slightly extends the head. The practitioner then places the hands on the top of the head and applies gentle but firm downward pressure on the head (Fig. 3-56). The practitioner asks if this maneuver is painful and if it reproduces the patient's pain. This test should not be performed on a patient in whom severe acute injury is suspected.

As stated earlier, in the vast majority of patients with radiculopathy, the underlying cause is lateral stenosis, herniated disc, or some combination of both these. The only way to know the underlying cause for certain is MRI. However, in the vast majority of cases, MRI is unnecessary, as it will not impact primary management of the condition.

In patients in whom significant pathology is suspected (i.e., patients in whom there are factors of concern related to diagnostic question #1) or in whom injection or surgery are being considered, MRI is indicated. However, this applies to the minority of patients. See Chapters 4 and 12 in Volume I of this series, and Chapter 2 in this volume, for further discussions on the indications for advanced imaging such as MRI.

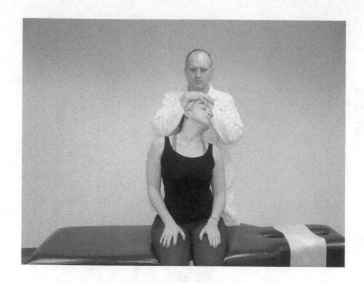

Figure 3-56. The Foraminal Compression Test, also known as Maximum Cervical Compression Test and Spurling's Test.

In the majority of patients with radiculopathy, whether from lateral canal stenosis, disc herniation or a combination of both, joint dysfunction will be found on the side and approximately at the level of the involved nerve root. It is likely that the joint dysfunction is the cause of the neck pain in these patients, with the radiculopathy causing the upper extremity pain. However, the presence of joint dysfunction should not be assumed; careful examination, as described above in the section on joint dysfunction, should be carried out.

Myofascial Pain

Myofascial pain is thought result from myofascial trigger points (TrPs). It was discussed in Volume I of this series that in patients with low back disorders (LBDs) myofascial pain usually occurs secondary to one of the other pain generators considered with diagnostic question #2. The same applies to patients with cervical disorders (CDs), although to a slightly lesser degree. That is, in most patients with CDs, any TrPs that are present are secondary. However, it is more common in CD patients than in LBD patients for TrPs to be a primary source of pain, with or without one of the other pain generators. In these patients the TrPs will often require treatment. This is particularly true of the headache patient.

TrPs can be identified through skilled palpation. In deciding what muscles to evaluate for the presence of TrPs it is useful to know the typical referred pain pattern that arises from the various muscles of the cervical spine. By having the patient specifically identify the location of the pain, the practitioner can determine what muscle or muscles should be examined for TrPs.

With the presence of a TrP, there is usually a taut band within the muscle that can be identified through palpation. This taut band will be tender to palpation but may not reproduce the patient's pain.

By moving along the taut band the practitioner will typically find the TrP, which will feel like a nodular formation. The TrP will be painful upon palpation and, if it is involved in the generation of the patient's pain, will reproduce the pain.

Discussed here are the muscles that are most commonly involved in patient with CDs.

Muscles that can contribute to neck, shoulder and upper extremity pain:

1. Cervical erector spinae: These include the iliocostalis cervicis, longissimus cervicis, semispinalis cervicis and seminspinalis capitis muscles. TrPs in this group of muscles typically cause local pain in the cervical spine that can occasionally extend into the upper thoracic spine (Fig. 3-57). Palpation can be performed with the patient in the supine or prone position (Fig. 3-58).

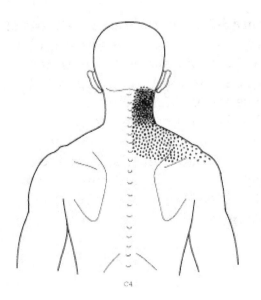

Figure 3-57. Referred pain pattern of trigger points in the cervical erector spinae muscles. Reprinted with permission from Murphy DR, ed. Conservative Management of Cervical Spine Syndromes. New York: McGraw-Hill, 2000.

2. Levator scapulae: TrPs in this muscle typically cause localized pain at the cervicothoracic junction, occasionally extending into the scapula. They are often found in conjunction with TrPs in the rhomboid muscles in patients with scapular pain (Fig. 3-59). The most common area for TrPs in this muscle is near the attachment point at the superior angle of the scapula. Palpation can be performed with the patient in the seated or prone position (Fig. 3-60).

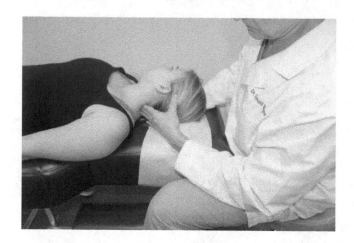

Figure 3-58. Palpation of the cervical erector spinae with the patient in the supine position.

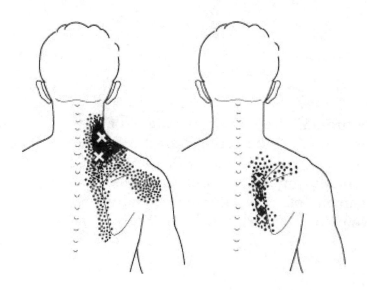

Figure 3-59. Referred pain patterns of trigger points in the levator scapulae and rhomboid muscles. Reprinted with permission from Murphy DR, ed. Conservative Management of Cervical Spine Syndromes. New York: cGraw-Hill, 2000. Adapted from Travell JG, Simons DG. Myofascial Pain and Dysfunction: The Trigger Point Manual. Vol. 1. 1983 Williams and Wilkens, Baltimore.

4. Scalenes: TrPs in the scalenes can cause pain to radiate into the upper extremity (Fig. 3-61). This can mimic radiculopathy or thoracic outlet syndrome in some patients, although the pain from scalene TrPs will typically not be as severe as that from neural entrapment conditions. Pain from scalene trigger points can also refer into the chest or scapular area. Palpation can be performed with the patient in the seated or supine position (Fig. 3- 62).

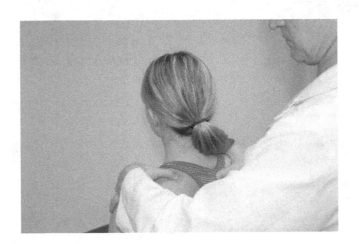

Figure 3-60. Palpation of the levator scapulae with the patient in the seated position.

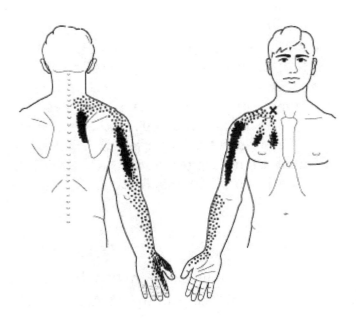

Figure 3-61. Referred pain pattern of trigger points in the scalenes. Reprinted with permission from Murphy DR, ed. Conservative Management of Cervical Spine Syndromes. New York: McGraw-Hill, 2000. Adapted from Travell JG, Simons DG. Myofascial Pain and Dysfunction: The Trigger Point Manual. Vol. 1. 1983 Williams and Wilkens, Baltimore.

Muscles that can contribute to headache:

1. Suboccipitals: TrP's in the suboccipals may refer pain over the side of the head and behind the eye (Fig. 3-63). Palpation is best performed with the patient in the supine position (Fig. 3-64).

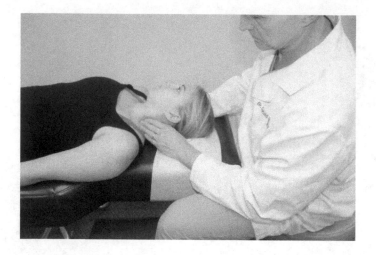

Figure 3-62. Palpation of the scalenes with the patient in the supine position.

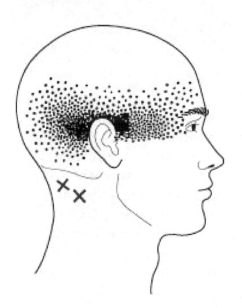

Figure 3-63. Referred pain pattern of trigger points in the suboccipals. Reprinted with permission from Murphy DR, ed. Conservative Management of Cervical Spine Syndromes. New York: McGraw-Hill, 2000. Adapted from Travell JG, Simons DG. Myofascial Pain and Dysfunction: The Trigger Point Manual. Vol. 1. 1983 Williams and Wilkens, Baltimore.

2. Sternoceidomastoid: This is perhaps the most common muscle involved in patients with facial pain, ear pain and headache. It often mimics pain from sinus infections and ear disorders. The referred pain pattern can include almost any part of the face and head (Fig. 3-65). Palpation is best performed with the patient in the supine position, using a pincer-type palpation (Fig. 3-66).

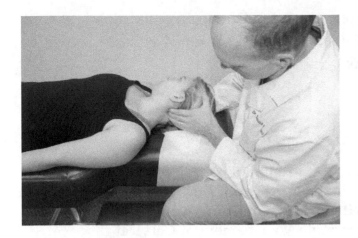

Figure 3-64. Palpation of the suboccipitals.

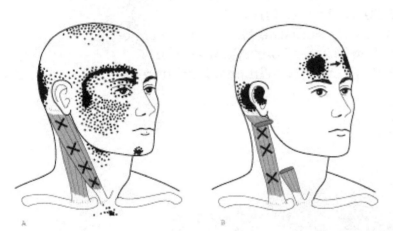

Figure 3-65. Referred pain pattern of trigger points in the sternocleido-mastoid. Reprinted with permission from Murphy DR, ed. Conservative Management of Cervical Spine Syndromes. New York: McGraw-Hill, 2000. Adapted from Travell JG, Simons DG. Myofascial Pain and Dysfunction: The Trigger Point Manual. Vol. 1. 1983 Williams and Wilkens, Baltimore.

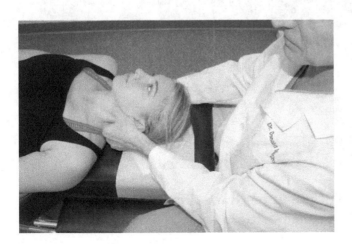

Figure 3-66. Palpation of the sternocleidomastoid.

3. Upper trapezius: TrPs in this muscle can cause localized pain in the muscle as well as temporal headaches (Fig. 3-67). Palpation can be performed with the patient in the supine or prone position (Fig. 3-68).

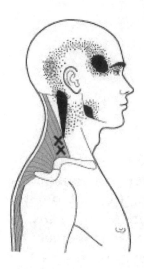

Figure 3-67. Referred pain pattern of trigger points in the upper trapezius. Reprinted with permission from Murphy DR, ed. Conservative Management of Cervical Spine Syndromes. New York: McGraw-Hill, 2000. Adapted from Travell JG, Simons DG. Myofascial Pain and Dysfunction: The Trigger Point Manual. Vol. 1. 1983 Williams and Wilkens, Baltimore.

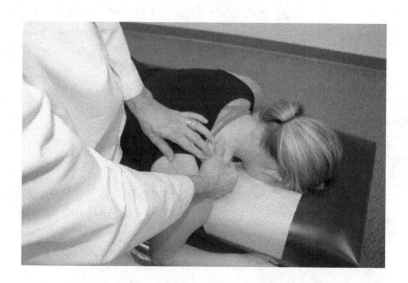

Figure 3-68. Palpation of the upper trapezius with the patient in the prone position

The purpose of diagnostic question #2 is to try to identify, with as much accuracy as possible, the source of the patient's pain. As has been stated before, diagnosis in the area of spine related disorders is, in the majority of cases, made clinically, based on history and examination. With regard to diagnostic questions #2 and 3, there are usually no definitive objective tests that provide the practitioner with absolute answers. However, in the majority of patients a careful history and skilled, evidence-based examination allows the practitioner to make a reasonably accurate diagnosis which allows for satisfactory patient education and helps drive management decisions. This will be explored further in the next chapter with regard to diagnostic question #3.

Recommended Reading

Aprill C, Dwyer A, Bogduk N. Cervical zygapophyseal joint plan patterns II: A clinical evaluation. Spine 1990;15(6):458-61.

Dreyfuss P, Michaelson M, Fletcher D. Atlanto-Occipital and Lateral Atlanta-Axial Joint Pain Patterns. Spine 1994; 19(10):1125-1131.

Dwyer A, Aprill C, Bogduk N. Cervical zygapophyseal joint pain patterns I: A study in normal volunteers. Spine 1990;15(6):453-457.

Farmer JC, Wisneski RJ. Cervical spine nerve root compression: An analysis of neuroforaminal pressures with varying head and arm positions. Spine 1994; 19(16):1850-1855.

Hall TM, Robinson KW, Fujinawa O, Akasaka K, Pyne EA. Intertester reliability and diagnostic validity of the cervical flexion-rotation test. J Manipulative Physiol Ther. 2008 May;31(4):293-300.

Hall TM, Briffa K, Hopper D, Robinson KW. The relationship between cervicogenic headache and impairment determined by the flexion-rotation test. J Manipulative Physiol Ther. 2010 Nov-Dec;33(9):666-71.

http://www.mckenziemdt.org/ [accessed 15 July 2016]

Laerum E, Indahl A, Skouen JS. What is "the good back consultation?" a combined qualitative and quantitative study of chronic low back pain patients' interaction with and perceptions of consultations with specialists. J Rehabil Med 2006;38(4):255-262.

Lohman CM, Gilbert KK, Sobczak S, Brismee JM, James CR, Day M, et al. 2015 Young Investigator Award Winner: Cervical Nerve Root Displacement and Strain During Upper Limb Neural Tension Testing: Part 1: A Minimally Invasive Assessment in Unembalmed Cadavers. Spine (Phila Pa 1976). 2015 Jun 1;40(11):793-800.

Manvell JJ, Manvell N, Snodgrass SJ, Reid SA. Improving the radial nerve neurodynamic test: An observation of tension of the radial, median and ulnar nerves during upper limb positioning. Man Ther. 2015 Dec;20(6):790-6.

McKenzie R, May S. The Cervical and Thoracic Spine: Mechanical Diagnosis and Therapy. 2nd ed. Raumati Beach, NZ: Spinal Publications; 2006.

Murphy DR, Hurwitz EL, Gerrard JK, Clary R. Pain patterns and descriptions in patients with radicular pain: Does the pain necessarily follow a specific dermatome? Chiropr Osteopat 2009;17(1):9.

Murphy DR, Hurwitz EL, Gregory AA, Clary R. A nonsurgical approach to the management of patients with cervical radiculopathy: A prospective observational cohort study. J Manipulative Physiol Ther 2006;29(4):279-87.

Rubio-Ochoa J, Benitez-Martinez J, Lluch E, Santacruz-Zaragoza S, Gomez-Contreras P, Cook CE. Physical examination tests for screening and diagnosis of cervicogenic headache: A systematic review. Man Ther. 2016 Feb;21:35-40.

Schneider GM, Jull G, Thomas K, Salo P. Screening of patients suitable for diagnostic cervical facet joint blocks--a role for physiotherapists. Man Ther 2012;17(2):180-3.

Schneider GM, Jull G, Thomas K, Smith A, Emery C, Faris P, et al. Intrarater and Interrater Reliability of Select Clinical Tests in Patients Referred for Diagnostic Facet Joint Blocks in the Cervical Spine. Arch Phys Med Rehabil 2013;94(8):1628-34.

Schneider GM, Jull G, Thomas K, Smith A, Emery C, Faris P, et al. Derivation of a clinical decision guide in the diagnosis of cervical facet joint pain. Arch Phys Med Rehabil. 2014 Sep;95(9):1695-701.

Simons DG, Travell JG, Simons LS. Myofascial Pain and Dysfunction: The Trigger Point Manual. Volume 1. Baltimore: Williams and Wilkens; 1999.

Verbeek J, Sengers M, Riemens L, Haafkens J. Patient expectations of treatment for back pain: a systematic review of qualitative and quantitative studies. Spine (Phila Pa 1976). 2004;29(20):2309-17.

Wainner RS, Fritz JM, Irrgang JJ, Boninger ML, Delitto A, Allison S. Reliability and diagnostic accuracy of the clinical and patient self report measures for cervical radiculopathy. Spine (Phila Pa 1976) 2003;28(1):52-62.

• Chapter 4 •

Diagnostic question #3: What has happened with this person as a whole that would cause the pain experience to develop and persist?

Introduction

Another way of asking this question is, "what factors are present that are perpetuating the ongoing pain, disability and suffering experience or are causing recurrent episodes?" There are several factors that can contribute to the perpetuation of cervical disorders (CDs). It should be noted that diagnostic question #3 is particularly important in the subacute or chronic patient, in addition to diagnostic questions #1 and 2. This is in contrast with the acute patient, in whom diagnostic questions #1 and 2 are most critical. Diagnostic question #3 is also important in the patient who initially presents in the acute stage but following a trial of primary spine care does not fully recover (or does not improve at all) from the acute episode.

It should be noted, however, that the psychological factors that are considered under diagnostic question #3 are *always* important, regardless of the stage of the disorder. However these are not generally included in the diagnosis in acute patients because in most cases they will improve with effective management of the factors related to diagnostic question #2, *provided this management occurs in the CBT/ACT context that is discussed throughout this book series.* In other words, most patients with an acute spine related disorder will improve through an approach that effectively addresses the primary pain generator with a focus on patient empowerment, self-care and functional independence, even if they initially exhibit elevated psychological perpetuating factors.

It should be noted that in this volume Cognitive-Behavioral Therapy is abbreviated "CBT". This is different from the "Cog-B" abbreviation that was used in Volume I of this series. Because the abbreviation "CBT" is more standard in the literature, this abbreviation will be used here.

The perpetuating factors that are considered with diagnostic question #3 in patients with cervical disorders are presented in Table 4-1.

Table 4-1. Perpetuating factors to be considered in diagnostic question #3 in patients with cervical disorders.

Somatic/ Neurophysiological factors	Psychological factors
Dynamic Instability	Fear
Passive Instability	Catastrophizing
Oculomotor dysfunction	Passive coping
Nociceptive system sensitization	Poor self-efficacy
	Depression
	Perceived injustice
	Cognitive fusion
	Hypervigilance for symptoms
	Anxiety

Dynamic Instability

While research in this area is relatively early in its development, it appears that in patients who are affected by dynamic instability in the cervical spine, the pattern of neuromuscular dysfunction is one in which there is inhibition of the deep cervical flexors and the lower cervical and upper thoracic extensors and hyperactivity of the sternocleidomastoids. The deep cervical flexors include the longus capitis, longus colli and rectus capitis anterior. The lower cervical and upper thoracic extensors include the multifidus, iliocostalis cervicis, longissimus cervicis, semispinalis cervicis and seminspinalis capitis.

Historical factors that may be suggestive of dynamic instability in the cervical spine include (see Cook, et al in Recommended Reading list):

- Increased pain and/or fatigue with prolonged static postures

- Less pain with external support, such as with the hands or a cervical collar

- Frequent need for self-manipulation (which can also be a factor in nociceptive system sensitization, as discussed below)

- A feeling of instability, shaking, or lack of control with movement

- Frequent acute episodes

- Pain with sudden movements such as turning in bed

The examination procedures that are designed to detect dynamic instability in the cervical spine primarily examine the activity of the deep cervical flexors.

1. Craniocervical Flexion Test: This test necessitates the use of a pressure biofeedback unit that can measure the amount of pressure applied by the deep cervical flexors. This unit can be obtained at **www.optp.com** [accessed 15 July 2016]. The patient lies supine and the pressure biofeedback unit is placed under the upper cervical spine (Fig. 4-1). The unit should come into contact with the occiput and maintain this contact throughout the test.

   The practitioner inflates the unit to a baseline pressure of 20 mm Hg. The practitioner shows the gauge to the patient and instructs the patient to nod the head, flexing the upper cervical spine, to increase the pressure to 22 mm Hg (Fig. 4-2).

   It is important for the patient to deliberately flex the upper cervical spine, rather than retracting or lifting the head. The practitioner should watch for activation of the superficial muscles, particularly the sternocleidomastoids. The practitioner should observe whether the movement is being carried out in a smooth fashion or if the movement is jerky. The patient holds the pressure at 22 mm Hg for 10 seconds. If the patient can do this successfully in a smooth fashion, the test is repeated at 24, 26, 28 and 30 mm Hg.

Normally an individual should be able to smoothly apply pressure to 26 mm Hg and hold that pressure for 10 seconds. Inability to attain and hold 26 mm Hg of pressure without jerking or shaking suggests the presence of dynamic instability (see Jull, et al in the Recommended Reading list).

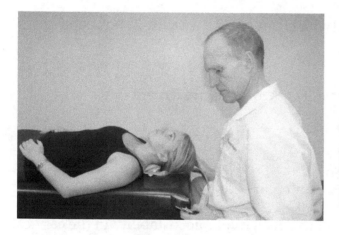 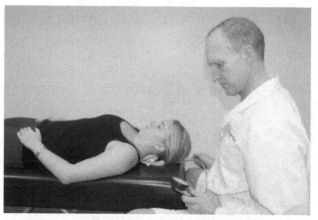

Figure 4-1. Positioning for the Cranio-cervical Flexion Test. Note that the pressure biofeedback unit is placed under the upper cervical spine, contacting the occiput.

Figure 4-2. Upper cervical flexion during the Craniocervical Flexion Test. Note that the movement is a pure "nodding" motion with no retraction or elevation of the head.

2. Cervical Stability Test: This is a quick screening test that is less precise than the Craniocervical Flexion Test but can be easily performed in the context of a busy clinic environment. The patient lies supine with the head beyond the edge of the table. The practitioner passively prepositions the head in the neutral position with the chin slightly tucked. The practitioner tells the patient that he or she is going to let go of the head and that the patient is to continue to hold this exact position for 10 seconds. The practitioner then slowly lets go of the head and observes (Fig. 4-3).

Normally, an individual should be able to hold the head in this position for 10 seconds. Inability to maintain this position suggests the presence of dynamic instability.

The most common findings that constitute a positive test are:

- Poking of the chin (Fig. 4-4)

- Excessive shaking

- Flexion of the cervical spine (Fig. 4-5)

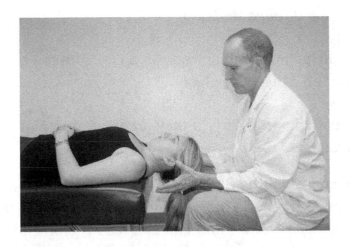

Figure 4-3. The Cervical Stability Test.

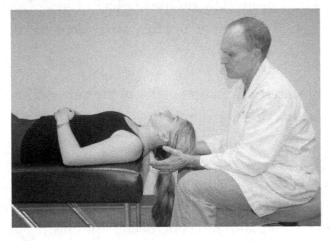

Figure 4-4. Chin poking during the Cervical Stability Test.

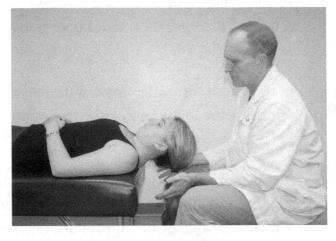

Figure 4-5. Flexion of the head during the Cervical Stability Test.

Passive Instability

Passive instability in the lower cervical spine should be suspected in patients who have had trauma severe enough to cause ligamentous disruption or who have degenerative spondylolisthesis.

Historical factors that may be suggestive of passive instability of the cervical spine include:

- Decreased pain with external support, such as with the hands or a cervical collar

- A feeling of instability, shaking, or lack of control with movement

- Increased pain after manipulation or end range stretching

- Increased pain after sleeping in an awkward position such as prone with the head twisted or falling asleep in a chair or on a bus or airplane

- Signs and/or symptoms of myelopathy, particularly if they are intermittent or induced by certain movements or positions

If there are clear reasons to suspect passive instability, flexion-extension radiographs are the preferred means of diagnosis. The standard criteria for determining segmental instability on flexion-extension radiographs are that of White and Panjabi (see Recommended Reading list) although more research is needed to investigate the clinical utility of these criteria. The criteria consider both translation of the segment and flexion/ extension of the segment.

In the lower cervical spine, sagittal plane translation >3.5 mm or 20% of the vertebral body width is considered excessive translation. Flexion or extension of the segment greater than 11 degrees is considered excessive movement.

It is important in patients with passive instability to consider not only biomechanical instability but also neurological "instability". That is, passive instability in the cervical spine, if it is of sufficient magnitude in the presence of spondylotic encroachment on the spinal cord, can lead to neurologic compromise, i.e., cervical spondylotic myelopathy. So it is important in the patient with passive instability of the cervical spine to carefully assess for signs and symptoms suggestive of cervical cord compression. See Chapter 2 for specifics regarding the clinical diagnosis of cervical spondylotic myelopathy. Important with regard to the patient with cervical spondylotic myelopathy who has associated passive instability is that the symptoms of cord compression can be intermittent. In patients with cervical spondylotic myelopathy without instability, the symptoms are more likely to be persistent.

Passive instability in the upper cervical spine can occur in pathological states such as rheumatoid arthritis and ankylosing spondylitis and in congenital conditions such as Down syndrome and Ehlers-Danlos syndrome. Rarely, it can occur after throat infection. Passive instability in the upper cervical spine in the absence of these disorders or very severe trauma (which would likely cause significant neurologic compromise and thus would fall under diagnostic question #1) is controversial.

White and Panjabi (see Recommended Reading list) suggest that anterior translation of the anterior arch of C1 of 3mm beyond the dens in the adult or 4mm beyond the dens in the child suggests instability. It has also been suggested that excessive lateral translation of C1 noted on anterior-to-posterior, open-mouth (APOM) radiographs during lateral bending suggests passive instability.

However most of the studies related to this involve patients with rheumatoid arthritis, not subacute or chronic neck pain, and there is no agreement on the amount of translation that should be considered to represent "instability". Further, it is difficult on an APOM radiograph to distinguish between pure lateral translation of C1 and rotational artifact, due to the fact that a three dimensional movement is being evaluated with a two dimensional static image.

Physical examination procedures have been proposed to assess the passive stability of the upper cervical spine (see Osmotherly, et al and Mathers, et al in the Recommended Reading list) however, again, it is unclear whether true passive instability exists in the non-pathologic patient in the absence of severe trauma. In addition, there no Gold Standard for the identification of passive instability of the upper cervical spine in these patients. Thus, the clinical utility of these examination procedures is unknown.

So it can be seen that the detection of passive instability in the cervical spine is not well-defined and represents the principle of "doing the best we can with the information we currently have."

Scapular Instability

It is thought that poorly coordinated movement of the scapula ("scapular instability", sometimes referred to as "scapular dyskinesis") can play a role in the perpetuation of chronic CDs. It appears that there is no typical pattern of muscular imbalance that consistently occurs with scapular instability. It is likely that, if alteration in scapular muscle activity is a factor in CD patients, the specific alteration is highly individual. Thus it best for the practitioner to look for general patterns of dysfunction rather than any particular altered pattern. It is also important to look for asymmetry from one side to the other, particularly in a patient whose CD is unilateral.

A simple examination procedure is presented can be applied in the primary spine care environment. This procedure is based on the work of McClure and Tate (see recommended reading list).

The patient stands with the scapulae exposed (i.e., shirtless or wearing a halter top or gown) while holding a three-pound weight in each hand. The patient slowly flexes the shoulders, raising the weight straight out in front, then lowers to the starting position (Fig. 4-6).

The patient then abducts the shoulders in the plane of the scapula (i.e., 30-45 forward of the coronal plane), then lowers to the starting position (Fig. 4-7).

The practitioner observes the movement of the scapula during both raising and lowering. Each test movement is repeated up to five times, as repetition is sometimes required to elicit or visualize the aberrant motion.

Normally the scapula remains stable, with minimal motion during the initial 30-60 degrees of movement, then smoothly and continuously rotates upward during elevation of the arms. The scapula then smoothly and continuously rotates downward as the patient returns to the starting position.

An abnormal finding is any combination of:

- Elevation or protraction of the scapula prior to 30-60 degrees of arm movement
- Excessive elevation of the scapula

- Erratic or stuttering motion of the scapula

- Rapid downward rotation of the scapula during arm lowering

- Winging of the medial border and/or inferior angle of the scapula

Oculomotor Dysfunction

Oculomotor dysfunction is a condition in which there is disruption of the reflexes that control the coordinated activity of the eyes, head and cervical spine. This is thought to result from cervical trauma. Specifically, it is thought that disturbance of normal afferent input from cervical muscles that arises after trauma leads to the alteration of oculomotor reflexes.

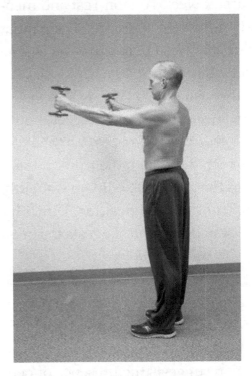

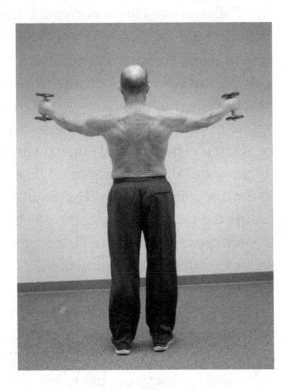

Figure 4-6. Flexion of the shoulders to examine scapular stability. Note the positioning is for purpose of illustration. During the actual examination the practitioner will be standing behind the patient.

Figure 4-7. Abduction of the shoulders to examine scapular stability.

Treleavan (see Recommended Reading List) has developed clinical examination procedures that the practitioner may find useful. As of this writing the first two tests have known reliability as well as construct and discriminative validity (see Jorgensen, et al in the Recommended Reading list). The other two tests are included for completeness and appear to at least have face validity.

1. Gaze Stability Test: This theoretically tests the cervico-ocular and vestibular-ocular reflexes. The patient is seated and the practitioner holds an object, such as a pen, at eye level. The patient is asked to move the head into flexion, extension and rotation while maintaining eye focus on the object (Fig. 4-8 a-d). Inability to maintain focus, awkward cervical motion or symptoms such as dizziness, blurred vision or nausea suggest the presence of oculomotor dysfunction.

2. Eye Follow Test: This is also called the Smooth Pursuit Neck Torsion Test and theoretically tests the smooth pursuit reflex, with and without neck torsion. The patient is seated and the practitioner again holds an object, such as a pen, at eye level. The patient is asked to maintain eye focus on the object while holding the head still. The practitioner moves the object horizontally across the visual field (Fig. 4-9). A visual angle of approximately 40 degrees is the maximum lateral distance the target should be moved. The patient is then positioned with the trunk rotated approximately 45 degrees and the test is repeated (Fig. 4-10). This is then done with the trunk rotated in the opposite direction. The practitioner compares the patient's ability to smoothly follow the target in the neutral position versus the trunk rotated position. Difficulty in keeping up with the moving target in the trunk rotated position suggests the presence of oculomotor dysfunction.

3. Saccadic Eye Movement Test: This theoretically tests the saccade reflex. The patient is seated and fixes the eyes on the object. The practitioner quickly moves the object, and then holds the object momentarily. This is repeated in various directions. Difficulty with quickly moving to the new target position suggests the presence of oculomotor dysfunction.

4. Eye-head Coordination Test: This tests the general ability to coordinate the movements of the eyes and head. The patient is again seated and the practitioner holds the object anywhere in the visual field other than in the neutral position. The patient

is asked to move the eyes to the target, then to move the head. This is repeated in various positions in the visual field. Difficulty with this coordinated movement suggests the presence of oculomotor dysfunction.

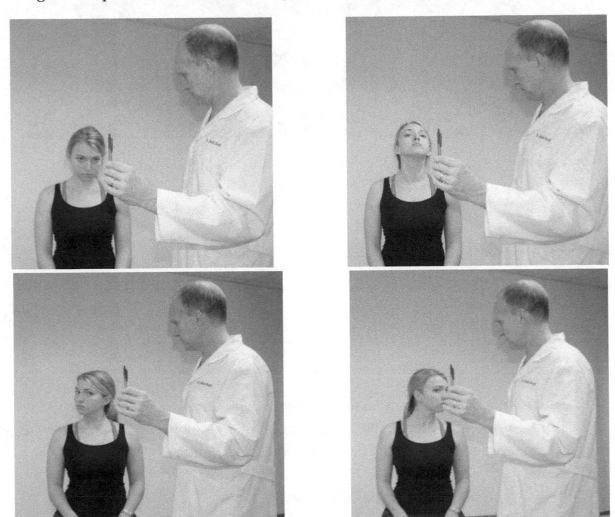

Figure 4-8 a-d. Movement of the head into flexion, extension and rotation while maintaining eye fixation during the performance of the Gaze Stability Test.

Oculomotor dysfunction is closely associated with neck pain that is located in the upper cervical spine and that began as a result of trauma (e.g. whiplash). So the practitioner should particularly suspect its presence in patients with upper cervical pain of traumatic onset.

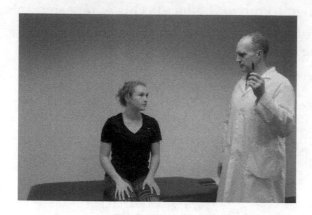

Figure 4-9. The Eye Follow test in the neutral position.

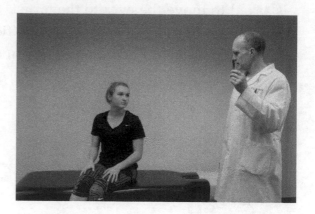

Figure 4-10. The Eye Follow Test with the trunk rotated approximately 45 degrees.

Nociceptive System Sensitization (NSS)

NSS should be suspected in any patient whose reported pain intensity is out of proportion to the clinical findings. Further investigation can then be carried out to support or refute the initial impression.

As discussed in Volume I, Smart, et al (see Recommended Reading list) developed the following criteria for the identification of NSS (though they do not use this particular term) through a Delphi process, and found good discriminative validity:

- Pain disproportionate to the tissue injury or pathology.

- Strong association with psychological factors.

- Disproportionate, non-mechanical and unpredictable exacerbating and remitting factors in the history.

- Diffuse, nonanatomic areas of pain and/ or tenderness.

The utilization of these criteria forms a good basis for screening for the presence of NSS. In most patients, no further investigation is necessary.

Nonorganic signs related to the cervical spine are likely to in part be reflective of the presence of NSS although it appears that nonorganic signs indicate a more complex picture. As has been discussed throughout this book series, NSS is part of a larger clinical picture of chronic spine related disorders in which somatic, neurophysiologic and psychological factors contribute to the overall pain, disability and suffering experienced by the patient. It appears that the presence of nonorganic signs is reflective of a particularly intense interaction between NSS and at least some of the psychological factors that contribute to the CD experience. Thus, nonorganic signs cannot be attributed purely to NSS.

A nonorganic sign examination has been presented by Vernon, et al (see Recommended Reading list) for use in patients with CDs. This examination consists of four tests designed to simulate a potential (but not actual) painful stimulus. The tests are:

Test 1: The patient is seated. The practitioner stands behind the patient and gently places his or her hands on the sides of the patient's head, with the elbows contacting the patients shoulders (Fig. 4-11). The practitioner then asks the patient to rotate both the head and shoulders as a unit, without inducing any cervical rotation. The practitioner guides the movement with the head and shoulder contacts. The practitioner asks the patient if this causes pain. If pain is reported, the test is positive.

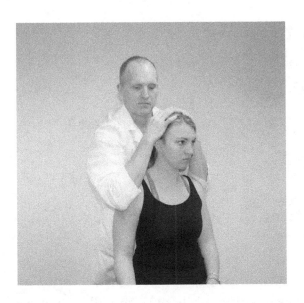

Figure 4-11.
Nonorganic test 1.

Test 2: The patient is lying supine and the practitioner asks the patient to rotate the head to one side to the point at which pain is experienced. The practitioner makes note of this point. The patient is then asked to do the same with rotation to the other side. The practitioner then gently performs passive rotation of the cervical spine to either side (Fig. 4-12) to the point at which either the patient reports pain or resistance is perceived by the practitioner. The test is positive if the passive range is less than 10% greater than the active range.

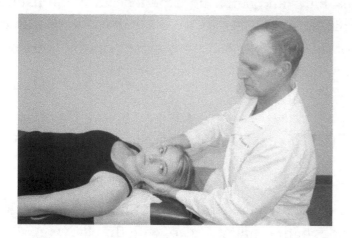

**Figure 4-12.
Nonorganic test 2.**

Test 3: This is also known as Libman's test. The patient is supine and the practitioner applies pressure to the mastoid process of approximately 3 kg/ cm2, or just enough pressure that causes the thumbnail to become lightly blanched (Fig. 4-13). The report of pain is a positive test.

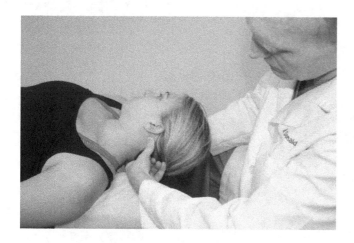

**Figure 4-13.
Nonorganic test 3.**

Test 4: The patient is in the side lying position and the practitioner gently places one hand over the lateral aspect of the cervical spine while with the other passively abducts the shoulder to approximately 120 degrees (Fig. 4-14). A report of neck pain is a positive test. A report solely of shoulder pain does not constitute a positive test.

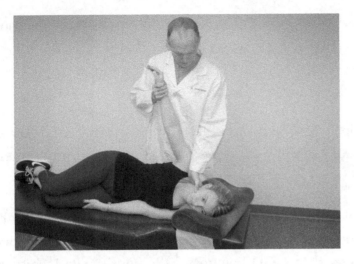

Figure 4-14.
Nonorganic test 4.

More research is required to determine the usefulness of these nonorganic signs. In the meantime, the Smart criteria are the best tool available thus far in identifying NSS.

Psychological Factors

There are a number of psychological factors that can perpetuate an ongoing pain, disability and suffering experience. These are sometimes referred to as "Yellow Flags." As was discussed in Chapter 2 of Volume I of this series, the "Big 5" psychological factors in patients with spine related disorders are fear, catastrophizing, passive coping, low self-efficacy and depression:

1. Fear: This typically relates to the perception that the CD is a serious condition that threatens the patient's ability to live a life that is fulfilling. Often the fear relates to activity, i.e., that activity must be limited or avoided because of the perception that the "damage" in the neck will "worsen" with movement, particularly movements that provoke pain. Thus, this is often referred to as "fear avoidance" because in many patients the fear leads to avoidance of activity. However the term "fear avoidance" should not be used universally because not all fearful patients avoid activities. In fact, in patients who are used to being active and who thrive (either adaptively or maladaptively) on activity may continue to pursue activities that are best avoided, at least temporarily, because of their "fear" of losing the ability be active.

2. Catastrophizing: This means dwelling on the most negative possible outcome of a problem, in this case, the CD. The CD is seen as a disaster that is reflective of something serious having happened in the neck that will have a major impact on the patient's life, with very little likelihood of resolution.

3. Passive coping: This means dealing with the problem by attempting, or desiring, to "make the pain go away", seeking relief of symptoms in lieu of improvement in functional abilities.

4. Low self-efficacy: Self-efficacy is how confident an individual is in his or her ability to perform a particular task or overcome a particular problem. Therefore a person with low self-efficacy with regard to a CD has very little confidence in his or her ability to deal effectively with the problem and return to a normal life.

5. Depression: This is a negative affect resulting from feelings of despair and hopelessness in the face of a problem, in this case, a CD.

In addition, other factors can be important in certain individuals, such as:

1. Perceived injustice: This is sometimes referred to as "the experience of injustice". It is particularly important in many patients with whiplash associated disorder or whose CD began following a slip-and-fall in which someone else is perceived to be "at fault". It is characterized by the perception that the patient's basic human rights have been unfairly violated, irreparable loss has occurred and people do not understand the severity of the patient's suffering.

2. Cognitive fusion: This is characterized by the fusion of the patient's assumptions, beliefs, and cognitions about the CD with his or her experience of the CD. So rather than experiencing the pain as an objective fact, the patient views it through the lens of his or her assumptions about the pain ("the pain is an indication of something seriously wrong"), beliefs about the nature of pain in general ("pain is always a reason to stop activity") and cognitions about the pain ("it feels like something is being pinched in my neck").

3. Hypervigilance for symptoms: This is when the patient continuously seeks for cues during daily activities that support his or her assumptions, beliefs and cognitions about the "fearsome catastrophe" that is occurring related to the CD. The individual scans the environment for threats to his or her wellbeing.

4. Anxiety: This is essentially the same as fear except that it is less specific and is future-oriented. That is, whereas fear relates to a particular event that is happening or is about to happen in the present, anxiety relates more generally to things that *might* happen in the future. Similar to fear, in many patients anxiety leads to avoidance of activity.

See Chapter 2 in Volume I of this series for a more detailed discussion of these psychological processes.

The astute and experienced spine practitioner can, in the vast majority of patients, get a good sense of the presence of many of these psychological factors simply by interacting with the patient; indeed, it is in establishing a relationship with the patient that allows the spine practitioner to gather the most important insights (see the discussion of Relationship-Centered Care in Chapter 1 of Volume I of this series). Simply by asking questions such as "are there certain activities that you would normally be engaging in but are avoiding because of the pain? If so, why are you avoiding them?" will often open the door for an understanding of the patient's beliefs, cognitions and assumptions about the pain.

There are also a variety of patient self-report questionnaires available that are useful in detecting clinically meaningful psychological factors that may potentially contribute to the perpetuation of the pain, disability and suffering experience. While it is probably important to measure more than one of the important psychological factors in CDs, it is not necessary to obtain a detailed quantitative assessment of all these factors. This would be burdensome to the patient and impractical in a busy practice environment. Described here are some of the more useful questionnaires. This is certainly not an exhaustive list, but the questionnaires discussed are ones that the busy spine practitioner may find useful in practice.

Neck Pain Screening Tool – short form

This is a modification of the Keele STarT Back 9-item Screening Tool* discussed in Volume I [http://www.keele.ac.uk/sbst/ accessed 5 April 2016]. It was modified by John Ventura, DC (data unpublished as of this writing) for use in neck pain patients. It contains a series of questions related to the patient's neck pain experience. The items that specifically relate to psychological factors are questions 5 (fear), 6 (anxiety), 7 (catastrophizing) and 8 (depression**) and 9 (overall "bothersomeness").

Extrapolating from studies on the Keele STarT Back 9-item Screening Tool, a combined score of 3 or more on items 5-9 may suggest the presence of clinically meaningful psychological factors that have the potential to perpetuate the CD, and thus are important diagnostic factors under diagnostic question #3. However, this requires independent verification which, as of this writing, as not yet occurred.

The Neck Pain Screening Tool – short form may also be useful in measuring risk of chronicity in the same way that the STarT Back 9-item Screening Tool is useful for this purpose in patients with low back disorders. As of this writing, data on this have not yet been published. Therefore, the potential for use as a screening tool will have to await these data.

Neck Pain Screening Tool – long form

This is a modification of the Keele STarT Back 9-item Clinical Tool*. The Neck Pain Screening Tool – long form contains the same questions as the short form, except items 3-8 have an 11-point ordinal scale (i.e., from 0 to 10). This questionnaire is discussed in Chapter 5 with regard to its potential role as an outcome measurement tool. However, it may also allow the practitioner to obtain, through questions 5-9, a deeper understanding of the fear, anxiety, catastrophizing, depression** and "bothersomeness" the patient is experiencing related to the CD.

The long form, because of the use of ordinal scales, can be used to monitor incremental changes in each the factors measured on each scale. This is especially useful for the scales that relate to psychological factors, i.e., items 5-9. Thus, this tool is more useful to the spine practitioner than the short form.

---

*While the STarT Back screening and clinical tools were developed at Keele University, the Neck Pain Screening tools were not. They are not endorsed by Keele University and as of this writing have not yet be validated for use as a risk stratifying tool.

It should be noted that the item related to depression on the Neck Pain Screening questionnaires applies to generalized depressive symptoms, as it asks, "In general I have **not enjoyed all the things I used to enjoy" (emphasis added). Therefore, it may be useful to separately ask, using an 11-point ordinal scale, a question that relates to depression that the patient may be experiencing specifically regarding their experience of the cervical disorder, such as "How depressed do you feel as a result of your current problem?"

The Tampa Scale for Kinesiophobia

This questionnaire is designed to evaluate and measure kinesiophobia, which literally translates as "fear of movement". The original questionnaire contained 17 items however an 11-item version has been developed and validated that is easier for patients as well as clinic staff. These questions focus on the patient's beliefs about the pain with regard to its overall meaning and its relationship with movement and activity. In addition, the instrument contains a question about the patient's perception of how seriously people are taking the pain.

The questionnaire is scored by totaling the responses to each question, with the score being expressed out of a total of 44 (e.g. 29/44). In general, a score of 27 or higher should be considered the threshold for clinically meaningful fear beliefs. So if a patient's score on this questionnaire is at or above this threshold, the practitioner should be concerned that fear beliefs are an important component to the 3rd question of diagnosis.

The full 11-item Tampa scale can be obtained at:
http://www.lni.wa.gov/ClaimsIns/Files/OMD/IICAC/FunctionalScales.pdf [accessed 5 April 2016].

The Fear Avoidance Beliefs Questionnaire

The Fear Avoidance Beliefs Questionnaire (FABQ) measures fear beliefs and was developed primarily for use in patients with low back disorders. There are two subscales of the FABQ – the Activity Subscale (questions 1 through 5) and the Work Subscale (questions 6 through 16). The Activity subscale is appropriate for use in all patients and the Work Subscale is specific to patients in whom the onset of the problem has been attributed to work. Therefore, the best use of the FABQ is for all patients to complete the Activity subscale and for patients with work related spine problem to complete both subscales.

As with the Tampa scale, the questionnaire is scored by adding the scores for each individual question, although with the FABQ not all the items are included in the total score. For the Activity subscale, only items 2-5 are scored while for the Work subscale items 6, 7, 9, 10, 11, 12, 15 are scored. This is expressed as the score out of a total of 24 for the Activity subscale and 42 for the Work subscale.

The threshold for clinically meaningful fear beliefs using the FABQ is a score of 15 or higher on the activity subscale.

The FABQ can be obtained at:

http://www.lni.wa.gov/ClaimsIns/Files/OMD/IICAC/FunctionalScales.pdf [accessed 5 April 2016]. Note that at this website the FABQ is identified as the "Functional Activity Back Questionnaire".

The Two-Question Coping Screen

This consists of two questions taken from the larger Coping Strategies Questionnaire. The questions address the patient's perception regarding the effectiveness of his or her coping strategies. The score of the two questions is totaled. The questions are:

Based on all the things you do to cope, or deal with, your neck pain, on an average day, how much control do you feel you have over it? Please circle the appropriate number. Remember, you can circle only one number along the scale.

No control   Some   Complete Control

0   1   2   3   4   5   6

Based on all the things you do to cope, or deal with, your neck pain, on an average day, how much are you able to decrease it? Please circle the appropriate number. Remember, you can circle only one number along the scale.

Can't   Can decrease   Can decrease
Decrease   it somewhat   it completely
it at all

0   1   2   3   4   5   6

A score less than 4 on the combined scales should be considered the threshold for clinically meaningful coping difficulties.

The Bournemouth Disability Questionnaire

This is a seven-item questionnaire that is primarily designed as a functional outcome measurement tool (see Chapter 5). However one of the items relates to depression and another relates to anxiety. So the scores on these two items can give the practitioner an idea as to the degree to which depression and/ or anxiety are contributing to the patient's pain, disability and suffering experience. There is no established threshold for the presence of clinically meaningful depression and anxiety using these scales.

The Bournemouth Disability Questionnaire can be obtained at:

http://9564e6cf93ec0c618a68-4f22a039f96a487025fe8e71cbbe8130.r40.cf3.rackcdn.com/Research/Publications/BQ%20ONLY%20%28NECK%29.pdf [accessed 5 April 2016].

Self-efficacy

The Chronic Pain Self-Efficacy scale and the Pain Self-Efficacy Questionnaire can be used to assess this important construct however these instruments include 22 and 10 questions, respectively. As such, they are not conducive to use in a busy clinical environment.

However a brief screening, involving two items from the Pain Self-Efficacy Questionnaire, has recently been validated and is more user-friendly for patients and clinic staff (see Nicholas, et al and Chiarotto, et al in Recommended Reading list).

The questions included in this screen are:

I can do some form of work, despite the pain ("work" includes housework and paid and unpaid work).

Not at all
Confident

Completely
confident

0   1   2   3   4   5   6

I can live a normal lifestyle, despite the pain.

Not at all   Completely
Confident   confident

0   1   2   3   4   5   6

The scores are totaled. A score of five or less is considered significant in terms of problematic self-efficacy that will likely need to be addressed. A score of eight or higher reflects a desirable level of self-efficacy regarding the patient's confidence in his or her ability to function in the presence of pain.

These questions measure the patient's self-efficacy with regard to functional abilities, which is critically important. However they do not measure patients' self-efficacy with regard to their ability to recover from the CD. This can be informally assess patients by simply asking:

How confident are you in your ability to overcome your problem?

Total   No
confidence   confidence

0   1   2   3   4   5   6   7   8   9   10

Perceived Injustice

Perceived injustice, sometimes referred to as "experience of injustice", is particularly important in the patient whose CD resulted (or is perceived by the patient as having resulted) from the actions or inactions of another person. In many patients perceived injustice is closely related to catastrophizing.

This construct is most applicable to the patient with whiplash associated disorder in whom another driver is perceived to be "at fault" or whose CD resulted from a slip-and-fall incident *that occurred on someone else's property* and thus is perceived to be the other person's "fault". These are situations that, both from a medicolegal perspective and in the mind of the patient, are considered to be a result of *someone else's negligence*. In these patients, perceived injustice can be the most important psychological perpetuating factor and in many cases, if it is not managed appropriately, it can cripple the patient's ability to recover.

The best instrument to measure perceived injustice is the **Injustice Experience Questionnaire**.

This instrument asks a series of questions related to the patient's perceptions of the impact that the CD has had on his or her life and the degree to which the patient perceives the pain, disability and suffering experience to be "unfair", that something important has been "taken away from me", that "nothing will make up for all that I have gone through", that the pain, disability and suffering experience is not being taken seriously by others, and similar perceptions.

The Injustice Experience Questionnaire can be obtained at:

http://sullivan-painresearch.mcgill.ca/ieq.php [accessed 6 April 2016].

Even if formal measurement is not made, the spine practitioner should be alert to statements made by the patient that provide clues to the presence of perceived injustice. Statements such as "I can't believe they did this to me", "I will never forgive them for this", "I can't believe this has happened to me" and "I will never be the same because of what they did to me" are critical in this regard.

In addition, observing the patient's pain behavior can be useful in suspecting the presence of perceived injustice. Essentially, there are two types of pain behavior (see Sullivan, et al in Recommended Reading list):

Communicative pain behavior – this includes facial expressions such as grimacing or wincing, grunting, sighing, moaning and verbal expressions of pain severity.

Protective pain behavior – this includes actions that appear to be intended to reduce irritation or further "injury" to the involved body part, including guarding, holding or rubbing the body part and moving gingerly in a protective manner.

Both types of pain behavior are associated with risk of chronicity, prolonged work loss and functional deficits. However, protective pain behavior is particularly associated with the presence of perceived injustice. So in in a patient who displays a great deal of protective pain behavior, perceived injustice should be considered a potential factor regarding diagnostic question #3.

The preceding questionnaires are probably the most useful scales currently available for use in the clinic.

There are other tools that a practitioner may find useful, such as the Pain Catastrophizing Scale, the Beck Depression Questionnaire and the Beck Anxiety Questionnaire.

However, it is not practical to use all of these patient self-report questionnaires in the clinical setting. It is much more efficient to take a streamlined approach that provides the most information with the least number of questions.

A great deal of information regarding psychological factors can be obtained by, first, taking a relationship-centered care approach, i.e., getting to know the patient and observing for clues in language and behavior that suggest significant psychological distress. This should be combined with the following tools:

- Neck Pain Screening Tool - long form

- Two-question coping screen

- Condition-specific depression question

- The single self-efficacy question.

This general approach is applicable to the vast majority of patients.

It is worth reiterating that while questionnaires and scales are very useful in measuring important psychological factors that can contribute to patients' pain, disability and suffering experience, they do not replace good one-on-one communication between the practitioner and the patient. The application of the principles of relationship-centered care (see Chapter 1 in Volume I of this series) is the most important tool in understanding the patient and his or her psychological and emotional reactions to the CD. This provides great insight into the impact these reactions have on perpetuating the pain, disability and suffering experience. A great deal can be learned through mindful observation of the way in which the patient talks about his or her CD and the patient's pain behavior. Developing skills in this area is at least as important as developing skills in all other areas of evaluation and management discussed in this book series.

The purpose of diagnostic question #3 is to identify important factors that may be perpetuating the ongoing pain, disability and suffering experience in patients whose CD has become subacute or chronic. This allows for decisions to be made as to the best management strategies to address these factors. These strategies are presented in Chapter 7.

Recommended Reading

Bolton JE, Humphreys BK. The Bournemouth Questionnaire: a short-form comprehensive outcome measure. II. Psychometric properties in neck pain patients. J Manipulative Physiol Ther 2002;25(3):141-8.

Chiarotto A, Vanti C, Cedraschi C, Ferrari S, de Lima ESRF, Ostelo RW, et al. Responsiveness and Minimal Important Change of the Pain Self-Efficacy Questionnaire and Short Forms in Patients With Chronic Low Back Pain. J Pain. 2016 Jun;17(6):707-18.

Cleland JA, Childs JD, Fritz JM, Whitman JM. Interrater reliability of the history and physical examination in patients with mechanical neck pain. Arch Phys Med Rehabil 2006;87(10):1388-95.

Cook C, Brismee JM, Fleming R, Sizer PS, Jr. Identifiers suggestive of clinical cervical spine instability: a Delphi study of physical therapists. Phys Ther 2005;85(9):895-906.

DeLeo JA. Basic science of pain. J Bone Joint Surg 2006;88-A(Suppl 2):58-62.

Edmondston SJ, Wallumrod ME, Macleid F, Kvamme LS, Joebges S, Brabham GC. Reliability of isometric muscle endurance tests in subjects with postural neck pain. J Manipulative Physiol Ther 2008;31(5):348-54.

Falla DL, Jull GA, Hodges PW. Patients with neck pain demonstrate reduced electromyographic activity of the deep cervical flexor muscles during performance of the craniocervical flexion test. Spine (Phila Pa 1976) 2004;29(19):2108-13.

Helgadottir H, Kristjansson E, Mottram S, Karduna AR, Jonsson H, Jr. Altered scapular orientation during arm elevation in patients with insidious onset neck pain and whiplash-associated disorder. J Orthop Sports Phys Ther 2010;40(12):784-91.

Hill JC, Dunn KM, Lewis M, Mullis R, Main CJ, Foster NE, et al. A primary care back pain screening tool: identifying patient subgroups for initial treatment. Arthritis and Rheumatism 2008;59(5):632-41.

Jorgensen R, Ris I, Falla D, Juul-Kristensen B. Reliability, construct and discriminative validity of clinical testing in subjects with and without chronic neck pain. BMC Musculoskelet Disord. 2014;15:408.

Jull G, Barrett C, Magee R, Ho P. Further clinical clarification of the muscle dysfunction in cervical headache. Cephalalgia 1999;19:179-85.

Jull G, Amiri M, Bullock-Saxton J, Darnell R, Lander C. Cervical musculoskeletal impairment in frequent intermittent headache. Part 1: Subjects with single headaches. Cephalalgia 2007;27(7):793-802.

Jull G, Kristjansson E, Dall' Alba P. Impairment in the cervical flexors a comparison of whiplash and insidious onset neck pain patients. Man Ther 2004;9(2):89-94.

Latremoliere A, Woolf CJ. Central sensitization: a generator of pain hypersensitivity by central neural plasticity. J Pain 2009;10(9):895-926.

Leeuw M, Goossens ME, Linton SJ, Crombez G, Boersma K, Vlaeyen JW. The fear-avoidance model of musculoskeletal pain: current state of scientific evidence. J Behav Med 2007;30(1):77-94.

Linton SJ, Shaw WS. Impact of psychological factors in the experience of pain. Phys Ther 2011;91(5):700-11.

Main CJ, Buchbinder R, Porcheret M, Foster N. Addressing patient beliefs and expectations in the consultation. Best Pract Res Clin Rheumatol 2010;24(2):219-25.

Main CJ, Foster N, Buchbinder R. How important are back pain beliefs and expectations for satisfactory recovery from back pain? Best Pract Res Clin Rheumatol 2010;24(2):205-17.

Mathers KS, Schneider M, Timko M. Occult hypermobility of the craniocervical junction: a case report and review. J Orthop Sports Phys Ther 2011;41(6):444-57

McClure P, Tate AR, Kareha S, Irwin D, Zlupko E. A clinical method for identifying scapular dyskinesis, part 1: reliability. J Athl Train. 2009 Mar-Apr;44(2):160-4.

Miles CL, Pincus T, Carnes D, Taylor SJ, Underwood M. Measuring pain self-efficacy. Clinical J Pain 2011; 27(5):461-70.

Murphy DR, Hurwitz EL. The Usefulness of Clinical Measures of Psychologic Factors in Patients with Spinal Pain. J Manipulative Physiol Ther 2011;34:609-13.

Nicholas MK, McGuire BE, Asghari A. A 2-item short form of the Pain Self-efficacy Questionnaire: development and psychometric evaluation of PSEQ-2. J Pain. 2015 Feb;16(2):153-63.

O'Leary S, Cagnie B, Reeve A, Jull G, Elliott JM. Is there altered activity of the extensor muscles in chronic mechanical neck pain? A functional magnetic resonance imaging study. Arch Phys Med Rehabil 2011;92(6):929-34.

Olson LE, Millar AL, Dunker J, Hicks J, Glanz D. Reliability of a clinical test for deep cervical flexor endurance. J Manipulative Physiol Ther 2006;29(2):134-8.

Osmotherly PG, Rivett DA, Rowe LJ. The anterior shear and distraction tests for craniocervical instability. An evaluation using magnetic resonance imaging. Man Ther 2012;17(5):416-21.

Osmotherly PG, Rivett DA, Rowe LJ. Construct validity of clinical tests for alar ligament integrity: an evaluation using magnetic resonance imaging. Phys Ther 2012;92(5):718-25.

Pelletier R, Higgins J, Bourbonnais D. Is neuroplasticity in the central nervous system the missing link to our understanding of chronic musculoskeletal disorders? BMC Musculoskelet Disord. 2015;16:25.

Robinson ME, Riley JL, Myers CD, Sadler IJ, Kvaal SA, Geisser ME, et al. The Coping Strategies Questionnaire: a large sample, item level factor analysis. Clin J Pain 1997;13:43–9.

Scott W, McCracken LM, Trost Z. A psychological flexibility conceptualisation of the experience of injustice among individuals with chronic pain. Br J Pain. 2014 May;8(2):62-71.

Smart KM, Blake C, Staines A, Doody C. Clinical indicators of 'nociceptive', 'peripheral neuropathic' and 'central' mechanisms of musculoskeletal pain. A Delphi survey of expert practitioners. Man Ther 2010;15(1):80-7.

Smart KM, Blake C, Staines A, Doody C. The Discriminative Validity of "Nociceptive," "Peripheral Neuropathic," and "Central Sensitization" as Mechanisms-based Classifications of Musculoskeletal Pain. Clin J Pain 2011;27(8):655-63.

Sullivan MJ, Adams H, Horan S, Maher D, Boland D, Gross R. The role of perceived injustice in the experience of chronic pain and disability: scale development and validation. J Occup Rehabil. 2008 Sep;18(3):249-61.

Sullivan MJL, Davidson N, Garfinkel B, Siriapaipant, N, Scott W. Perceived Injustice is Associated with Heightened Pain Behavior and Disability in Individuals with Whiplash Injuries. Psychol Inj Law. 2009;2(3-4):238-47.

Sullivan MJ, Adams H, Martel MO, Scott W, Wideman T. Catastrophizing and perceived injustice: risk factors for the transition to chronicity after whiplash injury. Spine (Phila Pa 1976) 2011;36(25 Suppl):S244-9.

Sullivan MJ, Scott W, Trost Z. Perceived injustice: a risk factor for problematic pain outcomes. Clin J Pain. 2012;28(6):484-8.

Tate AR, McClure P, Kareha S, Irwin D, Barbe MF. A clinical method for identifying scapular dyskinesis, part 2: validity. J Athl Train. 2009 Mar-Apr;44(2):165-73.

Treleaven J, Jull G, LowChoy N. The relationship of cervical joint position error to balance and eye movement disturbances in persistent whiplash. Man Ther 2006;11:99-106.

Treleaven J. Sensorimotor disturbances in neck disorders affecting postural stability, head and eye movement control. Man Ther 2008;13(1):2-11

Treleaven J, Clamaron-Cheers C, Jull G. Does the region of pain influence the presence of sensorimotor disturbances in neck pain disorders? Man Ther 2011;16(6):636-40.

Vernon H, Proctor D, Bakalovski D, Moreton J. Simulation tests for cervical nonorganic signs: a study of face validity. J Manipulative Physiol Ther 2010;33(1):20-8.

Vernon H, Guerriero R, Kavanaugh S, Soave D, Puhl A. Self-rated disability, fear-avoidance beliefs, nonorganic pain behaviors are important mediators of ranges of active motion in chronic whiplash patients. Disabil Rehabil 2013;35(23):1954-60.

Woby SR, Roach NK, Urmston M, Watson PJ. Psychometric properties of the TSK-11: a shortened version of the Tampa Scale for Kinesiophobia. Pain 2005;117(1-2):137-44.

Section III.
Outcome Assessment

•Chapter 5 •

Outcome Assessment in Patients with Cervical Disorders

Introduction

The purpose of outcome assessment is to measure the patient's perceived functional abilities. Stated another way, the purpose is to measure the degree to which the patient perceives the cervical disorder (CD) as impacting his or her ability to conduct and enjoy life. Baseline measures should be made on the initial visit and then repeated at each re-examination. This allows the practitioner to measure whether the management strategy that is being employed is impacting the patient's CD in a meaningful way.

Ideally, there should be simple means of outcome assessment that places minimum burden on the patient while providing maximum information to the practitioner. Fortunately, there are several outcome assessment tools (OATs) available for this purpose. These tools are known as Patient-Reported Outcome Measures because they allow the patients themselves to report how they are doing with regard to their CD and the results of clinical management.

This is what effective outcome assessment *is*, and details will be provided in this chapter regarding the assessment of outcomes in patients with CDs (see Chapter 7 in Volume I of this series for discussion of outcome assessment for patients with low back disorders). But it is also important to discuss here the *misconceptions* about outcome assessment.

There are a number of tests and procedures that are thought by many practitioners to be effective for outcome assessment but, in fact, are not.

One popular assumption is that measures of range of motion (ROM), in and of themselves, constitute effective outcome assessment. However it is known that ROM does not correlate well with functional abilities (see Chui, et al, Natrass, et al and Parks, et al in the Recommended Reading list). Further, a patient's range of motion can vary from day to day or even at different times on the same day. So, while there may be particular ranges of movement that are important for certain functional movements in an individual patient (cervical rotation for a patient who operates a back hoe, for example), ROM should not be used systematically as an outcome measure.

Many practitioners assume that "orthopedic tests" can serve as OATs. As has been discussed in Chapter 5 in Volume I of this series and in Chapter 3 of this volume, there are a number of pain provocation maneuvers that are reliable and valid in helping the practitioner seek the answer to diagnostic question #2 (Where is the pain coming from?). The purpose of these maneuvers is to help identify the pain producing tissue. Thus, they are diagnostic tests, *not* OATs.

For example, while the Cervical Extension-Rotation Test (see Chapter 3) may be useful as part of the examination for the presence of cervical joint dysfunction, this test does *not* provide information on the degree to which the CD is interfering with the patient's ability to conduct and enjoy life. The test may be helpful in the process of identifying one aspect of the *cause* of this interference, but it is not a *measure* of the interference itself.

This does not necessarily mean that pain provocation tests that were positive at initial examination should never be re-applied at re-examination, although it is important for the practitioner to seriously consider the value of this *versus* the potential detrimental effect of repeating pain provocation tests (see cases 5 and 13 in Chapters 9 and 10 for discussions of this). It means that changes in these tests do not necessarily reflect changes in the patient's functional abilities.

Threshold for Minimal Clinically Important Difference using OATs

Minimally Clinically Important Difference (MCID) is also referred to as clinically meaningful improvement (this latter term is the most common one used in this book series) and is the change in score from baseline to re-examination on a questionnaire that would represent the minimum amount of change that would be detectable by the patient as true improvement. In order to determine whether any improvement in the score on a questionnaire is clinically meaningful to the patient, the change would have to be equal to or surpass this threshold.

The generally agreed upon threshold for MCID for functional and pain questionnaires is a 30% change (see Ostelo, et al and Gatchel, et al in Recommended Reading list). That is, if the score on an OAT, when administered at re-examination, has decreased by at least 30% from the score at the initial visit (i.e., prior to the commencement of care), this change can be considered clinically meaningful.

It must be noted however, that this 30% change is the threshold for *minimal* improvement. So if a patient has improved by 30% on a particular instrument, this means, at least as it pertains to that instrument, their improvement has been meaningful and detectable, but has been *minimal*. This is not necessarily a bad thing, but clinical decisions with regard to next steps in the management strategy must be made with this in mind.

The concept of MCID has been criticized in recent years (see Copay in Recommended Reading list) however, in the absence of any other way to determine whether a patient is improving in a meaningful way, this remains the standard.

The Most Useful OATs for Patients with CDs

Neck Disability Index

This is a 10-item questionnaire based on the Oswestry Low Back Pain Disability Questionnaire (see Chapter 7 in Volume I of this series). It is perhaps the most widely used OAT in patients with CDs. It obtains information regarding pain intensity and the presence and intensity of headaches as well as interference with personal care, lifting, reading, concentration, work, driving, sleeping and recreation. The response to each item is scored from 0 to 5 and the total number of points from each item is added. This number is then doubled and expressed as a percentage.

The Neck Disability Index can be obtained at:

http://www.cmcc.ca/document.doc?id=53 [accessed 30 April 2016]

Bournemouth Disability Questionnaire

This is virtually identical to the Bournemouth Disability Questionnaire for patients with low back disorders (see Chapter 7 in Volume I of this series). It is a 7-item questionnaire with a 0-10 scale for each question.

The questionnaire covers pain intensity, interference with daily activities, interference with recreational, social and family activities, anxiety, depression, interference with work activities and control of symptoms. The score for each scale is added to calculate the total score for the questionnaire.

The Bournemouth Disability Questionnaire can be obtained at:

http://www.aecc.ac.uk/research-at-aecc/current-studies/outcome-measures-in-practice/ [accessed 20 July 2016]

Northwick Park Neck Pain Questionnaire

This is a 10-item questionnaire that obtains information about neck pain intensity and duration, numbness and paresthesia at night and interference with sleeping, carrying, driving, working, social activities, reading and watching television. It also contains a question regarding the degree of improvement since the last reassessment.

The Northwick Park Neck Pain Questionnaire can be obtained at:

http://rheumatology.oxfordjournals.org/content/33/5/469.abstract [accessed 30 April 2016]

Core Outcome Measure for Neck Pain

This is a 6-item questionnaire that obtains information regarding the "bothersomeness" of neck pain as well as interference with work/ school and general activities. It also asks questions about satisfaction with the patient's present symptoms and with medical care.

The Core Outcome Measure for neck pain can be obtained at:

http://journals.lww.com/spinejournal/Abstract/2004/09010/The_Core_Outcomes_for_Neck_Pain__Validation_of_a.17.aspx [accessed 30 April 2016]

Headache Disability Inventory

As the name implies, this questionnaire is specific to patients whose primary complaint is headache. It contains 25 items that ask various questions about the impact of the headache condition. The patient is asked to answer "Yes", "Sometimes" or "No" to each item. For scoring, a "Yes" answer is worth four points, a "Sometimes" answer two points and a "No" answer zero points. The score for all the questions is totaled and expressed as a percentage.

The Headache Disability Inventory can be obtained at:

http://onlinelibrary.wiley.com/doi/10.1111/j.1526-4610.1995.hed3509534.x/full   [accessed 30 April 2016]

All the above instruments are available in the English language. Some are also available in other languages, such as Spanish (see Murphy and Lopez in the Recommended Reading list).

Patient-Specific Functional Scale

The above questionnaires are very useful for obtaining detailed quantifiable information regarding the patient's general perception of his or her functional abilities. However it is also helpful to ascertain the patient's perception regarding the ability to engage in *specific activities that are important to the patient*. Useful for this is a modification of the Patient-Specific Functional Scale (see Stratford, et al in Recommended Reading list). The patient provides two or more activities that he or she has difficulty with but would like to participate in and rates the perceived ability to engage in each activity on a numerical scale:

What are two important activities that you cannot do or are having trouble doing? (i.e., "I can't get dressed without help," "I can't play golf," "I can't go to work.")

Activity 1._____

Please rate activity

0   1   2   3   4   5   6   7   8   9   10

Unable to perform   *Able to perform at same
level as before problem*

Activity 2._____

Please rate activity

0   1   2   3   4   5   6   7   8   9   10

Unable to perform   *Able to perform at same
level as before problem*

The full Patient-Specific Functional Scale can be obtained at:

http://www.tac.vic.gov.au/__data/assets/pdf_file/0020/27317/Patient-specific.pdf [accessed 30 April 2016]

Neck Pain Screening Tool – long form

This is adapted from the Keele STarT Back 9-Item Screening Tool* (see Chapter 4) and contains questions related to pain spreading down the arms from the neck, any back or hip pain the patient may be having, interference with dressing/ washing and sleeping as well as the degree of fear, anxiety, catastrophizing, depression and "bothersomeness" the patient is experiencing.

As of this writing, data are not yet available regarding its use as an OAT.

*While the STarT Back screening tools was developed at Keele University, the Neck Pain Screening Tool – Long Form was not. It is not endorsed by Keele University and as of this writing has not yet be validated for use as a risk stratifying tool or an OAT.

Numerical Pain Rating Scale

The Numeric Pain Rating scale (NRS) is a simple 0-10 scale that allows the patient to indicate the intensity of the pain, with 0 representing "no pain" and 10 representing "the worst pain imaginable."

Three- and four-level scales are sometimes used but it is adequate to use a single scale that measures the average pain intensity over the past week.

An example of such a scale is:

Over the past week, on average how would you rate your neck pain?

No pain   Worst possible pain

0   1   2   3   4   5   6   7   8   9   10

A reduction of 2 points is often used as the threshold for clinically meaningful change using the NRS. However, using percentage change, rather than change in the raw score, likely more accurate reflects true meaningful improvement. Sloman, et al (see Recommended Reading list) found the following correlations between percentage change in pre- and postoperative NRS
scores and the patients' actual experience of improvement:

35% reduction – "minimal" improvement
67% reduction – "moderate" improvement
70% reduction – "much" improvement
93% improvement – "complete" improvement

However, it should be noted that this study involved patients with postoperative pain. So it is not known whether these correlations can be generalized to non-surgical patients.

The practitioner should take a look at these tools and decide which ones seem most useful. It is recommended that the following set of instruments are currently the best way to measure the pain, disability and suffering experience and to monitor the outcome of care with minimum burden to the patient:

- Neck Disability Index or Bournemouth Questionnaire (one or the other - both are not necessary)

- Neck Pain Screening Tool – Long Form

- Numerical Pain Rating Scale

- Patient-Specific Functional Scale

As stated earlier, the purpose of outcome assessment is to measure the degree to which the CD is interfering with the patient's ability to conduct and enjoy life, and then to periodically measure the impact of the management strategy on this ability. The instruments should be completed on the first visit as well as at each re-examination.

It is important to note that these instruments do not replace good practitioner-patient communication and the application of relationship-centered care (see Chapters 1 and 8 in Volume I of this series). It is the combination of quantitative and relationship-centered information that should guide the management strategy.

In the next few chapters, we will discuss specific treatment approaches that can be utilized as part of an overall management strategy in helping patients overcome CDs.

Recommended Reading

Chiu TT, Lam TH, Hedley AJ. Correlation among physical impairments, pain, disability, and patient satisfaction in patients with chronic neck pain. Arch Phys Med Rehab 2005;86:534-540.

Copay AG. Commentary: The proliferation of minimum clinically important differences. Spine J. 2012 Dec;12(12):1129-31.

Fankhauser CD, Mutter U, Aghayev E, Mannion AF. Validity and responsiveness of the Core Outcome Measures Index (COMI) for the neck. Eur Spine J. 2012 Jan;21(1):101-14.

Gatchel RJ, Mayer TG, Choi Y, Chou R. Validation of a consensus-based minimal clinically important difference (MCID) threshold using an objective functional external anchor. Spine J 2013;13(8):889-93.

Gay RE, Madson TJ, Cieslak KR. Comparison of the Neck Disability Index and the Neck Bournemouth Questionnaire in a sample of patients with chronic uncomplicated neck pain. J Manipulative Physiol Ther. 2007 May;30(4):259-62.

Jacobson GP, Ramadan NM, Aggarwal SK, Newman CW. The Henry Ford Hospital Headache Disability Inventory (HDI). Neurology. 1994 May;44(5):837-42.

Leak AM, Cooper J, Dyer S, Williams KA, Turner-Stokes L, Frank AO. The Northwick Park Neck Pain Questionnaire, devised to measure neck pain and disability. Br J Rheumatol. 1994 May;33(5):469-74.

Murphy DR, Lopez M. Neck and back pain specific outcome assessment questionnaires in the Spanish language: a systematic literature review. Spine J. 2013 Nov;13(11):1667-74.

Nattrass CL, Nitschke JE, Disler PB, Chou MJ, Ooi KT. Lumbar spine range of motion as a measure of physical and functional impairment: an investigation of validity. Clin Rehabil 1999;13(3):211-8.

Ostelo RW, Deyo RA, Stratford P, et al. Interpreting change scores for pain and functional status in low back pain: towards international consensus regarding minimal important change. Spine. 2008;33(1):90-4.

Parks KA, Crichton KS, Goldford RJ, McGill SM. A comparison of lumbar range of motion and functional ability scores in patients with low back pain: assessment for range of motion validity. Spine. 2003;28(4):380-384.

Sim J, Jordan K, Lewis M, Hill J, Hay EM, Dziedzic K. Sensitivity to change and internal consistency of the Northwick Park Neck Pain Questionnaire and derivation of a minimal clinically important difference. Clin J Pain. 2006 Nov-Dec;22(9):820-6.

Stratford PW, Gill C, Westaway MD, Binkley JM. Assessing disability and change on individual patients: a report of a patient specific measure. Physiother Can 1995;47:258-262.

Vernon H, Mior S. The Neck Disability Index. A study of reliability and validity. J Manipulative Physiol Ther. 1991;14:409-15.

White P, Lewith G, Prescott. The core outcomes for neck pain: validation of a new outcome measure. Spine (Phila Pa 1976). 2004;29(17):1923-9.

DR. DONALD R. MURPHY

Section IV.

Management Based on the Clinical Reasoning in Spine Pain® Protocols

• Chapter 6 •

Treatment Approaches for Diagnostic Question #2

Introduction

The second question of diagnosis is, "Where is the pain coming from?" Another way to ask this question is, "Are there characteristics of the pain generating tissue or tissues that can be identified and that allow treatment decisions to be made?"

Recall that, in most cases, there are no completely objective means to unequivocally know the exact tissue that is the pain generator in patients with cervical disorders (CDs). However, in the majority of patients it is possible for the practitioner to:

- Develop a reasonable assessment as to what the most likely pain generator is, based on current best evidence;

- Communicate this to the patient in a way that is satisfactory for his or her desire to know "why am I hurting?" and;

- Develop a management strategy based on the diagnosis.

In the context of Clinical Reasoning in Spine Pain® (the CRISP® protocols) there are four possibilities under diagnostic question #2:

1. Disc derangement

2. Joint dysfunction

3. Radiculopathy

4. Myofascial pain

The identification of each of these possible diagnoses was presented in Chapter 3. Each requires a different treatment approach.

Disc Derangement

As discussed in detail in Chapter 3, disc derangement is identified through historical factors suggestive of cervical disc pain and the end range loading (ERL) examination. In patients with disc derangement with antalgia the treatment is inherent in the examination process. In patients with disc derangement without antalgia, the ERL examination is used to identify the Direction of Benefit, i.e., the direction in which the patient (with or without the assistance of the practitioner) repetitively moves the cervical spine for the purpose of "reducing" the derangement. Thus, the ERL examination not only allows the practitioner to answer diagnostic question #2 (i.e., rule in or out disc derangement as the primary pain generator) but also to determine the treatment.

Importantly, in the vast majority of cases the treatment can largely be *self-applied by the patient*. Providing the patient with self-care strategies is at the heart of effective spine care because it not only helps to rapidly reduce the generation of pain, it builds self-efficacy, one of the most important aspects of spine care (see Chapters 8 and 11 in Volume I of this series).

Because the treatment of disc derangement is inherent in the examination process, treatment is covered in Chapter 3.

Joint Dysfunction

The treatment of choice for joint dysfunction is manipulation combined with self-mobilization exercises. The purpose of manipulation is to introduce movement to the zygapophyseal joints. As of this writing research to determine the mechanisms by which manipulation works is ongoing. But what is known now is that this form of treatment has both segmental mechanical and segmental neurophysiological effects, as well as effects in the central nervous system.

Manipulation is an effective treatment approach in patients with CDs however, as emphasized by the CRISP® protocols, appropriate patient selection is paramount. In addition, manipulation should always be accompanied by self-mobilization strategies on the part of the patient that mimic, as closely as possible, the manipulative procedure. This establishes active patient participation from the very beginning, which helps build self-efficacy and allows transition from practitioner-driven care to patient-driven care.

Manipulation requires great skill that cannot be obtained from a book. Principles and methods for manipulation are presented here and these should only be applied by practitioners with appropriate training in this form of treatment.

Several general principles that are important in the proper application of manipulation were presented in Chapter 10 in Volume I of this series, and are equally applicable to the cervical spine as to the lumbopelvic spine. As such, they are reproduced in part here.

The methods of cervical manipulation will be divided into high-velocity, low amplitude (HVLA) techniques (sometimes referred to a "thrust" techniques) and low velocity, low amplitude techniques (LVLA) (sometime referred to as "mobilization" techniques). The LVLA techniques will be further divided into muscle energy technique (MET) and oscillatory mobilization (OM) technique. In the majority of cases the practitioner and patient positioning is the same with HVLA and LVLA techniques. The difference is in the application of the therapeutic movement.

The Barrier

All tissues, when lengthened, allow for a certain amount of length increase while providing little or no resistance. There then reaches a point at which internal resistance can be perceived by the practitioner. This point is known as the *barrier of resistance*, or simply *the barrier*. When applying manipulation it is important to move the involved joint to the barrier and then to apply the manipulative maneuver, be it HVLA or LVLA, at the point of the barrier, for the purpose of moving the segment just past the barrier. While the importance of the barrier has not been specifically subjected to rigorous scientific investigation, it is likely that attention to the barrier during manipulation maximizes the therapeutic benefit of this method.

High-Velocity, Low Amplitude Manipulation

With HVLA manipulation, the patient is positioned in a manner that allows the practitioner to bring the targeted joint to the barrier. At that point the practitioner applies a quick (high-velocity) and short (low amplitude - some have estimated this to be about 3 millimeters) maneuver designed to move the joint just beyond the barrier. Most commonly, this maneuver is accompanied by an audible release, or "click" sound although this sound is not always necessary for therapeutic benefit. Typically only one maneuver is necessary in a given treatment session.

Muscle Energy Technique for Joint Manipulation

Muscle energy technique (MET) is a general term for a method that uses reflexes to elicit relaxation of muscles and, where appropriate, allow for the lengthening of tissues (see Chaitow in Recommended Reading list). Described here is the application of MET to joint manipulation. The theory behind the use of MET for joint manipulation is that the MET procedure relaxes the muscles that would limit joint movement, thus allowing for easier mobilization of the involved joint.

The practitioner and patient positioning with MET is the same as with HVLA manipulation and OM (see below). The joint is moved to the barrier as with the other methods. But with MET an isometric contraction is elicited in a direction opposite that in which the joint is being moved. When using MET for manipulation of a cervical joint, the isometric contraction can be brought about by movements of the eyes (see below). The patient then inhales. During this time, the practitioner maintains the positioning of the joint at the barrier. The patient then ceases the isometric contraction, relaxes and exhales. At this point the practitioner continues to feel the barrier and as the barrier releases, the practitioner gently guides the joint to a position in which the barrier is again met. The maneuver is then repeated. Typically, three repetitions of the maneuver are sufficient.

The use of eye movements with MET

In the cervical spine, isometric contraction and subsequent relaxation during an MET maneuver can be brought about through eye movements. With lateral flexion maneuvers, when the patient looks superiorly (moving the eyes toward the forehead) this facilitates muscular activity that would oppose lateral flexion (thereby creating an isometric contraction). The patient looking inferiorly (moving the eyes toward the cheekbones) facilitates muscular activity that would enhance lateral flexion (thereby assisting the practitioner in inducing lateral flexion in the joint).

With rotation maneuvers, looking away from the direction movement is being induced (i.e., moving the eyes to the left when manipulating into right rotation; moving the eyes right when manipulating into left rotation) facilitates muscular activity that would oppose the maneuver (isometric contraction).

Looking toward the direction in which movement is being induced (moving the eyes to the right when manipulating into right rotation; moving the eyes left when manipulating left rotation) facilitates muscular activity that would then facilitate the practitioner's ability to move the joint in the desired rotational direction.

Oscillatory Mobilization

With Oscillatory Mobilization (OM) the practitioner and patient positioning is the same as with HVLA manipulation and MET. The targeted joint is moved to the barrier as with the other methods. However with OM, instead of the practitioner applying a high-velocity, low-amplitude maneuver or an MET procedure, an oscillatory motion is applied to the joint. To do this the practitioner moves the joint away from the barrier, and then returns to the barrier. This is done repeatedly. As the repetitions are being applied the practitioner feels the barrier.

It is expected that the barrier will gradually be perceived later in the movement, i.e., it will take longer to reach the point of the perceived barrier. However, the important thing is for the practitioner to continually engage the barrier on each repetition of the oscillatory maneuver, regardless of at what point in the movement the barrier is reached.

The specificity of manipulation

As of this writing, research on the mechanics of manipulation is still in its infancy. Physiologic and anatomical evidence, at least in the lumbar spine, does not support the contention that a practitioner can consistently target an individual joint with manipulation. In addition, it is not known whether the therapeutic effect of manipulation is to "correct" a "lesion" in the spine or whether there is another explanation for this effect.

There is good evidence, however, that manipulation is a useful tool in patients with CDs, that it causes gapping of the zygapophyseal joints and that it has segmental and central nervous system neurologic effects.

Further research should shed light on the mechanisms by which manipulation is helpful. In the meantime, it is sensible for the practitioner to try to be as precise as possible when applying manipulation while realizing that absolute specificity may not be realistic.

Another important point about manipulation is that it is unlikely that directional specificity is necessary. In other words, the therapeutic benefit of manipulation likely comes from inducing movement in the joint in any direction that is comfortable for the patient.

Deciding whether to use a HVLA or LVLA technique

A number of factors help guide the decision to use a HVLA or LVLA technique. This decision should be a shared one between the practitioner and the patient, with the practitioner providing leadership and guidance while respecting the desires and preferences of the patient.

The decision factors include:

1. Patient preference: This is the most important and commonly-applied factor in the decision. There are many patients who are "manipulophobic", i.e., afraid of "being cracked". This is particularly true in relation to cervical manipulation. While HVLA manipulation to the cervical spine is exceedingly safe compared to the vast majority of health care procedures, patients often view the cervical spine as a delicate part of the body. Of course, this is not helped by images from action movies in which the hero effortlessly "snaps" a bad guy's neck, killing him instantly. As fantastical as that image is, it sticks in the minds of many people.

   Another reason manipulophobia is particularly acute with regard to cervical manipulation is that, because the cervical spine is so close to the ears, and bone conduction of sound is so efficient, audible releases from the cervical spine appear to be much louder than from the thoracic or lumbar spine. The anxiety related to the application of a HVLA technique to the cervical spine in a manipulophobic patient will likely decrease the effectiveness of the treatment, therefore, a LVLA technique is preferable.

   On the other hand, there are patients who feel as if "nothing really happened" unless they hear and feel an audible release. This is especially true among patients who have had prior beneficial experiences with HVLA manipulation. In these patients, a LVLA technique is less likely to be of benefit, and a HVLA is preferred.

2. Acute radiculopathy: The majority of patients with radiculopathy, whether related to lateral canal stenosis or disc herniation, have joint dysfunction on the side and approximately at the level of the lesion. In these patients, manipulation will likely be part of the treatment process. Acute radiculopathy can be quite volatile and it is often easy to temporarily exacerbate the pain with HVLA manipulation. Therefore, a LVLA technique is often useful. It is important to note that this does not mean that HVLA manipulation is *contraindicated* in the presence of acute radiculopathy. Many patients with acute radiculopathy accompanied by joint dysfunction will tolerate, and benefit from, an HVLA technique quite well. It simply means that the practitioner should consider the potential volatility of the condition in the acute stage when deciding which type of technique to use.

Another advantage of using a LVLA technique in these patients is that the practitioner can monitor the pain and sensory symptoms during the application of the maneuver, asking the patient about increase or peripheralization of symptoms. If this occurs, the maneuver should be stopped and a different direction of movement should be pursued.

3. Neurologic deficit: This applies to patients with radiculopathy as well as patients with *mild, gradually developing* cervical spondylotic myelopathy who do not have significant no risk factors for progression (see Chapter 2). In these patients, the practitioner should consider using a LVLA technique. As stated earlier regarding acute radiculopathy, using a LVLA technique allows the practitioner to carefully monitor the effect of the manipulative maneuver on the patient's symptoms and to alter or abandon the method if potentially adverse responses are noted.

   In patients with acute myelopathy, such as from an acute central disc herniation, or advanced myelopathy, such as those with severe spasticity or bowel/ bladder involvement, manipulation is not indicated and surgical consult should be sought.

   It must be noted that appropriate management of patients with neurologic deficit requires great manual skill as well as keen diagnostic acumen. Therefore, it is essential that the spine practitioner only manage these patients if he or she has great confidence in his or her abilities in this regard, and that this confidence is realistic.

   Manipulation is a treatment for joint dysfunction, i.e., for a painful zygapophyseal joint.
   Manipulation is not a treatment *per se* for radiculopathy or for cervical spondylotic myelopathy. However, some patients with these conditions also have concomitant neck pain that is caused by joint dysfunction. The discussion here relates specifically to those patients.

4. Post-surgical patients: Manipulation is not typically a key element of post-surgical rehabilitation but many patients who have had previous surgery will have subsequent neck pain – either related or unrelated to the surgery – for which joint dysfunction may be a component. In many patients who have had previous surgery, the tissues in the area are more sensitive than "normal" tissue. More specifically, the

nociceptive system as it relates to those tissues is more sensitive. Sometimes the tissues in the area of previous surgery are less robust than "normal" tissue. Thus, the spine practitioner might want to consider a LVLA technique in these patients.

5. Osteopenia or osteoporosis: Decreased bone density should not be considered an absolute contraindication to HVLA manipulation. However, there may be some patients in whom the spine practitioner might want to use a LVLA method.

6. Nociceptive system sensitization (NSS): As has been discussed through this book series, NSS is a condition in which the nociceptive system has become hypersensitive and hyper-responsive to incoming stimuli. It very common for NSS to coexist with important psychological factors such as fear, catastrophizing, hypervigilance for symptoms and anxiety. Because of this, LVLA methods are often better tolerated by patients with NSS than are HVLA methods.

Self-mobilization exercises

Patients with joint dysfunction should always be given self-mobilization exercises to compliment and augment the manipulative treatment. This allows the patient to apply repetitive movements to the involved joint. Importantly, it also promotes self-efficacy – one of the most important aspects of patient care.

The self-mobilization exercises should be simple enough to maximize compliance and should target the involved joint as closely as possible. In addition, it should be made clear to the patient that the purpose of the manipulative treatment is to facilitate the application of self-mobilization exercises – the exercises are the essential aspect of management and are the key to sustained recovery.

As was discussed in Chapter 8 in Volume I of this series, it is essential that the patient is placed at the center of the management process. The patient must be the "hero of the story", with the practitioner serving in the role of facilitator, coach and guide to recovery. Therefore, it is important for the practitioner to always be mindful of the tendency to want to be *practitioner-focused*, rather than *patient-focused* and, as a result, place the greatest focus on manual treatments rather than self-treatments.

If the practitioner realizes that he or she has taken on a practitioner-focused, rather than patient-focused orientation, the best thing to do is forgive oneself for being human and shift the focus back to the patient.

This message, as with the CBT/ ACT messages discussed in detail in Volume I of this series, should permeate *every* practitioner-patient encounter.

Presented here are some common maneuvers that have wide application in a variety of patients with cervical joint dysfunction. However, it is essential for the spine practitioner to be familiar with a vast array of manipulative procedures for each area of the spine. A full presentation of the breadth of methods available is beyond the scope of this book. Again, it is assumed that any practitioner who would attempt this form of treatment would already have extensive experiential training, including various techniques for each spinal area.

For more extensive reading in this area, the reader is directed to the book by Bergmann and Peterson in the Recommended Reading list.

The presentation of manipulative techniques is broken up into maneuvers for the occipito-atlantal joint, the atlanto-axial joint, the mid- to lower cervical joints and the upper thoracic and first costotransverse joints.

Occipito-atlantal joint

The patient is lying supine and the practitioner sits at the head of the table. The practitioner places one hand on the occiput on the opposite side of involvement and rotates the head toward that side (Fig. 6-1). The practitioner then places the pisiform of the opposite hand on the occiput on the side of involvement. Placement should be just posterior to the mastoid process. The head is laterally flexed slightly, limiting the movement to the upper cervical spine, and movement is induced in the long axis direction to the point at which the barrier is engaged (Fig. 6-2). At that point the practitioner applies a HVLA or OM maneuver.

A MET maneuver can be used for manipulation of the occipito-atlantal joint. The setup is exactly the same as when using a HVLA or OM maneuver except that from the point of the barrier the practitioner asks the patient to look upward toward the forehead and breathe in, then look downward toward the cheeks (with the eyes only and without flexing the head) and breathe out. The practitioner waits to perceive the release of the barrier, then gently moves the segment further into the direction in which the barrier was first engaged. When a new barrier is met the practitioner maintains engagement at the barrier and again asks the patient to look upward and breathe in, then look downward and breathe out. When the barrier releases the practitioner again moves the segment until a new barrier is met. This process is then repeated for a third time.

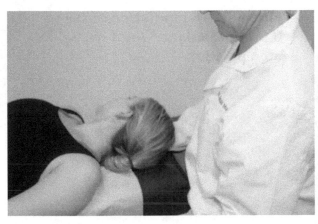

Figure 6-1. Rotation of the head away from the side of involvement for manipulation of the left occipito-atlantal joint.

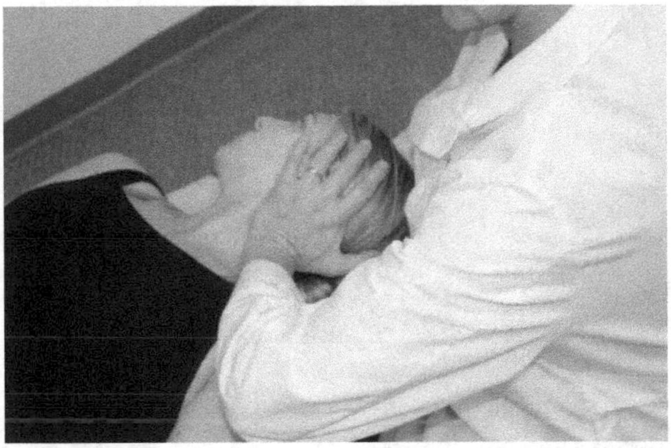

Figure 6-2. Meeting the barrier for manipulation of the left occipito-atlantal joint.

The occipito-atlantal joint can also be manipulated with the patient in the seated position. The patient is seated and the practitioner stands behind the patient. The patient's head is rotated so that the side of involvement is away from the practitioner. The practitioner makes contact with the middle finger on the occiput just posterior to the mastoid. The practitioner's thenar eminence contacts the zygomatic process. It is important that pressure is not placed on the temporomandibular joint. The practitioner's opposite hand supports the contact hand (Fig. 6-3). The practitioner supports the side of the patient's head with his or her sternum. The patient's upper cervical spine is laterally flexed toward the side of involvement and then long axis traction is applied to the point at which the barrier is engaged. At that point the practitioner can apply a HVLA, OM or MET maneuver in the same way as was described for the supine method.

Atlanto-axial joint

The patient is supine and the practitioner sits at the head of the table. The practitioner rotates the cervical spine so that the involved side is up. The practitioner makes contact with the proximal portion of the index finger as close as possible to the vicinity of the posterior arch of the atlas. The upper cervical spine is laterally flexed to the point at which the barrier is perceived (Fig. 6-4). From the point of the barrier the practitioner can provide a HVLA or OM maneuver.

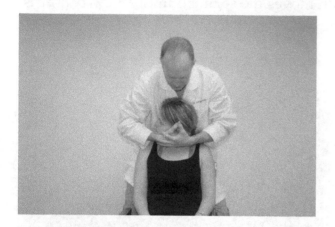

Figure 6-3. Manipulation of the left occipito-atlantal joint in the seated position.

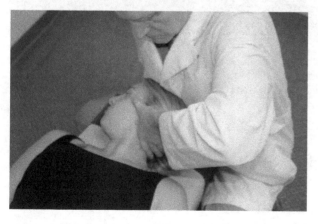

Figure 6-4. Meeting the barrier for manipulation of the atlanto-axial joint.

If the practitioner wants to use MET, the patient is asked to look superiorly and breathe in, then look inferiorly and breathe out. The practitioner waits for the barrier to release, then moves the joint further into lateral flexion until another barrier is met. This procedure is repeated two more times.

C2-3 through C6-7

The patient is supine and the practitioner sits at the head of the table. The practitioner holds the cervical spine with the hand on the uninvolved side and makes contact with the proximal aspect of the index finger as close to the involved joint as possible (Fig. 6-5). The segment is laterally flexed toward the side of involvement to the point at which the barrier is met. It is important that this movement is segmental, i.e., focused at the targeted segment (Fig. 6-6) rather than involving the entire cervical spine (Fig. 6-7). From the point of the barrier a HVLA or OM maneuver can be applied.

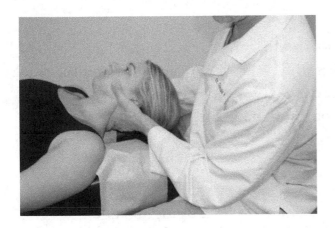
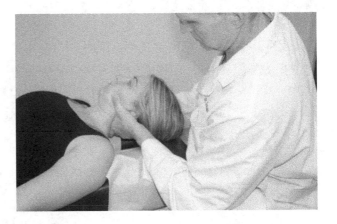

Figure 6-5. Segmental contact for manipulation of a left-sided segment from C2-3 through C6-7.

Figure 6-6. Segmentally-focused lateral flexion for manipulation of a left-sided segment from C2-3 through C6-7.

For MET, the segment is moved to the barrier as described above and at that point the patient is asked to look upward toward the forehead and breathe in, then look downward toward the cheeks and breathe out. During the exhalation the practitioner feels for the release of the barrier. When this occurs the practitioner gently moves the segment further into lateral flexion until a new barrier is met. This procedure is then repeated two more times.

To manipulate the joint into rotation, the setup and contact are the same except the segment is moved into rotation away from the side of involvement (Fig. 6-8). The practitioner

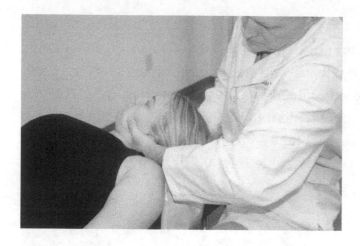

Figure 6-7. Incorrect technique in applying lateral flexion for manipulation of a segment from C2-3 through C6-7.

engages the barrier and can apply a HVLA, OM or MET procedure. For MET, the patient looks toward the side of involvement and breathes in, then looks away from the side of involvement and breathes out. When the practitioner feels the release of the barrier and the segment is gently moved further into rotation until a new barrier is met. This procedure is then repeated two more times.

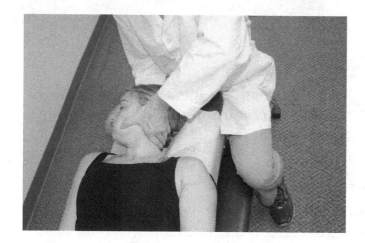

Figure 6-8. Manipulation of a left-sided segment from C2-3 through C6-7 into rotation.

The atlanto-axial and C2-3 though C6-7 joints can also be manipulated in the seated position. This maneuver is attributed to a chiropractor named Gonstead. The patient is seated and the practitioner stands behind the patient. The patient should sit in a slightly "slumped" position by sliding the buttocks forward somewhat. The practitioner makes contact with the proximal aspect of the index finger as close to the involved joint as possible, with the palm facing upward (Fig. 6-9). The practitioner's opposite hand makes a similar contact at the same segment on the opposite side. The segment is moved into long axis extension, ipsilateral lateral flexion, slight extension and contralateral rotation until the barrier is met (Fig. 6-10). It is important that this movement is segmental, i.e., focused at the targeted segment rather than involving the entire cervical spine.

From the point of the barrier an HVLA or OM maneuver can be applied. MET can be applied by having the patient look upward toward the forehead and breathe in, then look downward toward the cheeks and breathe out. During the exhalation the practitioner feels for the release of the barrier. When this occurs the practitioner gently moves the segment further into lateral flexion until a new barrier is met. This procedure is then repeated two more times.

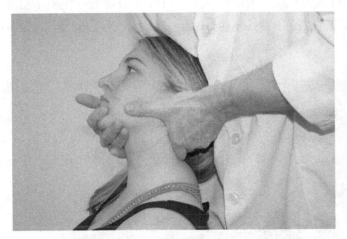

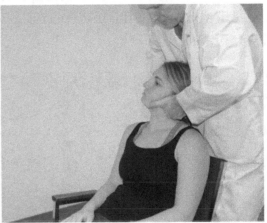

Figure 6-9. Segmental contact on the side of involvement for seated manipulation of a left-sided segment between C2-3 and C6-7. The same maneuver can be applied to the antlanto-axial joint by making contact at that segment.

Figure 6-10. Meeting the barrier during seated manipulation of a left-sided segment between C2-3 and C6-7. The same maneuver can be applied to the antlanto-axial joint by making contact at that segment.

Patients with cervical radiculopathy, whether from disc herniation or spinal stenosis, often have concomitant joint dysfunction at the level and on the side of radiculopathy. A manipulative maneuver that is often most comfortable in these patients is one that purports to move the ipsilateral facet joint into an anterior-to-posterior direction. This is best performed with the patient in the supine position.

The patient is supine and the practitioner sits at the head of the table. The practitioner reaches underneath the cervical spine and makes initial contact with the index or middle finger *just below and well anterior to* the segment to which the manipulation is to be directed. The practitioner's opposite hand supports the head in a slightly flexed position (Fig. 6-11). The cervical spine is then moved toward the barrier while at the same time the contact finger takes up tissue slack obliquely cephalad and medial, with the tip of the finger ending approximately at the spinous process. The movement of the cervical spine is in the direction of flexion, lateral flexion away from the side of involvement and rotation toward the side of involvement (Fig. 6-12).

It is essential that the movement of the finger taking up tissue slack occurs simultaneously with the movement of the cervical spine. This enables the practitioner to use the tissue slack to meet the barrier of the involved joint. Once the barrier is met, a HVLA or OM maneuver can be applied.

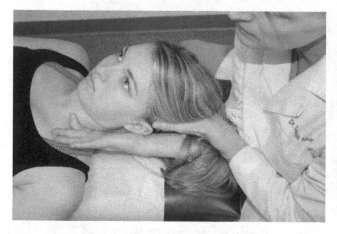

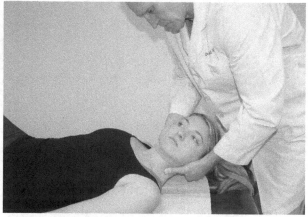

Figure 6-11. Initial finger contact for anterior-to-posterior manipulation of a lower cervical segment. Note the finger contact starts in the anterolateral aspect of the cervical spine.

Figure 6-12. Meeting the barrier by simultaneously taking up tissue slack in an obliquely cephalad direction and moving the cervical spine into flexion, lateral flexion away from the side of involvement and rotation toward the side of involvement.

For MET to manipulate in an anterior-to-posterior rotational direction, the setup is exactly the same. At the point of the barrier the MET procedure is applied as described above, with the patient looking away from the side of involvement during inhalation, and toward the side of involvement during exhalation. When the practitioner feels the release of the barrier the segment is moved further into rotation until a new barrier is met. This procedure is then repeated two more times.

The cervicothoracic junction and upper costotransverse joints

The patient is prone and the practitioner stands on the side of involvement or on the opposite side, depending on the practitioner's preference. The practitioner makes contact with the proximal aspect of the index finger as close to the involved joint as possible (Fig. 6-13). The practitioner then places the patient's head and cervical spine in slight extension, slight lateral flexion toward the side of involvement and slight rotation away from the side of involvement, with the patient's cheek resting on the headrest (Fig. 6-14). Gentle pressure is applied to the segment until the barrier is engaged. From the point of the barrier a HVLA or OM maneuver can be applied.

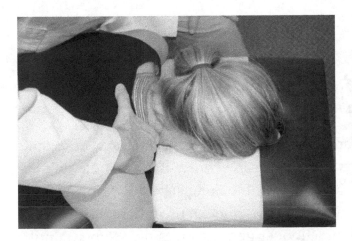

Figure 6-13. Hand contact for manipulation of the cervicothoracic junction and upper costotransverse joints on the right. The precise contact will depend on which segment is being targeted.

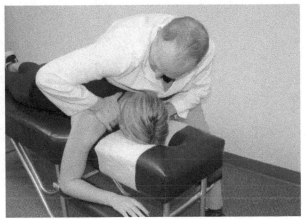

Figure 6-14. Meeting the barrier for manipulation of the cervicothoracic junction and upper costotransverse joints on the right.

Manipulation of the cervicothoracic junction and upper costotransverse joints can be applied with the patient in the seated position. The practitioner stands behind the patient and makes contact as close the involved segment as possible in the same manner as described for prone manipulation. The patient's head and cervical spine are again moved into slight extension, slight lateral flexion toward the side of involvement and slight rotation away from the side of involvement (Fig. 6-15). The barrier is engaged and a HVLA or OM maneuver is applied.

To attempt to direct the manipulation to the upper thoracic segments (T1 though T3) the practitioner can set up the maneuver in the same way and apply the tip of the thumb to the spinous process of the desired segment. Once the barrier is met, a HVLA, OM or MET maneuver can be applied.

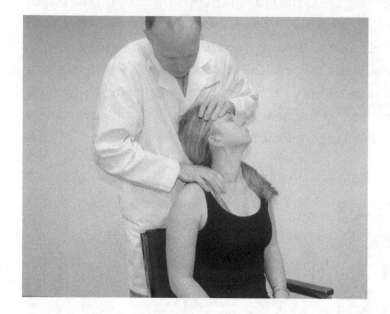

Figure 6-15. Manipulation of the cervicothoracic junction and upper costotransverse joints in the seated position.

For MET for manipulation of the cervicothoracic junction and upper costotransverse joints in the prone or supine position, the setup is the same as described above. At the point of the barrier the MET procedure is applied with the patient looking superiorly during inhalation, and inferiorly during exhalation. During the exhalation the practitioner feels for the release of the barrier. When this occurs the practitioner gently moves the segment until a new barrier is met. This procedure is then repeated two more times.

There is some controversy regarding the rare association between cervical manipulation, particularly involving the upper cervical spine, and stroke related to vertebral artery dissection (VAD). A line of research has investigated this purported relationship. At the time of this writing the current best evidence is that in patients who are reported to experience VAD following manipulation, it is not the treatment that causes the VAD but rather the VAD is pre-existing and incidental to the treatment.

However, because many people remain uninformed about this, the end of this chapter contains an appendix that discusses the evolution of knowledge related to the association between cervical manipulation and stroke related to VAD and the current state of the science in this area. It is excerpted from a paper written by the lead author of this book (DRM).

Patient-Generated Self-Mobilization Exercises

General Cervicothoracic Self-Mobilization

The cervical retraction maneuver was discussed in Chapter 3 with regard to its utilization as part of the examination and treatment of cervical disc derangement. This maneuver can also be used as a general self-mobilization exercise for the upper and lower cervical spine as well as the cervicothoracic junction.

The patient is seated and first moves the cervical spine into protrusion (unless this direction of movement has been found to peripheralize the patient's symptoms) (Fig. 6-16). The patient then moves the cervical spine into retraction (Fig. 6-17). Finally, the patient self-applies overpressure to further retract the cervical spine (Fig. 6-18). Depending on the patient's sensitivity, the spine practitioner might want to start with active protrusion and retraction movements for the first few days and progress to the application of overpressure after the patient has adapted to the movement.

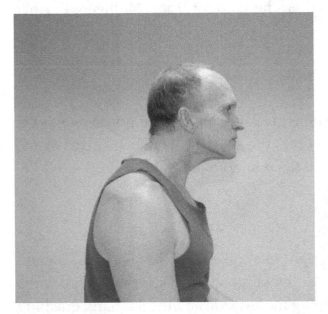

Figure 6-16. Protrusion of the cervical spine for general cervicothoracic self-mobilization.

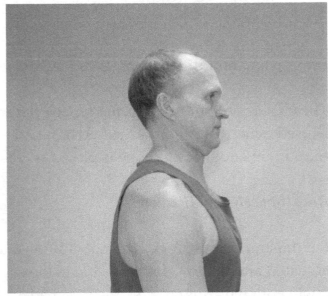

Figure 6-17. Retraction of the cervical spine for general cervicothoracic self-mobilization.

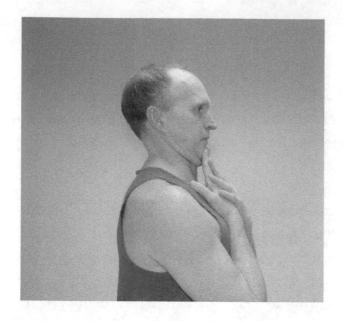

**Figure 6-18.
Applying overpressure for
general cervicothoracic self-
mobilization.**

Cervical Joints

The following self-treatment methods are based on the work of Brian Mulligan. Further information can be found at:

http://www.bmulligan.com/ [accessed 10 June 2016]

These exercises can be performed using a strap or a towel. For illustration purposes a towel is used here. It is important when using a towel that the edge of the towel is used as the focal point and that this edge is placed as close to the point of pain as possible.

Rotation self-mobilization

For illustration purposes, self-mobilization into right rotation is described here. The patient is seated and the towel is placed with the edge at the point of pain. The patient holds the towel with the arms crossed, the right had grasping the left side and the left hand grasping the right side.

To address right rotation, the left hand applies gentle but firm tension downward toward the floor to anchor the opposite side of the cervical spine while the right hand applies gentle but firm tension straight forward (Fig. 6-19). The patient then actively rotates to the right while guiding the segment into rotation with the right hand as far as is comfortable (Fig. 6-20). The patient returns to the starting position and repeats for 10-20 repetitions.

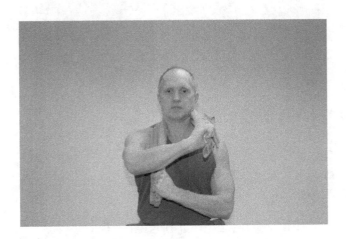

Figure 6-19. Starting position for rotation self-mobilization to the right.

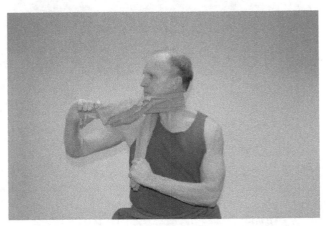

Figure 6-20. End position for rotation self-mobilization to the right.

Some people emphasize that the tension on the strap or towel on the mobilizing side should be directed diagonally upward, toward the eyes, so that the tension is applied in the same plan as the orientation of the cervical facet joints. However, recent evidence suggests that the movement of the cervical facet joints is exactly the same regardless of the direction in which the tension is applied (see Kawchuk and Perle in Recommended Reading list).

The exercise should be pain-free or cause no more than mild discomfort in most patients. If there is significant pain, it may be necessary to have the patient apply less firm pressure with one or both hands. If significant pain remains after this change, it may be useful to try mobilizing in extension first (see below), with progression to rotation as the patient improves.

Extension self-mobilization

The patient is seated and the towel is placed with edge at the point of pain. The patient holds the towel with each hand and applies gentle but firm tension straight forward on both sides (Fig. 6-21). The patient maintains this pressure while actively extending the cervical spine as far as is comfortable. While the patient is doing this, the hands move upward as the cervical spine extends, while maintaining forward tension (Fig. 6-22). The patient returns to the starting position and repeats for 10-20 repetitions.

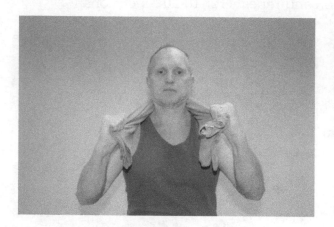 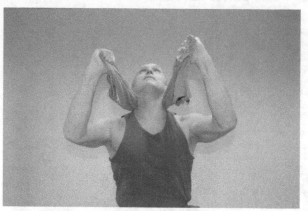

Figure 6-21. Starting position for extension self-mobilization.

Figure 6-22. End position for extension self-mobilization.

Again, the exercise should be pain-free or cause mild discomfort in most patients. If there is significant pain, it may be necessary to have the patient apply less firm pressure with the hands. If significant pain occurs after this change, the patient should be reassessed.

Cervicothoracic Junction and Upper Costotransverse Joints

Self-mobilization with a towel

This self-mobilization maneuver may necessitate a longer towel than was used for self-mobilization of the cervical joints. The patient is seated and a towel is placed so that the edge is as close to the involved joint as possible. The ends of the towel are held with one hand in front and the other behind the back (Figs. 6-23 and 6-24). Each hand applies gentle but firm tension diagonally toward the opposite hip.

The patient rotates and laterally flexes the head toward the side of involvement to relax the scalene muscles and to allow for mobilization of the involved joint (Fig. 6-25). As the patient does this, he or she applies increased tension with each hand on the towel toward the opposite hip. The patient then returns to the starting position while reducing tension on the towel. This movement is repeated for 10-20 repetitions.

As with self-mobilization of the cervical joints, this maneuver should be pain-free or cause mild discomfort in most patients. If there is significant pain, it may be necessary to have the patient apply less firm pressure with the hands. If significant pain occurs after this change, the patient should be reassessed.

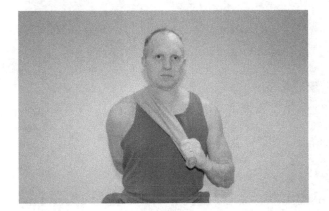
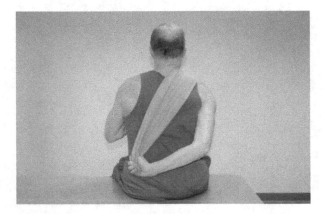

Figures 6-23 and 6-24. Starting position for self-mobilization of the cervicothoracic and upper costotransverse joints.

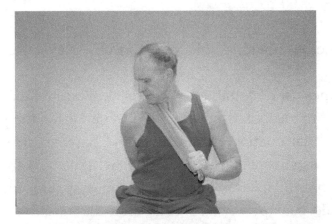

Figure 6-25. Rotation and lateral flexion toward the side of involvement for self-mobilization of the cervicothoracic and upper costotransverse joints.

Self-mobilization with the upper extremities

This is a self-mobilization originally presented by Karel Lewit (see recommended reading list). Clinical experience suggests that it is quite helpful but the mechanism is unknown. The patient is seated with arms spread out to each side. The patient rotates the arms so that the thumb points downward on one side and upward on the other side. At the same time the patient turns the head to look at the down-thumb side (Fig. 6-26). The patient then reverses this, rotating the arms in the opposite direction and again turning the head to look at the down-thumb side (Fig. 6-27). This movement is repeated for 10-20 repetitions.

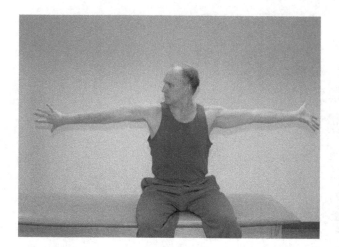 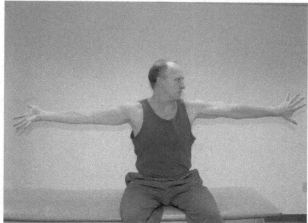

Figures 6-26 and 6-27. Self-mobilization of the cervicothoracic junction and upper costotransverse joints.

The vast majority of patients should be able to perform these exercises without difficulty.

Joint injection is sometimes used for patients with cervical facet pain. With this procedure, anesthetic, with or without steroid, is injected into the joint for the purpose of relieving pain and/ or suspected inflammation. As discussed in Chapter 3, these are useful at times for diagnostic purposes, as substantial temporary relief (i.e., 80% improvement in pain) after injection suggests that the injected joint is the primary pain source. If this is the case, pain improvement should be experienced shortly after the injection, during the period in which the anesthetic is expected to exert its anesthetic effect. Occasionally, longer lasting improvement occurs as a result of the steroid. Lasting benefit is "hit or miss" – some patients experience improvement in pain for extended periods of time. However, most do not.

While complications, including allergic reaction, infection and bleeding, are rare, the limited benefit of joint injections for *therapeutic* purposes is such that they should be used judiciously and sparingly.

Joint injections should be avoided in patients with systemic or local infection, history of allergy to anesthetic or steroid, bleeding disorder or who are on anticoagulants. Some patients with severe degenerative changes in the facet joint are not candidates for joint injection. In these patients the primary spine practitioner (PSP) should discuss the case with the interventionalist who would be performing the procedure.

In those patients who do experience substantial temporary relief from joint injection, manipulation under joint analgesia may be worthwhile. The theory behind this approach is that a joint that is resistant to manipulation due to pain-related muscle tension may respond better to manipulation after injection-induced pain reduction. It is useful for the interventionalist and PSP to coordinate their activities in this regard.

In patients who do not experience substantial improvement with an adequate trial of primary spine care, and who experience at least 80% temporary improvement in facet pain after joint injection, medial branch block is indicated to confirm the diagnosis of facet pain. If this is positive, radiofrequency neurotomy can be considered. As with injections, radiofrequency neurotomy is "hit or miss", that is, some patients experience benefit and others do not. In addition, the duration of improvement is variable and is not usually permanent. Typically, patients can expect durations of benefit that last from eight months to a year, and sometimes longer.

Careful clinical reasoning and shared decision making, in light of the entire clinical picture presented by the CRISP® protocols as well as the patient's values, should be used in making the recommendation.

Radiculopathy

Acute – anti-inflammatory measures

With acute radiculopathy, the pathophysiology is primarily related to acute inflammation. Therefore, anti-inflammatory measures are most important. This can be in the form of non-steroidal anti-inflammatory medications (NSAIDs), oral steroid medications or epidural steroid injection. Many NSAIDs can be obtained by patients over-the-counter.

For spine practitioners who are not licensed to prescribe medications and/or do not perform injections, having a referral relationship with practitioners who can provide these interventions is necessary. The following discussion regarding medications is for information purposes only.

Oral medications

The oral medications most commonly used to treat an acute inflammatory process such as acute radiculopathy are non-steroidal anti-inflammatory drugs (NSAIDs) and oral steroids. NSAIDs include medications that can be obtained over-the-counter such as aspirin, ibuprofen and naproxen and prescription-only medications such as diclofenac, etodolac, fenoprofen, flurbiprofen, oxaprozin and celecoxib. Side effects and complications of NSAIDs include gastrointestinal (GI) disorders such as ulcers and high blood pressure. A type of NSAID known as a Cox-II inhibitor (celecoxib) reduces the likelihood of GI disturbance but this medication carries a risk of myocardial infarction and stroke.

Oral steroids are more powerful anti-inflammatory medications and are designed to be used for a brief period. Examples of oral steroids include prednisone, cortisone, methylprednisolone and triamcinolone. They are commonly administered in a tapered fashion, with a gradually decreasing dosage schedule over the course of days. Side effects and complications of oral steroids include glaucoma, fluid retention, elevated blood pressure, mood swings, weight gain and elevated blood sugar.

Both NSAIDs and oral steroids should only be used under close supervision. Particularly in the case of prescription medications, the patient must be under the supervision of a practitioner who is licensed to prescribe these medications.

Epidural steroid injection

Epidural steroid injection (ESI), as with joint injection, is a procedure most commonly performed by anesthesiologists or physiatrists although some spine surgeons perform them as well. ESI usually involves injection of a combination of a steroid such as cortisone and either a short-acting analgesic, such as lidocaine or a long-acting analgesic, such as bupivacaine. Sometimes saline is included for the purpose of "flushing" the area or diluting chemicals around the nerve root that promote inflammation. The injection needle is inserted into the epidural space in order to place the injectate as close to the involved nerve root as possible. This procedure is best performed under fluoroscopic guidance to ensure proper placement. Typically a contrast dye is injected first to confirm that the needle is properly placed. This is followed by injection of the solution.

In the lumbar spine the transforaminal approach, in which the needle is placed directly into the lateral canal for maximal proximity to the nerve root, is preferred. However, in the cervical spine it is less clear that this approach is superior to the interlaminar approach. What is more, the transforaminal approach is carries a greater risk due to the presence of the vertebral artery and radicular arteries. Therefore, most interventionalists use the interlaminar approach in the cervical spine. For the PSP, the most important thing is to establish a relationship with one or more reputable interventionalists, preferably with a documented record of good outcomes and appropriate utilization of injections, and to trust their shared decision making process with the patient regarding the application of the procedure.

Serious complications of ESIs are very uncommon. Infection can occur in approximately 0.1% to 0.01% of ESIs and dural puncture in approximately 0.5%. Bleeding or nerve root injury, as a result of the needle contacting the nerve root itself, can also occur. Less severe side effects may also occur, including temporary local pain, temporary headache, nausea and vomiting, temporary fever, facial flushing, anxiety, sleep disturbance, blood sugar elevation and temporary immunosuppression. Other side effects have been reported as well.

ESI should be avoided in patients with systemic or local infection, a bleeding disorder or anticoagulant use or a history of allergy to contrast material, anesthetic or corticosteroid.

Subacute or chronic – neural mobilization

In subacute and chronic cases of radiculopathy, acute inflammation plays a less prominent role in the pathophysiology. At this stage, congestion, ischemia, intraneural edema and periradicular fibrosis, along with sensitization, dominate the pathophysiological picture.

Therefore, in patients with subacute or chronic radiculopathy, neural mobilization should be incorporated into the management strategy. This involves applying maneuvers that are designed to improve the mobility of the involved nerve root and theoretically to improve circulation in and around the nerve root.

In addition, neural mobilization is designed to desensitize the involved nerve root (or more specifically, to desensitize the central nervous system as it relates to the involved nerve root).

Neural mobilization is applied via manual procedures and exercises. Virtually all of the exercises can be performed by the patient at home.

General principles regarding neural mobilization

A number of descriptions of neural mobilization can be found in various books and seminars (see Recommended Reading list). Presented here is a streamlined approach that can be applied in virtually any patient with subacute or chronic cervical radicular pain.

Of course, the nerve root cannot be moved in isolation. Any mobilization maneuver applied to neural structures moves an entire neural tract. As was discussed in Chapter 3, the Brachial Plexus Tension Test (BPTT) is part of the diagnostic test cluster in identifying radiculopathy. This test is designed to apply tension to the cervical nerve roots. It does this via maneuvers applied to the upper extremity that create tension on the peripheral nerves, the brachial plexus and, ultimately, the nerve roots.

Variation in patient and practitioner position allows greater emphasis to be placed on certain peripheral nerves, and thus on certain nerve roots. Likewise, with neural mobilization, the practitioner can focus the maneuvers on the involved nerve root(s) through strategic positioning.

In general there are two different types of maneuvers involved in neural mobilization:

1. Flossing (sometimes called gliding) maneuvers: These are maneuvers that are designed to move the nerve root back and forth within the lateral canal. This is done by slackening the neural tract at one end and tensioning the neural tract on the other.

2. Tensioning maneuvers: These are maneuvers that are designed to apply tension to the nerve root. This is done by keeping one end of the neural tract stationary and applying tension to the other end.

Flossing and tensioning maneuvers can be applied both by the practitioner and by the patient. It is important to emphasize patient-generated neural mobilization maneuvers in all cases. This allows the maneuvers to be applied daily and also promotes self-efficacy and active coping.

Both flossing and tensioning maneuvers can be performed from three different locations:

1. Distal: The emphasis of the movement is on the distal end of the neural tract.

2. Intermediate: The emphasis of the movement is somewhere in the middle of the neural tract.

3. Proximal: The emphasis of the movement is on the proximal end of the neural tract.

All three flossing or tensioning locations (distal, intermediate and proximal) can be performed on the same visit. Because flossing maneuvers are generally better tolerated than tensioning maneuvers, it is often useful to start with flossing maneuvers and later transition to tensioning maneuvers.

Neural mobilization maneuvers are to be done repetitively with little or no pause. These are *mobilization* maneuvers, not *stretches*. In most cases, 10-30 repetitions of the movement is adequate although the number may vary based on patient comfort, symptom production and relative acuteness of the condition.

The barrier phenomenon as it applies to neural mobilization

The barrier phenomenon that was discussed in the section on joint manipulation should be applied to neural mobilization as well. Mobilization maneuvers should be performed at the barrier. This means that when setting up the neural mobilization maneuver the practitioner should move the extremity in the direction required to elicit tension on the neural structure being targeted and should feel for the initial onset of resistance to this movement. This serves as the starting point for neural mobilization, be it flossing or tensioning.

In most cases, it can be expected that the point at which the practitioner perceives the barrier will also be the point at which the patient initially perceives symptoms. This will be felt by the patient as mild tension or "pulling", or sometimes mild discomfort. However, there are some patients who will report significant discomfort before the point at which the barrier is perceived by the practitioner. It is best in these patients for the practitioner to start neural mobilization at the point at which initial symptom production is reported by the patient rather than trying to start at the barrier.

Generally, as desensitization occurs it will be easier for the practitioner to work from the barrier. However, patient symptoms should take priority over the practitioner's perception of the barrier – it is better to work at a level that is well tolerated by the patient than to attempt to work at the barrier.

It is important that the practitioner carefully monitor symptoms while performing neural mobilization. A certain amount of mild pain and/or paresthesia is normal and should not cause alarm or lead to alteration of the technique. If significant pain and/or paresthesia should occur, particularly if the elicited symptoms cause the patient distress, the amplitude of the movement should be reduced, i.e., tension should be taken off the involved neural structure so the maneuver can be applied with minimal to mild symptoms.

The principle of centralization and peripheralization, as discussed with regard to end range loading (see Chapter 3) should apply to neural mobilization. That is, if the pain or paresthesia that is elicited gradually moves toward the axial spine (i.e., "centralizes") with repeated movements, even if the central pain increases, the maneuver should be continued, with careful monitoring of symptoms.

However, if the pain or paresthesia moves farther down the upper extremity (i.e., "peripheralizes") with repeated movements, the maneuver should be stopped or the amplitude should be reduced.

A wide variety of practitioner-generated and patient-generated maneuvers can be used for neural mobilization. Presented here are a number of manual procedures and exercises that are widely applicable to the vast majority of patients with cervical radiculopathy. In general, patient-generated maneuvers should be performed for 10-30 repetitions twice per day.

This is by no means an exhaustive examination of all the various maneuvers that are available. Readers who are interested in learning additional maneuvers are directed to the work of Butler, Shacklock, Neurodynamic Solutions and the NOI Group, provided in the Recommended Reading list.

The position in which neural mobilization is performed is determined by the "bias" position that reproduced the patient's pain on examination (see Chapter 3). The three potential positions, in order of how commonly they present, are:

Median bias

Ulnar bias

Radial bias

Median bias position flossing – practitioner-generated movement

Proximal flossing: The patient is supine and the practitioner sits facing the superior. The practitioner places the patient in the same position as during the examination using the median bias position of the BPTT (see Figs 3-29 through 3-34 in Chapter 3) – the patient's arm is placed in 90 degrees of shoulder abduction and 90 degrees of elbow flexion. The practitioner depresses the shoulder girdle by pressing downward on the shoulder except that the practitioner does this by hand rather than with the elbow (for reasons that will become clear). The practitioner then extends the wrist and fingers, supinates the forearm, externally rotates the shoulder and extends the elbow to the point at which the practitioner and/or patient feels tension develop, (i.e., to the barrier) (Fig. 6-28).

The patient is asked to depress the opposite shoulder, tensioning the involved nerve root from its proximal end, while the practitioner simultaneously allows the shoulder on the involved side to elevate (Fig. 6-29).

This maneuver theoretically causes movement of the nerve root inward within the lateral canal. The patient then elevates the opposite shoulder while the practitioner simultaneously depresses the shoulder on the involved side (Fig. 6-30). This theoretically causes the nerve root to move outward within the lateral canal. This flossing movement is performed repetitively.

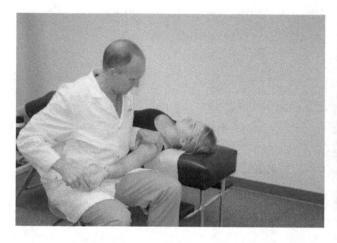

Figure 6-28. Starting position for practitioner-generated flossing and tensioning in the median bias position.

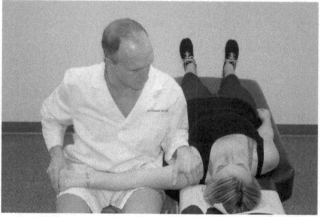

Figure 6-29. Depression of the opposite shoulder with elevation of the shoulder on the involved side for practitioner-generated proximal flossing in the median bias position.

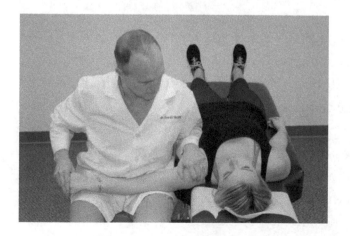

Figure 6-30. Elevation of the opposite shoulder with depression of the shoulder on the involved side for practitioner-generated proximal flossing in the median bias position.

Lateral glide proximal flossing: Another maneuver that can provide proximal flossing is one in which the cervical spine is moved while the nerve root remains stationary. The practitioner sits at the head of the table. The patient's upper extremity is placed in a position that mimics the median bias position of the BPTT. If possible, an assistant can be used to maintain this position.

The practitioner places one hand on the shoulder to prevent it from rising during the maneuver. With the other hand the practitioner reaches underneath the cervical spine to make contact on the lateral aspect on the side of involvement. The hand placement should be just superior to the involved cervical segment.

The practitioner glides the cervical spine laterally away from the side of involvement while holding the shoulder in position, preventing elevation (Fig. 6-31). The spine is then moved back to the starting position. This flossing movement is performed repetitively.

 It is important that the movement of the cervical spine is one of lateral translation (x axis translation) above the level of involvement as opposed to lateral flexion (z axis rotation).

Intermediate flossing: The patient is supine and the practitioner sits facing the superior. The practitioner again places the patient in the same position as during the examination using the median bias position of the BPTT to the point at which the practitioner and/or patient feels tension develop (i.e., to the barrier) (Fig. 6-28).

The patient is asked to depress the opposite shoulder, tensioning the involved nerve root from its proximal end, while the practitioner simultaneously flexes the elbow on the involved side (Fig. 6-32).

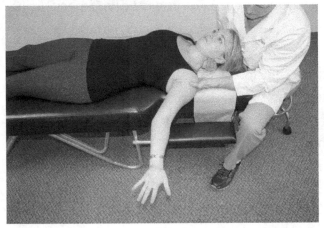

Figure 6-31. Lateral translation of the cervical spine during practitioner-generated lateral glide flossing in the median bias position.

This maneuver theoretically causes movement of the nerve root inward within the lateral canal. The patient then elevates the opposite shoulder while the practitioner simultaneously extends the elbow on the involved side (Fig. 6-33). This theoretically causes the nerve root to move outward within the lateral canal. This flossing movement is performed repetitively.

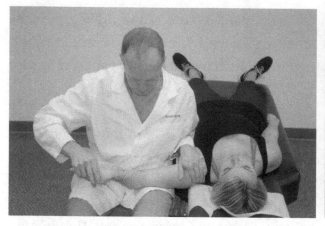 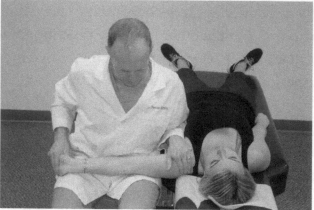

Figure 6-32. Depression of the opposite shoulder with flexion of the elbow for practitioner-generated intermediate flossing in the median bias position.

Figure 6-33. Elevation of the opposite shoulder with extension of the elbow for practitioner-generated intermediate flossing in the median bias position.

Distal flossing: The patient is supine and the practitioner sits facing the superior. The practitioner again places the patient in the same position as during the examination using the median bias position of the BPTT to the point at which the practitioner and/or patient feels tension develop (i.e., to the barrier) (Fig. 6-28).

The patient is asked to depress the opposite shoulder, tensioning the involved nerve root from its proximal end, while the practitioner simultaneously flexes the wrist and fingers on the involved side (Fig. 6-34). This maneuver theoretically causes movement of the nerve root inward within the lateral canal. The patient then elevates the opposite shoulder while the practitioner simultaneously extends the wrist and fingers on the involved side (Fig. 6-35). This theoretically causes the nerve root to move outward within the lateral canal. This flossing movement is performed repetitively.

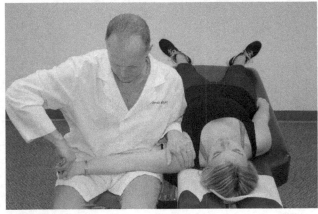

Figure 6-34. Depression of the opposite shoulder with flexion of the wrist and fingers for practitioner-generated distal flossing in the median bias position.

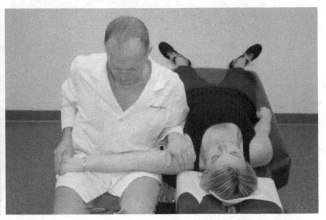

Figure 6-35. Elevation of the opposite shoulder with extension of the wrist and fingers for practitioner-generated distal flossing in the median bias position.

Median bias position flossing – patient-generated movement

Proximal flossing: The patient can be standing or sitting. The upper extremity on the involved side is placed in external rotation and elbow extension with the wrist neutral and the fingers spread wide (Fig. 6-36).

To perform the proximal flossing maneuver the shoulder on the opposite side is depressed while the shoulder on the involved side is simultaneously elevated (Fig. 6-37). The shoulder on the opposite side is then elevated while the shoulder on the involved side is simultaneously depressed (Fig. 6-38). This flossing movement is performed repetitively.

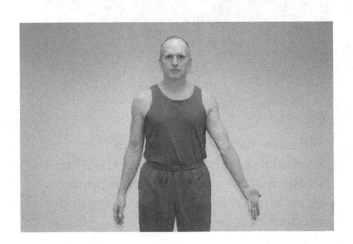

Figure 6-36. Starting position for patient-generated proximal flossing in the median bias position.

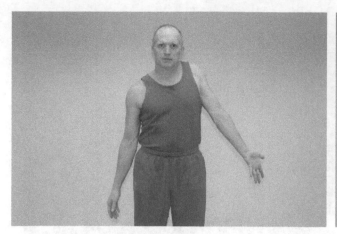

Figure 6-37. Depression of the contralateral shoulder with elevation of the ipsilateral shoulder for patient-generated proximal flossing in the median bias position.

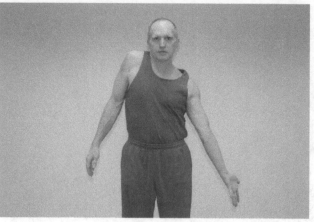

Figure 6-38. Elevation of the contralateral shoulder with depression of the ipsilateral shoulder for patient-generated proximal flossing in the median bias position.

Intermediate flossing: The patient can be standing or sitting. The upper extremity on the involved side is placed in external rotation and elbow extension with the wrist neutral and the fingers spread wide (Fig. 6-36). The shoulder on the opposite side is depressed while the elbow on the involved side is simultaneously flexed (Fig. 6-39). The shoulder on the opposite side is then elevated while the elbow on the involved side is simultaneously extended (Fig. 6-40). This flossing movement is performed repetitively.

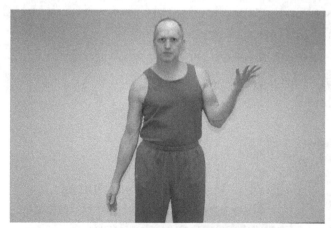

Figure 6-39. Depression of the contralateral shoulder and flexion of the ipsilateral elbow for patient-generated intermediate flossing in the median bias position.

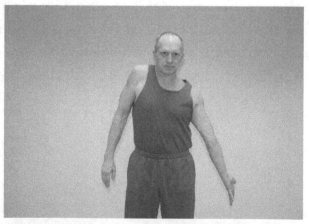

Figure 6-40. Elevation of the contralateral shoulder and extension of the ipsilateral elbow for patient-generated intermediate flossing in the median bias position.

Distal flossing: The patient can be standing or sitting. The upper extremity on the involved side is placed in external rotation and elbow extension with the wrist neutral and the fingers spread wide (Fig. 6-36). The shoulder on the opposite side is depressed while the wrist and fingers on the involved side are simultaneously flexed (Fig. 6-41). The shoulder on the opposite side is then elevated while the wrist and fingers on the involved side are simultaneously extended (Fig. 6-42). This flossing movement is performed repetitively.

Median bias position tensioning – practitioner-generated movement

The practitioner-generated tensioning maneuvers are identical the flossing maneuvers (other than the lateral glide proximal flossing maneuver) with the exception that the patient remains stationary and only the practitioner applies the movement.

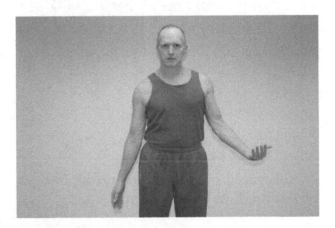

Figure 6-41. Depression of the contralateral shoulder and flexion of the ipsilateral wrist and fingers for patient-generated distal flossing in the median bias position.

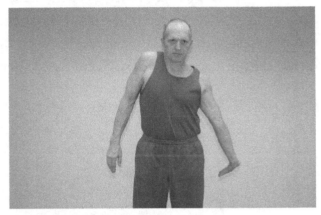

Figure 6-42. Elevation of the contralateral shoulder and extension of the ipsilateral wrist and fingers for patient-generated distal flossing in the median bias position.

Proximal tensioning: The patient is supine and the practitioner sits facing the superior. The practitioner places the patient in the same position as during practitioner-generated flossing in the median bias position. The practitioner depresses the shoulder girdle by pressing downward on the shoulder by hand, then extends the wrist and fingers, supinates the forearm, externally rotates the shoulder and extends the elbow to the point at which the practitioner and/or patient feels tension develop, (i.e., to the barrier) (Fig. 6-28).

To apply the tensioning maneuver the practitioner allows the shoulder to rise, moving just away from the barrier (Fig. 6-43), then depresses the shoulder to return to the barrier. This movement is performed repetitively, with the practitioner always moving the shoulder just to the barrier and then away from the barrier.

Intermediate tensioning: The patient is supine and the practitioner sits facing the superior. The practitioner places the patient in the same position as during practitioner-generated flossing in the median bias position. The practitioner depresses the shoulder girdle by pressing downward on the shoulder by hand, then extends the wrist and fingers, supinates the forearm, externally rotates the shoulder and extends the elbow to the point at which the practitioner and/or patient feels tension develop, (i.e., to the barrier) (Fig. 6-28).

To apply the tensioning maneuver the practitioner slightly flexes the elbow, moving just away from the barrier (Figure 6-44), then extends the elbow to return to the barrier. This movement is performed repetitively, with the practitioner always moving the elbow just to the barrier and then away from the barrier.

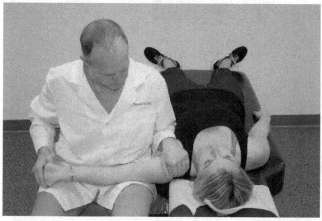

Figure 6-43. Moving away from the barrier for practitioner-generated proximal tensioning in the median bias position.

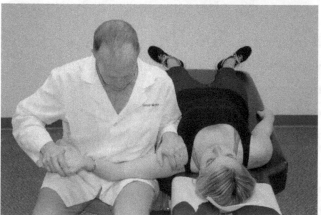

Figure 6-44. Moving away from the barrier for practitioner-generated intermediate tensioning in the median bias position.

176

Distal tensioning: The patient is supine and the practitioner sits facing the superior. The practitioner places the patient in the same position as during practitioner-generated flossing in the median bias position. The practitioner depresses the shoulder girdle by pressing downward on the shoulder by hand, then extends the wrist and fingers, supinates the forearm, externally rotates the shoulder and extends the elbow to the point at which the practitioner and/or patient feels tension develop, (i.e., to the barrier) (Fig. 6-28).

To apply the tensioning maneuver the practitioner slightly flexes the wrist and fingers, moving just away from the barrier (Fig. 6-45), then extends the wrist and fingers to return to the barrier. This movement is performed repetitively, with the practitioner always moving the wrist and fingers just to the barrier and then away from the barrier.

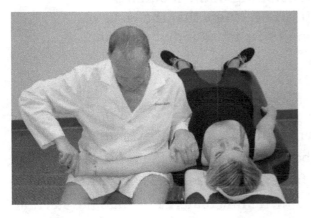

Figure 6-45. Moving away from the barrier for practitioner-generated distal tensioning in the median bias position.

Median bias position tensioning – patient-generated movement

Proximal tensioning: The patient can be standing or sitting. The upper extremity on the involved side is placed in external rotation and elbow extension with the wrist neutral and the fingers spread wide (Fig. 6-36). The head is laterally flexed away from the side of involvement, applying tension to the neural tract (Fig. 6-46) and then immediately returns to the starting position. This tensioning movement is performed repetitively for 10-30 repetitions.

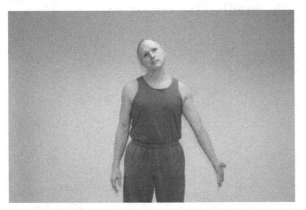

Figure 6-46. Lateral flexion of the head away from the side of involvement for patient-generated proximal tensioning in the median bias position.

Intermediate tensioning: The patient can be standing or sitting. The upper extremity on the involved side is placed in external rotation and elbow extension with the wrist neutral and the fingers spread wide (Fig. 6-36). The wrist is first extended to apply tension to the neural tract and then the elbow on the involved side is flexed (Fig. 6-47). The elbow then immediately returns to the starting position. This tensioning movement is performed repetitively for 10-30 repetitions, maintaining wrist extension during the exercise.

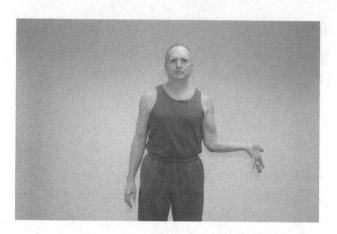

Figure 6-47. Flexion of the elbow away from the barrier for patient-generated intermediate tensioning in the median bias position. Note that the wrist remains in an extended position.

Distal tensioning: The patient can be standing or sitting. The upper extremity on the involved side is placed in external rotation and elbow extension with the wrist neutral and the fingers spread wide (Fig. 6-36). The wrist and fingers on the involved side are extended, applying tension to the neural tract (Fig. 6-48) and then immediately return to the starting position. This tensioning movement is performed repetitively for 10-30 repetitions.

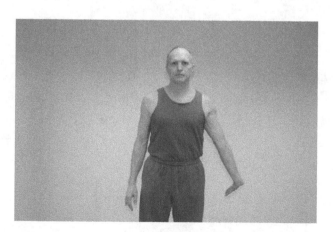

Figure 6-48. Extension of the wrist and fingers for patient-generated distal tensioning in the median bias position.

Ulnar bias position flossing – practitioner-generated movement

Proximal flossing: The patient is supine and the practitioner sits facing the superior. The practitioner places the patient in the same position as during the examination using the ulnar bias position of the BPTT (see Figs 3-38 through 3-41 in Chapter 3) – the patient's arm is placed in 90 degrees of shoulder abduction and 90 degrees of elbow flexion. The practitioner depresses the shoulder girdle by pressing downward on the shoulder. The practitioner extends the wrist and 4th and 5th fingers. The practitioner then pronates the forearm, externally rotates the shoulder and flexes the elbow and shoulder so that the patient's hand moves toward the ear. The movement is carried out to the point at which the practitioner and/or patient feels tension develop (i.e., to the barrier) (Fig. 6-49).

The patient is asked to depress the opposite shoulder, tensioning the involved nerve root from its proximal end, while the practitioner allows the shoulder on the involved side to elevate (Fig. 6-50). This maneuver theoretically causes movement of the nerve root inward within the lateral canal. The patient then elevates the opposite shoulder while the practitioner depresses the shoulder on the involved side (Fig. 6-51). This theoretically causes the nerve root to move outward within the lateral canal. This flossing movement is performed repetitively.

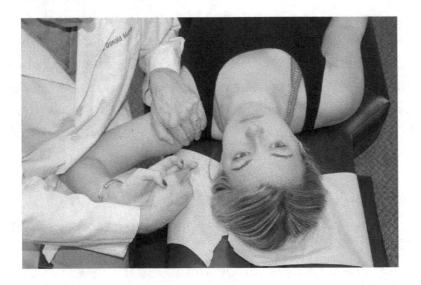

Figure 6-49. Starting position for practitioner-generated flossing and tensioning in the ulnar bias position.

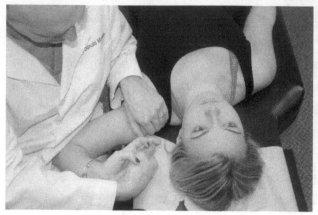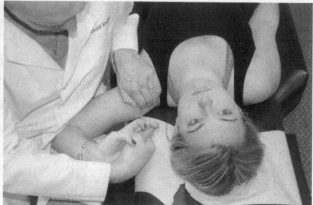

Figure 6-50. Depression of the opposite shoulder with elevation of the shoulder on the involved side for practitioner-generated proximal flossing in the ulnar bias position.

Figure 6-51. Elevation of the opposite shoulder with depression of the shoulder on the involved side for practitioner-generated proximal flossing in the ulnar bias position.

Lateral glide proximal flossing: The practitioner sits at the head of the table. The patient's upper extremity is placed in a position that mimics the ulnar bias position of the BPTT. If possible, an assistant can be used to maintain this position. The practitioner uses one hand to maintain the position and to prevent the shoulder from rising during the maneuver. With the other hand the practitioner reaches underneath the cervical spine to make contact on the lateral aspect on the side of involvement (Fig. 6-52). The hand placement should be just superior to the involved cervical segment. The practitioner glides the cervical spine laterally away from the side of involvement while holding the shoulder in position, preventing elevation. The spine is then moved back to the starting position. This flossing movement is performed repetitively.

It is important that the movement of the cervical spine is one of lateral translation (x axis translation) above the level of involvement as opposed to lateral flexion (z axis rotation).

Intermediate flossing: The patient is supine and the practitioner sits facing the superior. The practitioner again places the patient in the same position as during the examination using the ulnar bias position of the BPTT to the point at which the practitioner and/or patient feels tension develop (i.e., to the barrier) (Fig. 6-49). The patient is asked to depress the opposite shoulder, tensioning the involved nerve root from its proximal end, while the practitioner moves the elbow away from the barrier toward extension on the involved side (Fig. 6-53). This maneuver theoretically causes movement of the nerve root inward within the lateral canal. The patient then elevates the opposite shoulder while the practitioner flexes the elbow on the involved side (Fig. 6-54). This theoretically causes the nerve root to move outward within the lateral canal. This flossing movement is performed repetitively.

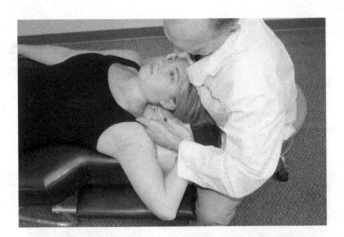

Figure 6-52. Lateral glide translation of the cervical spine during practitioner-generated lateral glide flossing in the ulnar bias position.

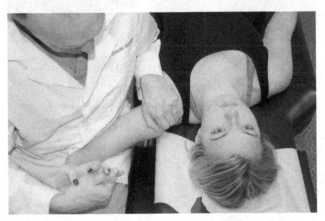

Figure 6-53. Depression of the opposite shoulder with movement of the elbow away from the barrier for practitioner-generated intermediate flossing in the ulnar bias position.

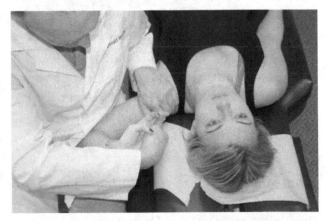

Figure 6-54. Elevation of the opposite shoulder with flexion of the elbow for practitioner-generated intermediate flossing in the ulnar bias position.

Distal flossing: The patient is supine and the practitioner sits facing the superior. The practitioner again places the patient in the same position as during the examination using the ulnar bias position of the BPTT to the point at which the practitioner and/or patient feels tension develop (i.e., to the barrier) (Fig. 6-49). The patient is asked to depress the opposite shoulder, tensioning the involved nerve root from its proximal end, while the practitioner moves the wrist and fingers on the involved side away from the barrier toward flexion (Fig. 6-55). This maneuver theoretically causes movement of the nerve root inward within the lateral canal. The patient then elevates the opposite shoulder while the practitioner extends the wrist and fingers on the involved side (Fig. 6-56). This theoretically causes the nerve root to move outward within the lateral canal. This flossing movement is performed repetitively.

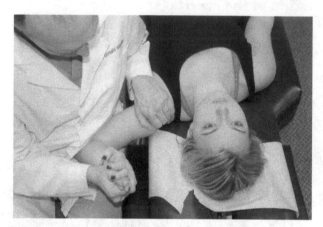

Figure 6-55. Depression of the opposite shoulder with flexion of the wrist and fingers for practitioner-generated distal flossing in the ulnar bias position.

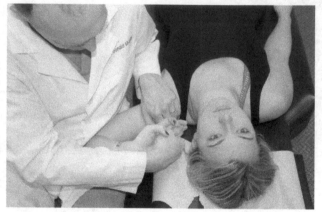

Figure 6-56. Elevation of the opposite shoulder with extension of the wrist and fingers for practitioner-generated distal flossing in the ulnar bias position.

Ulnar bias position tensioning – practitioner-generated movement

Proximal tensioning: The patient is supine and the practitioner sits facing the superior. The practitioner places the patient in the same position as during the examination using the ulnar bias position of the BPTT (Fig. 6-49) – the patient's arm is placed in 90 degrees of shoulder abduction and 90 degrees of elbow flexion. The practitioner depresses the shoulder girdle by pressing downward on the shoulder. The practitioner extends the wrist and 4th and 5th fingers. The practitioner then pronates the forearm, externally rotates the shoulder and flexes the elbow and shoulder so that the patient's hand moves toward the ear. The movement is carried out to the point at which the practitioner and/or patient feels tension develop (i.e., to the barrier).

To apply the tensioning maneuver the practitioner allows the shoulder on the involved side to rise, moving just away from the barrier (Fig. 6-57). The practitioner then depresses the shoulder to the point at which the barrier is engaged (Fig. 6-58). This movement is performed repetitively, with the practitioner always moving the shoulder just to the barrier and then away from the barrier.

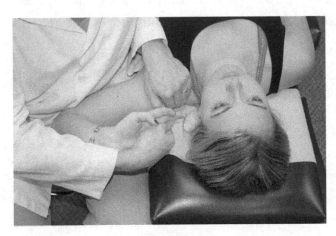 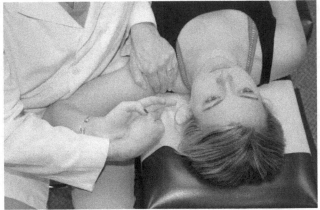

Figure 6-57. Elevation of the shoulder on the involved side for practitioner-generated proximal tensioning in the ulnar bias position.

Figure 6-58. Depression of the shoulder on the involved side for practitioner-generated proximal tensioning in the ulnar bias position.

Intermediate tensioning: The patient is supine and the practitioner sits facing the superior. The practitioner places the patient in the same position as during the examination using the ulnar bias position of the BPTT to the point at which the practitioner and/or patient feels tension develop (i.e., to the barrier) (Fig. 6-49).

To apply the tensioning maneuver the practitioner moves the elbow toward extension, moving just away from the barrier (Fig. 6-59). The practitioner then flexes the elbow to the point at which the barrier is engaged (Fig. 6-60). This movement is performed repetitively, with the practitioner always moving the elbow just to the barrier and then away from the barrier.

Distal tensioning: The patient is supine and the practitioner sits facing the superior. The practitioner again places the patient in the same position as during the examination using the ulnar bias position of the BPTT to the point at which the practitioner and/or patient feels tension develop (i.e., to the barrier) (Fig. 6-49).

To apply the tensioning maneuver the practitioner flexes the wrist and fingers, moving just away from the barrier (Fig. 6-61). The practitioner then extends the wrist and fingers to the point at which the barrier is engaged (Fig. 6-62). This movement is performed repetitively, with the practitioner always moving the wrist and fingers just to the barrier and then away from the barrier.

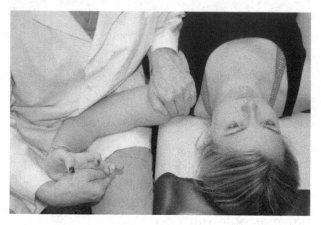

Figure 6-59. Moving the elbow away from the barrier for practitioner-generated intermediate tensioning in the ulnar bias position.

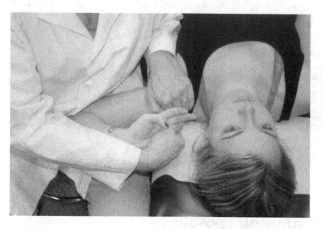

Figure 6-60. Flexion of the elbow to the barrier for practitioner-generated intermediate tensioning in the ulnar bias position.

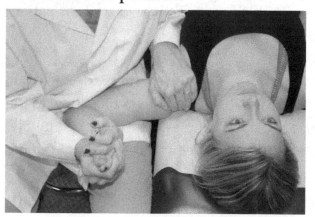

Figure 6-61. Moving the wrist and fingers away from the barrier for practitioner-generated distal tensioning in the ulnar bias position.

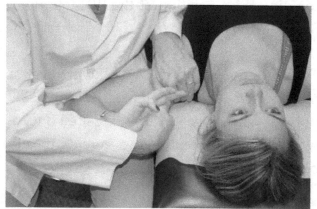

Figure 6-62. Extension of the wrist and fingers to the barrier for practitioner-generated distal tensioning in the ulnar bias position.

Ulnar bias position neural mobilization – patient-generated movement

Patient generated movements in cases in which the ulnar bias position is involved are not separated into flossing and tensioning maneuvers. The following two exercises are useful in the vast majority of patients.

General ulnar nerve mobilization: The patient can be standing or sitting. The patient places the hand on the uninvolved side onto the shoulder of the involved side, attempting to prevent the shoulder from rising during the exercise. The upper extremity on the involved side is placed in a position that mimics the ulnar bias position of the BPTT, the patient placing the hand against the side of the head (or as near to this as possible) with the fingers pointing toward the floor (Fig. 6-63).

The patient laterally flexes the head away from the side of involvement while maintaining contact on the head with the hand and raising the elbow toward the ceiling (Fig. 6-64), and then returns to the starting position. Using the hand that is placed on the shoulder, the patient attempts to prevent the shoulder from rising if possible.

The movement is performed repetitively for 10-30 repetitions. If range of motion or nerve sensitivity limits the patient's ability to bring the hand to the side of the head, the maneuver can still be performed with the hand and head moving simultaneously (Fig. 6-65).

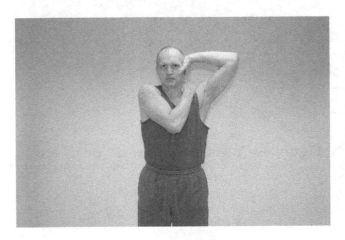

Figure 6-63. Starting position for general ulnar nerve mobilization.

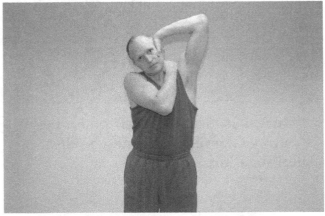

Figure 6-64. Lateral flexion of the head away with maintenance of hand contact with the head and elevation of the elbow.

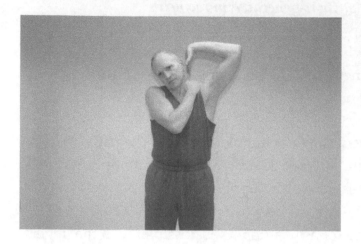

Figure 6-65. Alternate method in patients whose range of motion or nerve sensitivity limits their ability to make contact with the hand on the side of the head.

"Funny Glasses" ulnar nerve self-mobilization: This maneuver can be performed bilaterally and is another general ulnar nerve mobilization exercise. The patient can be standing or sitting. The patient contacts the tips of the index finger and thumb as if making an "OK" sign (Fig. 6-66), then raises the hands to the face so that the hole created by the finger contact moves over the eyes as if creating fake glasses (Fig. 6-67). The patient then returns to the starting position. This maneuver is performed repetitively for 10-30 repetitions.

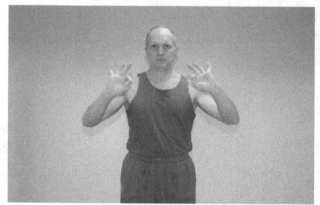

Figure 6-66. Starting position for the "Funny Glasses" ulnar nerve self-mobilization.

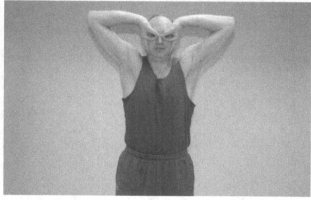

Figure 6-67. "Funny Glasses" position.

Radial bias position flossing – practitioner-generated movement

Proximal flossing: The patient is supine and the practitioner sits facing the inferior. The practitioner places the patient in the same position as during the examination using the radial bias position of the BPTT (see Figs 3-45 through 3-49 in Chapter 3) – the patient's arm is placed in 90 degrees of shoulder abduction and 90 degrees of elbow flexion. The practitioner depresses the shoulder girdle by pressing downward on the shoulder. The practitioner then flexes the wrist and fingers, pronates the forearm, internally rotates the shoulder and extends the elbow to the point at which the practitioner and/or patient feels tension develop (i.e., to the barrier) (Fig. 6-68).

The patient is asked to depress the opposite shoulder, tensioning the involved nerve root from its proximal end, while the practitioner allows the shoulder on the involved side to rise (Fig. 6-69). This maneuver theoretically causes movement of the nerve root inward within the lateral canal. The patient then elevates the opposite shoulder while the practitioner depresses the shoulder on the involved side (Fig. 6-70). This theoretically causes the nerve root to move outward within the lateral canal. This flossing movement is performed repetitively.

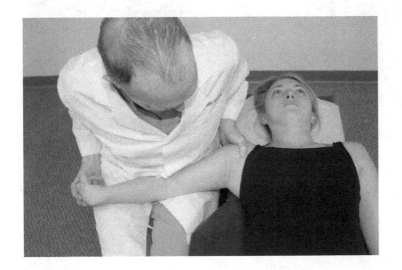

Figure 6-68. Starting position for practitioner-generated flossing and tensioning in the radial bias position.

Lateral glide proximal flossing: The practitioner sits at the head of the table. The patient's upper extremity is placed in a position that mimics the radial bias position of the BPTT. If possible, an assistant can be used to maintain this position. The practitioner places one hand on the shoulder to prevent the shoulder from rising during the maneuver. With the other hand the practitioner reaches underneath the cervical spine to make contact on the lateral aspect of the cervical spine on the side of involvement. The hand placement should be just superior to the involved cervical segment. The practitioner glides the cervical spine laterally away from the side of involvement while holding the shoulder in position, preventing elevation (Fig. 6-71). The spine is then moved back to the starting position. This flossing movement is performed repetitively. It is important that the movement of the cervical spine is one of lateral translation (x axis translation) above the level of involvement as opposed to lateral flexion (z axis rotation).

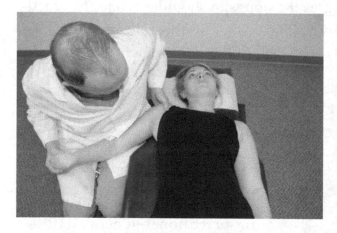

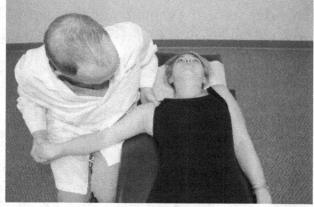

Figure 6-69. Depression of the opposite shoulder with elevation of the shoulder on the involved side for practitioner-generated proximal flossing in the radial bias position.

Figure 6-70. Elevation of the opposite shoulder with depression of the shoulder on the involved side for practitioner-generated proximal flossing in the radial bias position.

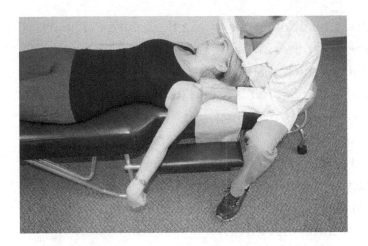

Figure 6-71. Lateral translation of the cervical spine during practitioner-generated lateral glide flossing in the radial bias position.

Intermediate flossing: The patient is supine and the practitioner sits facing the inferior. The practitioner places the patient in the same position as during the examination using the radial bias position of the BPTT to the point at which the practitioner and/or patient feels tension develop (i.e., to the barrier) (Fig. 6-68). The patient is asked to depress the opposite shoulder, tensioning the involved nerve root from its proximal end, while the practitioner flexes the elbow on the involved side (Fig. 6-72). This maneuver theoretically causes movement of the nerve root inward within the lateral canal. The patient then elevates the opposite shoulder while the practitioner extends the elbow on the involved side (Fig. 6-73). This theoretically causes the nerve root to move outward within the lateral canal. This flossing movement is performed repetitively.

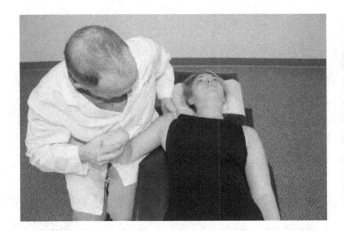

Figure 6-72. Depression of the opposite shoulder with flexion of the elbow for practitioner-generated intermediate flossing in the radial bias position.

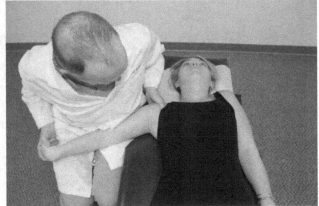

Figure 6-73. Elevation of the opposite shoulder with extension of the elbow for practitioner-generated intermediate flossing in the radial bias position.

Distal flossing: The patient is supine and the practitioner sits facing the inferior. The practitioner again places the patient in the same position as during the examination using the radial bias position of the BPTT to the point at which the practitioner and/or patient feels tension develop (i.e., to the barrier) (Fig. 6-68). The patient is asked to depress the opposite shoulder, tensioning the involved nerve root from its proximal end, while the practitioner extends the wrist and fingers on the involved side (Fig. 6-74). This maneuver theoretically causes movement of the nerve root inward within the lateral canal. The patient then elevates the opposite shoulder while the practitioner flexes the wrist and fingers on the involved side (Fig. 6-75). This theoretically causes the nerve root to move outward within the lateral canal. This flossing movement is performed repetitively.

Radial bias position flossing – patient-generated movement

Proximal flossing: The patient can be standing or sitting. The upper extremity on the involved side is placed in internal rotation and elbow extension with the wrist and fingers flexed (Fig. 6-76). The shoulder on the opposite side is depressed while the shoulder on the involved side is elevated (Fig. 6-77). The shoulder on the opposite side is then elevated while the shoulder on the involved side is depressed (Fig. 6-78). This flossing movement is performed repetitively for 10-20 repetitions.

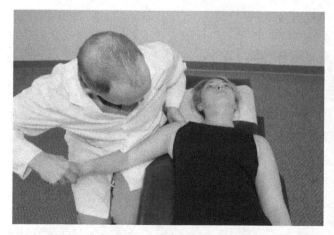 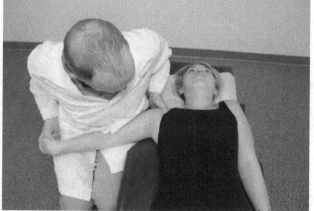

Figure 6-74. Depression of the opposite shoulder with extension of the wrist and fingers for practitioner-generated distal flossing in the radial bias position.

Figure 6-75. Elevation of the opposite shoulder with flexion of the wrist and fingers for practitioner-generated distal flossing in the radial bias position.

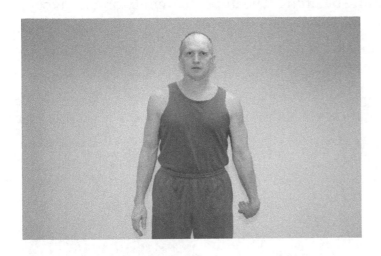

Figure 6-76. Starting position for patient-generated flossing and tensioning in the radial bias position.

Intermediate flossing: The patient can be standing or sitting. The upper extremity on the involved side is placed in internal rotation and elbow extension with the wrist and fingers flexed (Fig. 6-76). The shoulder on the opposite side is depressed while the elbow on the involved side is flexed (Fig. 6-79). The shoulder on the opposite side is then elevated while the elbow on the involved side is extended (Fig. 6-80). This flossing movement is performed repetitively for 10-30 repetitions

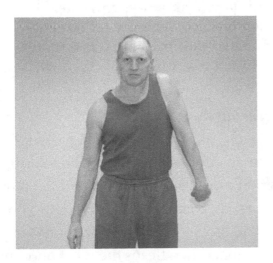

Figure 6-77. Depression of the contralateral shoulder with elevation of the ipsilateral shoulder for patient-generated proximal flossing in the radial bias position.

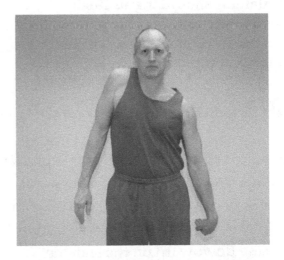

Figure 6-78. Elevation of the contralateral shoulder with depression of the ipsilateral shoulder for patient-generated proximal flossing in the radial bias position.

Distal flossing: The patient can be standing or sitting. The upper extremity on the involved side is placed in internal rotation and elbow extension with the wrist and fingers flexed (Fig. 6-76). The shoulder on the opposite side is depressed while the wrist and fingers on the involved side are extended (Fig. 6-81). The shoulder on the opposite side is then elevated while the wrist and fingers on the involved side are flexed (Fig. 6-82). This flossing movement is performed repetitively for 10-20 repetitions.

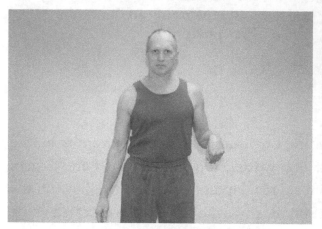

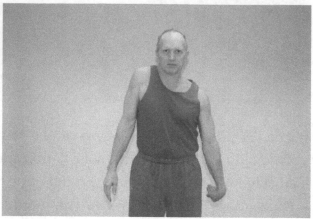

Figure 6-79. Depression of the contralateral shoulder and flexion of the ipsilateral elbow for patient-generated intermediate flossing in the radial bias position.

Figure 6-80. Elevation of the contralateral shoulder and extension of the ipsilateral elbow for patient-generated intermediate flossing in the radial bias position.

Radial bias position tensioning – practitioner-generated movement

Proximal tensioning: The patient is supine and the practitioner sits facing the inferior. The practitioner places the patient in the same position as during the examination using the radial bias position of the BPTT – the patient's arm is placed in 90 degrees of shoulder abduction and 90 degrees of elbow flexion. The practitioner depresses the shoulder girdle by pressing downward on the shoulder. The practitioner then flexes the wrist and fingers, pronates the forearm, internally rotates the shoulder and extends the elbow to the point at which the practitioner and/or patient feels tension develop (i.e., to the barrier) (Fig. 6-69). To apply the tensioning maneuver the practitioner allows the shoulder on the involved

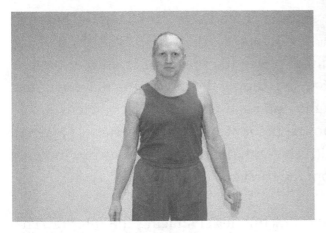

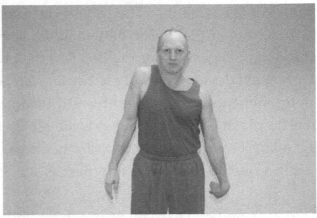

Figure 6-81. Depression of the contralateral shoulder and extension of the ipsilateral wrist and fingers for patient-generated distal flossing in the radial bias position.

Figure 6-82. Elevation of the contralateral shoulder and flexion of the ipsilateral wrist and fingers for patient-generated distal flossing in the radial bias position.

side to rise, moving just away from the barrier (Fig. 6-83). The practitioner then depresses the shoulder to the point at which the barrier is engaged (Fig. 6-84). This movement is performed repetitively, with the practitioner always moving the shoulder just to the barrier and then away from the barrier.

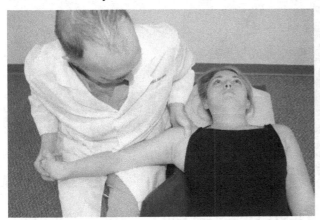

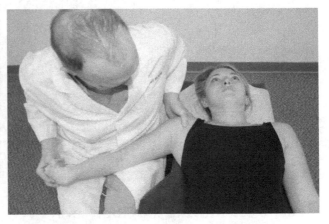

Figure 6-83. Elevation of the shoulder on the involved side for practitioner-generated proximal tensioning in the radial bias position.

Figure 6-84. Depression of the shoulder on the involved side for practitioner-generated proximal tensioning in the radial bias position.

Intermediate tensioning: The patient is supine and the practitioner sits facing the inferior. The practitioner places the patient in the same position as during the examination using the radial bias position of the BPTT to the point at which the practitioner and/or patient feels tension develop (i.e., to the barrier) (Fig. 6-69). To apply the tensioning maneuver the practitioner moves the elbow toward flexion, moving just away from the barrier (Fig. 6-85). The practitioner then extends the elbow to the point at which the barrier is engaged (Fig. 6-86). This movement is performed repetitively, with the practitioner always moving the elbow just to the barrier and then away from the barrier.

Distal tensioning: The patient is supine and the practitioner sits facing the inferior. The practitioner places the patient in the same position as during the examination using the radial bias position of the BPTT to the point at which the practitioner and/or patient feels tension develop (i.e., to the barrier) (Fig. 6-69). To apply the tensioning maneuver the practitioner moves the wrist and fingers toward extension, moving just away from the barrier (Fig. 6-87). The practitioner then flexes the wrist and fingers to the point at which the barrier is engaged (Fig. 6-88). This movement is performed repetitively, with the practitioner always moving the wrist and fingers just to the barrier and then away from the barrier.

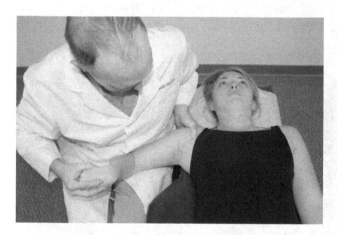

Figure 6-85. Moving the elbow away from the barrier for practitioner-generated intermediate tensioning in the radial bias position.

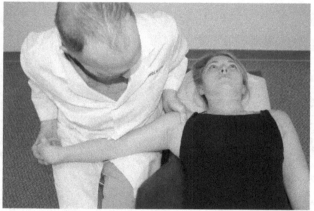

Figure 6-86. Extension of the elbow to the barrier for practitioner-generated intermediate tensioning in the radial bias position.

Radial bias position tensioning – patient-generated movement

Proximal tensioning: The patient can be standing or sitting. The upper extremity on the involved side is placed in internal rotation and elbow extension with the wrist and fingers flexed (Fig. 6-76). The head is laterally flexed away from the side of involvement, applying tension to the neural tract (Fig. 6-89) and then immediately returns to the starting position. This tensioning movement is performed repetitively for 10-30 repetitions.

Intermediate tensioning: The patient can be standing or sitting. The upper extremity on the involved side is placed in internal rotation and elbow extension with the wrist and fingers flexed (Fig. 6-76). The elbow on the involved side is flexed (Fig. 6-90) and then immediately returns to the starting position. This tensioning movement is performed repetitively for 10-30 repetitions.

Distal tensioning: The patient can be standing or sitting. The upper extremity on the involved side is placed in internal rotation and elbow extension with the wrist and fingers flexed (Fig. 6-76). The wrist and fingers on the involved side are moved toward extension, slackening the neural tract (Fig. 91) and then immediately return to the starting position. This tensioning movement is performed repetitively for 10-30 repetitions.

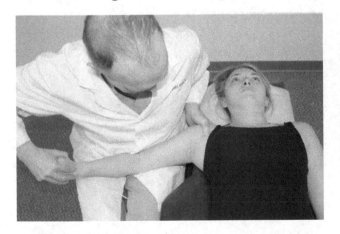 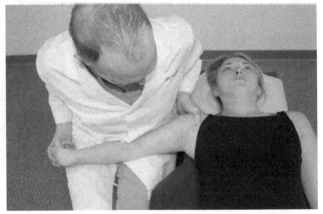

Figure 6-87. Moving the wrist and fingers away from the barrier for practitioner-generated distal tensioning in the radial bias position.

Figure 6-88. Flexion of the wrist and fingers to the barrier for practitioner-generated distal tensioning in the radial bias position.

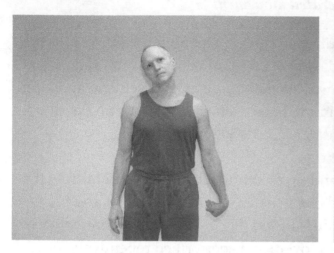

Figure 6-89. Lateral flexion of the head away from the side of involvement for patient-generated proximal tensioning in the radial bias position.

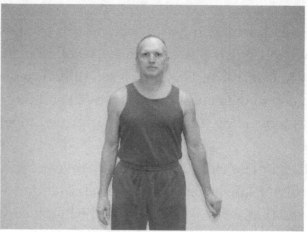

Figure 6-90. Extension of the wrist and fingers for patient-generated distal tensioning in the radial bias position.

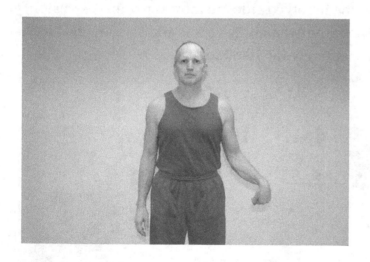

Figure 6-91. Flexion of the elbow patient-generated intermediate tensioning in the radial bias position.

Home traction

Patients with radiculopathy can self-treat with a home traction unit. There are several such units on the market and it is not likely that any particular type is clinically superior to the others. A simple over-the-door unit can be both useful and cost-effective. While traction in and of itself might not have a tremendous impact on the end result of treatment, it gives the patient an opportunity to provide temporary self-relief and, importantly, helps build self-efficacy by placing the patient in control. And, of course, it should not be used as a stand-alone treatment. It is best to test the patient with manual traction in the clinic to determine his or her response before providing a home traction unit.

It is essential that the patient is instructed carefully about the proper use of the home traction unit and that it is clear that the patient understands this proper use before being given the unit. The patient should sit facing the door (Fig. 6-92) with the head angulated 20-25 degrees. The amount of weight will vary according to the patient. It is recommended that for female patients 3.5 kg (~8 pounds) should be initially tried. For males, the initial weight should be 4.5 kg (~10 pounds). The weight can be gradually increased at 1 kg (~2 pounds) intervals to a maximum of 9-14 kg (~20-30 pounds), depending on patient tolerance and therapeutic benefit. Care should be taken to monitor the patient when first performing the procedure and it should be terminated immediately if there is any significant increase or peripheralization of pain or neurological symptoms. The traction should be applied for 15-20 minutes at a time, at least once to twice per day, depending on patient tolerance.

Myofascial Pain

It was discussed in Volume I of this series that while myofascial trigger points (TrPs) are very common in patients with low back disorders (LBDs), they usually develop in response to one of the other pain generators and are seldom the primary pain generator. Thus, in most cases, it is not necessary to treat the TrPs as they generally resolve following successful treatment of the primary pain generator (as well as the perpetuating factors covered in diagnostic question #3). The same is true in patient with CDs, however, to a somewhat lesser degree. That is, it is somewhat more common for patients with CDs to have clinically relevant TrPs than it is with LBD patients. This is particularly the case in patients with headaches related to the cervical spine.

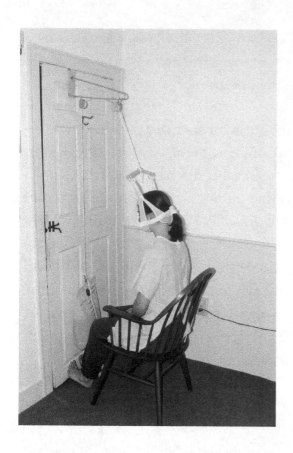

Figure 6-92. Over-the-door traction. The patient should be facing the door and the head should be angulated 20-25 degrees. Reprinted with permission from Murphy DR, ed. Conservative Management of Cervical Spine Syndromes. New York: McGraw-Hill, 2000.

There are a variety of methods available to treat TrPs and it is beyond the scope of this book to provide an exhaustive examination of all methods. There is no shortage of resources for the practitioner to learn further details regarding myofascial treatments (see the books by Simons, et al and Chaitow in the Recommended Reading list). Presented here is a basic approach that is applicable to nearly all patients with CDs who have clinically relevant TrPs contributing to their pain.

Myofascial treatments can generally be separated into three types: manual or instrumented pressure release techniques, muscle lengthening techniques and methods that apply a combination of pressure release and muscle lengthening. In keeping with one of the prevailing themes throughout this book, the patient should be taught to self-treat their TrPs in addition to (or in some cases, instead of) the practitioner generated treatments.

Manual or instrumented pressure release techniques

TrP palpation was described in detail in Chapter 3. Once the practitioner becomes skilled in palpation, the application of pressure release techniques becomes easy. The simplest method of pressure release is ischemic compression.

With this method the TrP is identified via palpation and pressure is applied, by a finger and/or thumb or with an instrument, to the point at which pain is reproduced at an intensity that the patient identifies as similar to the chief complaint, but that does not cause the patient to tense or become distressed. The practitioner maintains the pressure and asks the patient to report when the pain begins to diminish or centralize (i.e., occupy a smaller area). The pressure is maintained until the pain centralizes to just under the palpating finger or resolves, or for approximately one minute, whichever comes first.

Patients can easily be taught to self-treat TrPs using the same pressure release technique as practitioner-generated treatment. Cervical muscles are particularly well-suited for self-treatment given their easy accessibility. In most cases, the fingers can be used for self-treatment, but sometimes an instrument can be used. There are a number of instruments on the market that can be used for this purpose but often a simple tennis ball is more than adequate. However, the patient's own hands are usually preferable.

The practitioner can teach the patient to palpate the TrP by first identifying it him- or herself and then having the patient place a finger on the same spot. The patient can be taught to apply sustained pressure or to gently massage the TrP for a minute or so. The amount of pressure applied is not critical but in general the right amount of pressure is that which allows the patient to feel the pain associated with the TrP but that creates what patients often describe as "a good pain" rather than pain that causes the patient to tense up or become distressed.

Patients should be instructed to spend up to a total of five minutes treating the various relevant TrPs that are found. It is important that the patient is taught to stop at that point and not spend any more time trying to treat the TrPs or even think about them. It is best to spend a few minutes treating the TrPs and then move on with the important activities of the day.

Muscle lengthening procedures

A number of muscle lengthening techniques are available that can be useful for TrPs. One simple and widely applicable method is postisometric relaxation (PIR). This is similar to muscle energy technique that was described previously for LVLA joint manipulation. With PIR, the principles of MET are applied to muscle lengthening. Isometric contraction is used to tense the involved muscle and this is followed by cessation of the isometric contraction, resulting in relaxation of the muscle. This allows for gentle lengthening of the muscle as a whole, as well as the taut band within the muscle that contains the TrP. Eye movements are applied to aid with muscle activation and relaxation. A full description of the theoretical mechanism of PIR is beyond the scope of this book but can be found in the books by Chaitow in the Recommended Reading list. It should be pointed out that recent evidence suggests that the therapeutic benefit of muscle "lengthening" procedures may well result from reduction of the sensitivity of the muscle (or, more specifically, the nociceptive system) as much as or more than actual elongation of the muscle (see Konrad, et al in the Recommended Reading list).

Sternocleidomastoid

The patient is supine with the head off the end of the table. The practitioner places the middle finger of the hand opposite the side of involvement under the occipital ridge. The head is then moved into lateral flexion away from the side of involvement, slight rotation toward the side of involvement, extension of the lower cervical spine and flexion of the upper cervical spine to the point at which the barrier is met. The thumb of the hand on the involved side is then placed onto the forehead just above the patient's eye and the rest of that hand is placed on the side of the head (Fig. 6-93). The patient is asked to push upward against the thumb, move the eyes as if looking at the forehead, and take a deep breath in for the contraction phase. The patient then stops pushing, looks downward toward the cheeks and breathes out for the relaxation phase. The practitioner waits to feel the release of the barrier. When the barrier releases the practitioner gently guides the muscle to lengthen by moving the cervical spine into extension, keeping the upper cervical spine flexed, until a new barrier is met. This is repeated two more times.

Self-treatment of the sternocleidomastoid is best done with muscle lengthening procedures rather than with manual release procedures. This can be done with the patient in the seated or standing position. The patient first places one hand on the clavicle to anchor it in position. The patient then laterally flexes slightly away from the involved side, rotates slightly toward the involved side, flexes the upper cervical spine by slightly nodding the head and extending to the point at which the barrier is perceived (Fig. 6-94). The patient holds this position for 30-60 seconds.

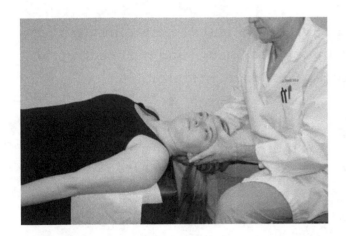

Figure 6-93. Positioning for PIR of the sternocleidomastoid muscle.

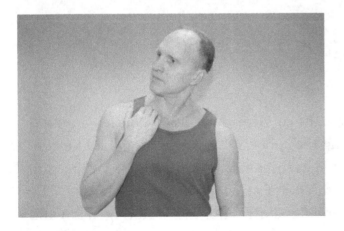

Figure 6-94. Self-treatment of the right sternocleidomastoid muscle.

Suboccipitals

The patient is supine and the practitioner blocks the C2 articular pillar (as close as possible) with one hand and rotates and laterally flexes a few degrees away from the side being treated to place focus on that side. The practitioner then flexes the upper cervical spine with the other hand to take up slack and meet the barrier (Fig. 6-95). It is important to limit the movement to the upper cervical spine. This can be done by placing slight pressure caudally on the head while taking up slack. The patient is asked to look upward with to the forehead and breathe in for the contraction phase and look downward and breathe out for the relaxation phase. The practitioner waits to feel for the release of the barrier and when this occurs, gently guides the muscle to lengthen into upper cervical flexion.

Posterior cervical

There are a number of muscles in the posterior cervical spine and it is very difficult, if not impossible, to distinguish them with certainty during examination and treatment. Fortunately, distinguishing these muscles is not necessary for proper treatment.

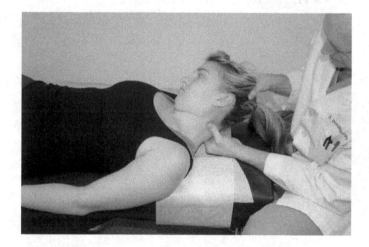

Figure 6-95. Positioning for PIR of the suboccipital muscles.

The patient is supine and the practitioner moves the cervical spine as a whole (as opposed to just the upper cervical spine as when treating the suboccipitals) into combined flexion, slight rotation away from the side being treated and lateral flexion away from the side being treated. The cervical spine is moved to the point at which the barrier is met. The practitioner then places one hand on the posterolateral aspect of the head (Fig. 6-96) and asks the patient to gently press against that hand, look up and breathe in for the contraction phase. The patient is then asked to stop pushing, breathe out and look down for the relaxation phase. The practitioner waits to feel for the release of the barrier and when this occurs, gently guides the muscle to lengthen into flexion and lateral flexion.

Levator scapulae

The patient is supine and the practitioner places the hand on the side of involvement on the superior angle of the scapula as close as possible to the attachment point of the levator scapulae. With the other hand the practitioner moves the cervical spine as a whole into combined flexion, rotation away from the side being treated and lateral flexion away from the side being treated. The cervical spine is moved to the point at which the barrier is met (Fig. 6-97). The practitioner then asks the patient to gently try to shrug the shoulder, attempting to press the superior angle of the scapula against the practitioner's hand and breathe in for the contraction phase. It is important for the practitioner to hold the superior angle of the scapula in place. The patient is then asked to stop pushing and breathe out for the relaxation phase. The practitioner waits to feel for the release of the barrier and when this occurs, gently guides the muscle to lengthen by moving the superior angle of the scapula inferiorward.

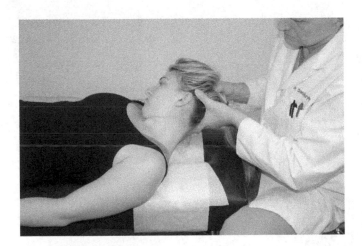

Figure 6-96. Positioning for PIR of the posterior cervical muscles.

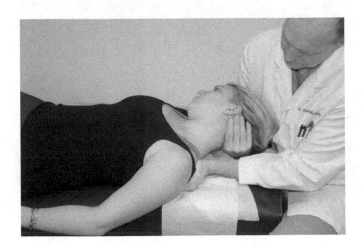

Figure 6-97. Positioning for PIR of the levator scapulae muscle.

Upper trapezius

The patient is supine and the practitioner places the hand on the side of involvement on the acromion process of the scapula. With the other hand the practitioner moves the cervical spine as a whole into combined flexion, slight rotation toward the side being treated and lateral flexion away from the side being treated. The cervical spine is moved to the point at which the barrier is met (Fig. 6-98). The practitioner then asks the patient to gently try to shrug the shoulder, attempting to press the acromion process against the practitioner's hand while the practitioner holds the shoulder in place, and breathe in for the contraction phase. The patient is then asked to stop pushing and breathe out for the relaxation phase. The practitioner waits to feel for the release of the barrier and when this occurs, gently guides the muscle to lengthen into shoulder depression.

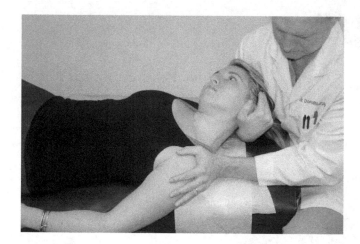

Figure 6-98. Positioning for PIR of the upper trapezius muscle.

Scalenes

The patient is supine with the hand on the involved side under the buttock. The purpose of this is to hold the shoulder in position. As with the SCM, the patient's head is off the end of the table. The practitioner's hand opposite the side of involvement is placed under the occipital ridge. The practitioner moves the cervical spine into lateral flexion away from the side of involvement, rotation slightly away that side and extension of the entire cervical spine. It is essential to maintain a neutral lordosis so that the extension does not occur solely at the upper cervical spine. The hand on the side of involvement is placed on the temporal bone (Fig. 6-99). The practitioner asks the patient to press the head against this hand and breathe in for the contraction phase and then stop pushing and breathe out for the relaxation phase. The practitioner waits to feel the release of the barrier and then gently guides the muscle to lengthen into lateral flexion and extension.

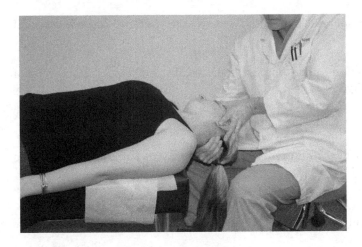

Figure 6-99. Positioning for PIR of the scalene muscles.

Treatment for factors related to diagnostic question #2 is designed to rapidly reduce nociception. This not only can decrease the patient's pain but often improves or resolves factors related to diagnostic question #3 (dynamic instability, nociceptive system sensitization, oculomotor dysfunction, psychological factors), as in many cases these factors are maintained in part by nociceptive input. However, in other cases, the factors related to diagnostic question #3 have to be addressed separately. This will be the topic of the next chapter.

Recommended Reading

Bergmann T, Peterson D. Chiropractic Technique Principles and Procedures; 3rd Ed. St. Louis: Elsevier, Mosby, 2011.

Butler DS. The Sensitive Nervous System. Adelaide, Australia: Noigroup Publications; 2000.

Chaitow. Modern Neuromuscular Techniques. 3rd ed. Edinburgh: Churchille Livingstone; 2011

Chaitow. Muscle Energy Techniques. 4th ed. Edinburgh: Churchille Livingstone; 2013.

Kawchuk GN, Perle SM. The relation between the application angle of spinal manipulative therapy (SMT) and resultant vertebral accelerations in an in situ porcine model. Man Ther. 2009 Oct;14(5):480–3.

Konrad A, Tilp M. Increased range of motion after static stretching is not due to changes in muscle and tendon structures. Clin Biomech 2014 Jun;29(6):636-42.

Lewit K. Manipulative Therapy in the Rehabilitation of the Locomotor System. 3rd Ed. Oxford: Butterworth-Heinemann Ltd., 1999

McKenzie R, May S. The Cervical and Thoracic Spine: Mechanical Diagnosis and Therapy. 2nd ed. Raumati Beach, NZ: Spinal Publications; 2006.

Murphy DR, Hurwitz EL, Gregory AA. Manipulation in the presence of cervical spinal cord compression: a case series. J Manipulative Physiol Ther. 2006;29(3):236-44.

Neurodynamic Solutions: http://www.neurodynamicsolutions.com [accessed 7 May 2016]

Prushansky T, Pevzner E, Gordon C, Dvir Z. Cervical radiofrequency neurotomy in patients with chronic whiplash: a study of multiple outcome measures. J Neurosurg Spine. 2006 May;4(5):365-73.

Raney NH, Petersen EJ, Smith TA, Cowan JE, Rendeiro DG, Deyle GD, et al. Development of a clinical prediction rule to identify patients with neck pain likely to benefit from cervical traction and exercise. Eur Spine J 2009;18(3):382-91

Shacklock M. Clinical Neurodynamics. A New System of Musculoskeletal Treatment. Edinburgh: Elsevier; 2005.

Simons DG, Travell JG, Simons LS. Myofascial Pain and Dysfunction: The Trigger Point Manual. Volume 1. Baltimore: Williams and Wilkens; 1999.

Smith AD, Jull G, Schneider G, Frizzell B, Hooper RA, Dunne-Proctor R, et al. Cervical radiofrequency neurotomy reduces psychological features in individuals with chronic whiplash symptoms. Pain Physician. 2014 May-Jun;17(3):265-74.

Smith AD, Jull G, Schneider G, Frizzell B, Hooper RA, Sterling M. Cervical radiofrequency neurotomy reduces central hyperexcitability and improves neck movement in individuals with chronic whiplash. Pain Med. 2014 Jan;15(1):128-41.

The McKenzie Institute International: http://www.mckenziemdt.org/ [accessed 7 May 2016]

The NOI Group: http://www.noigroup.com [accessed 7 May 2016]

Appendix

The Relationship between Cervical Manipulation and Stroke: The State of the Science

This appendix is excerpted and adapted from a paper written by the lead author this book (DRM) and published in the journal Chiropractic and Osteopathy (now known as Chiropractic and Manual Therapies). The original paper can be obtained at **http://www.chiromt.com/content/18/1/22** [accessed 7 May 2016]. The information presented has been updated to reflect recent literature on the topic.

When the paper was originally written, the primary target audience was the chiropractic profession. This is reflected in the text. However, in certain places in the text, where in the original paper the words "chiropractor" or "chiropractic profession" had appeared, the words "primary spine practitioner" ("PSP") or "primary spine care field" have been substituted.

The full citation of this paper is:
Murphy DR. Current understanding of the relationship between cervical manipulation and stroke: what does it mean for the chiropractic profession? Chiropr Osteopat. 2010;18:22.

Abstract

The understanding of the relationship between cervical manipulative therapy (CMT) and vertebral artery dissection and stroke (VADS) has evolved considerably over the years. In the beginning, the relationship was seen as simple cause-effect, in which CMT was seen to cause VADS in certain susceptible individuals. This was perceived as extremely rare by chiropractic physicians, but as far more common by neurologists and others. Recent evidence has clarified the relationship considerably, and suggests that the relationship is not causal, but that patients with VADS often have initial symptoms which cause them to seek care from a chiropractic physician and have a stroke sometime after, independent of the chiropractic visit.

This new understanding has shifted the focus for the primary spine practitioner from one of attempting to "screen" for "risk of complication to manipulation" to one of recognizing, if possible, the patient who may be having VADS so that early diagnosis and intervention can be pursued. In addition, this new understanding presents the primary spine care field with an opportunity to change the conversation about CMT and VADS by taking a proactive, public health approach to this uncommon but potentially devastating disorder.

Introduction

Cervical manipulative therapy (CMT) and vertebral artery dissection and stroke (VADS) have been linked in controversy for at least 75 years [1]. At the center of the controversy have been neurologists and other medical practitioners who have often perceived VADS to be a relatively frequent complication to CMT [2, 3] and chiropractors, who have generally perceived VADS after manipulation to be exceedingly rare [4-6]. Others have been involved as well [7, 8]. Starting with isolated case reports and culminating in four case-control studies, our understanding of the relationship between CMT and VADS has evolved considerably. The purpose of this commentary is to present an overview of the history of this relationship and to discuss how the chiropractic profession and other professionals who use manual therapy can move forward and focus on the wellbeing of patients and the public while avoiding defensiveness.

There are several pathophysiologic processes that can lead to stroke, such as atherosclerosis, hemorrhage secondary to aneurism or arteriovenous malformation, and arterial dissection. Arterial dissection is a specific process in which a tear occurs in the wall of the involved artery [9]. Cervical artery dissection is a general term for dissection that involves either the carotid artery (carotid artery dissection) or vertebral artery (vertebral artery dissection). As vertebral artery dissection has been found to have an association with visits to chiropractic physicians, this commentary primarily focuses on vertebral artery dissection. However, the terms cervical artery dissection and carotid artery dissection are used in certain instances in which both carotid artery dissection and vertebral artery dissection or carotid artery dissection alone is being referred to.

The evolution of our understanding of the relationship between cervical manipulation and vertebral artery dissection – case reports, surveys, biomechanical studies, case reviews

The awareness of a temporal relationship between cervical CMT and VADS began with a series of case reports published over a period of several years [10-22]. In a number of these studies, the treating practitioner was incorrectly identified as a chiropractor [23]. These studies reported on cases of patients who developed VADS sometime after receiving CMT, although in the majority no confirmation or details of the manipulative procedure were provided [24]. Generally in these reports the CMT was described as the cause of the dissection. In addition to CMT, a number of reports attributed the cause of VADS episodes to other mechanical events which preceded the VADS [25].

Later came a series of retrospective surveys. The first of these was a survey of the 367 members of the Swiss Society for Manual Medicine who were asked to recall over the course of their career (minimum 2 years, maximum 33 years, mean 8.1 years) how many CMTs they had provided and how many complications had occurred following CMT [26]. They estimated the rate of "slight neurological complications" to be 1:40,000 and the rate of "important complication" to be 1:400,000. Next was a survey of California neurologists who were members of the American Academy of Neurology [2]. In this study, recipients of the survey were asked to recall over the previous two years how many "neurologic complications following chiropractic adjustment", including radiculopathy, myelopathy and VADS, they had encountered. The authors reported a 37% response rate. Twenty-one percent reported at least one case of stroke. This was followed by a 10-year retrospective survey of chiropractors [27] in which the then-226 members of the Danish Chiropractors Association were surveyed (response rate 54%) in an effort to determine the incidence of "cerebrovascular incidents" between 1978-1988. From these data they estimated an incidence of one case per 362 chiropractor years and one case per 1.3 million cervical treatment sessions.

Later, a biomechanical study was performed by Symons, et al [28]. They used five unembalmed cadavers and exposed their cervical spines to movements similar to those that occur during clinical examination of range of motion as well as high-velocity, low amplitude CMT. This CMT was applied separately to the upper, middle and lower cervical spine. They measured the strain on the vertebral artery during these maneuvers. The arteries were then harvested and stretched to mechanical failure. They found that during ROM testing the strain to the vertebral artery was 1.2% to 12.5% greater than that at rest (the amount of strain varied according to the direction of movement applied). During CMT the average strain was 6.2% greater than that at rest. Finally, they found that mechanical failure did not occur until average strains of 139%-162% greater than that at rest. The authors concluded that the strain applied to the vertebral artery during CMT was unlikely to tear or otherwise mechanically disrupt a normal vertebral artery [28].

Other notable studies during this time period were published as well. Haldeman, et al [29] retrospectively reviewed 23 cases of VADS that occurred following CMT, utilizing data from a Canadian chiropractic malpractice insurance carrier over a 10-year period. From these cases they estimated the number of neurologists and chiropractors who were directly involved in each case. They calculated that one in 48 chiropractors was exposed to such cases, in comparison to one in two neurologists. They concluded that this selection or referral bias likely explained why neurologists tend to perceive VADS after CMT to be far more common than do chiropractors. Haldeman, et al [30] performed a retrospective review of 64 cases of VADS temporally related to CMT. They found no factors in the history or examination that would assist the physician in identifying the individual at risk of VADS after CMT. These authors concluded "Cerebrovascular accidents after manipulation appear to be unpredictable and should be considered an inherent, idiosyncratic, and rare complication of this treatment approach" [30]. This statement represented the prevailing thought at the time that study was published (2002).

However, none of the study designs discussed above are adequate to assess risk and to investigate a causal relationship between CMT and VADS. Descriptive studies such as case reports and case series are limited due to the absence of a comparison group [31, 32]. For example, in a case study in which a patient's headaches are reported to have improved after CMT, there is no way to determine whether the headaches would have improved without the CMT. Likewise, if an individual experiences an adverse event (e.g. VADS) following a treatment (e.g. CMT) or any other exposure there is no way to determine from a case report or case series whether that adverse event would have happened regardless of the treatment or exposure. To undertake an assessment of risk one must use one of three study designs:

1. Randomized, controlled trial (RCT): this is a design in which individuals are randomly assigned to one of two or more groups. Each group is provided a treatment, placebo, sham or no treatment and the outcomes of the groups are compared. The RCT is considered the Gold Standard for assessing treatment efficacy but is rarely used for risk assessment [33].

2. Prospective cohort study: this is a study that follows two or more groups over time, one of which is exposed to a certain treatment or exposure of interest and the other of which is not, and compares them for a particular outcome [33, 34]. This design works well if the condition of interest is relatively common, such as heart disease. Perhaps the most well-known cohort study is the Framingham Heart Study, which has prospectively tracked over time the rate of heart disease and its association with various risk profiles in an original cohort of 5,209 people since 1948. The prospective cohort design does not work well for studying a rare disease such as VADS, because one could follow thousands of patients for many years and potentially never come across a case of VADS.

3. Case-control study: this is the best research design for assessing the risks associated with a rare disorder such as VADS [32-34]. The case-control design compares a group of people who already have the outcome of interest to a similar group of people who do not. The researchers compare the two groups for exposures to a certain treatment or other factor prior to development of disease.

Using the case-control study design allows researchers to gain insight into whether the apparent relationship between an exposure (e.g., CMT) and an outcome (e.g., VADS) that is observed in case reports or case series is a true association, and, when properly designed, allows causal inferences to be made [33]. It does this in the case of the relationship between CMT and VADS by identifying individuals who already have VADS and comparing them to a matched control group of individuals without VADS with regard to exposures to CMT prior to developing VADS. Essential to minimizing bias in case-control studies is appropriate matching of cases and controls [34]. That is, the control group should be comparable to the "case" group. Reduction of bias in this regard is sometimes addressed by using a case-crossover design [35] in which cases serve as their own controls. This helps to better match the groups which reduces bias by better controlling for confounding variables [35].

However, case control studies can potentially be subject to a phenomenon known as protopathic bias [36]. Protopathic bias occurs when a therapeutic agent is applied for the early manifestations of a disease and, when the patient later develops the full manifestation of the disease, the therapeutic agent is mistakenly assumed to have been its "cause" [36]. To appropriately use a case control study to make causal inferences, it is important to include in the methodology factors that control for protopathic bias. This will be further discussed below with regard to case control studies on the association between CMT and VADS.

Case-Control Studies on the Association between CMT and VADS

Five case-control studies have investigated the association between CMT and VADS. The first was by Rothwell, et al. [37] This was a six year study performed in Ontario that compared 582 individuals who experienced vertebral artery-related stroke (cases) with 2328 individuals with no history of stroke (controls). They found that cases aged under 45 were five times more likely to have had a visit to a chiropractor within one week of their stroke. In individuals 45 or older, there was no difference between cases and controls.

The second case-control study was that of Smith, et al. [38] This was a six year study performed in two academic stroke centers. They compared 51 patients with stroke related to cervical artery dissection (25 involving the vertebral artery, 26 involving the carotid artery) with 100 patients with other types of stroke. Multivariate analysis found that patients with vertebral artery-related stroke were six times more likely than controls to recall having seen a chiropractor within 30 days of stroke. They concluded that CMT is an independent risk factor for vertebral artery-related stroke.

This was followed by a study by Dittrich, et al [39] in which 47 cases of either VADS or stroke related to carotid artery dissection were compared to 47 controls with other types of stroke. They looked at a variety of "mild" mechanical events that were potential risk factors (heavy lifting, mild direct neck trauma, mild indirect neck trauma, sexual intercourse, jerky or abnormal head movement, athletic activity, CMT) and their relationship to cervical artery dissection. They used seven days as the time period between the mechanical event and stroke for all the potential risk factors except CMT, for which they used a 30 day cutoff. They did not explain the reason for their use of different cutoffs. They found no statistically significant association between any individual mechanical event, including CMT, and cervical artery dissection. They did report a significant association between the mechanical factors as a group and cervical artery dissection. They also stated "our results indicate only a weak association of CMT with CAD, which might, however, be important in the pathogenesis". Unlike the previous studies, they included patients with VADS and stroke related to carotid artery dissection as a group and did not specifically assess the relationship between CMT and VADS.

Two of these three case control studies indicated a clear association between visits to a chiropractor and vertebral artery-related stroke (though not between visits to a chiropractor and carotid artery dissection). Three possible explanations emerged from these data with regard to the association between CMT and VADS:

1. CMT can cause VADS in certain susceptible individuals, and there is no way to predict, or screen for, the individual who was at risk of "post-manipulative stroke" [40-42].

2. Patients with early symptoms of VADS (neck pain and/or headache) seek care from a chiropractor or other practitioner of CMT and, subsequent to the visit, go on to experience a stroke, independent of the application of CMT [25]. If this explanation were true, explanation #1 would be reflective of protopathic bias.

3. CMT and VADS are simply unexplained epiphenomena.

These case-control studies were not able to substantiate any of these theories.

These studies were followed by a case-control study by Cassidy, et al. [43] These authors attempted to respond to the need for more rigorous research in this area by adding two elements that were not utilized in previous case-control studies. First, they used a standard case-control design but added a case-crossover design in which cases served as their own controls. Second, they attempted to, in effect, provide insight into which of the above three possible explanations for the association between CMT and VADS was most likely the correct one. They did this by including not only visits to chiropractors within 30 days of stroke but also visits to primary care physicians within the same time period.

This study involved 109,020,875 person-years of observation over a period of nine years. The cases were 818 patients with vertebral artery-related stroke and the controls were 3164 individuals without stroke. The case-crossover involved four random control periods amongst the individuals in the stroke group prior to their stroke.

As with the Rothwell, et al study, [37] they found an increased association between visits to a chiropractor within 30 days and vertebral artery-related stroke (OR 1.37; 95% CI 1.04–1.91 from the case crossover analysis) in individuals under 45 years of age, but no association in individuals 45 years of age or older. However, they also found an association between visits to primary care physicians and vertebral artery-related stroke. This association was found both in patients under 45 (OR 1.34; 95% CI 0.94–1.87 from the case crossover analysis) and in those 45 and older (OR 1.52; 95% CI 1.36–1.67 from the case crossover analysis).

Another difference between this study and previous case-control studies is that Cassidy, et al compared the association of visits to chiropractors and primary care physicians for complaints related to neck pain or headache with those without neck pain or headache. They found substantially greater associations between visits to both practitioners and vertebral artery-related stroke when the visits involved neck pain or headache.

It is commonly assumed that if VADS occurs immediately or soon after CMT a clear causal relation is established [44, 45]. Cassidy, et al [43] examined this assumption as well and found that the odds of stroke occurring within 24 hours of a visit to a primary care physician was virtually the same as stroke occurring within 24 hours of a visit to a chiropractor [43].

Cassidy, et al [43] pointed out the limitation of their use of administrative data and investigated this by performing a sensitivity analysis using various positive predictive values for stroke diagnosis. They found that this did not change the study's conclusions.

Since the publication of the Cassidy, et al [43] study, two additional case-control studies on this topic have been published. The first was that of Engelter, et al [46]. They compared 966 patients who had experienced stroke related to cervical artery dissection with 651 patients who had experienced ischemic stroke unrelated to cervical artery dissection as well as with 280 healthy controls. They assessed the relationship between stroke and a number of different potential mechanical triggers, including CMT, over the prior 30 days. They found an increased association between CMT and stroke related to cervical artery dissection as compared to the other two groups. However, because there were no other comparisons, such as visits to primary care practitioners, this study did not add anything to the discussion of cause and effect (i.e., distinguishing between the three possible explanations presented above), as did the Cassidy, et al study [43].

The second study was by Kosloff, et al. [47] This study attempted to replicate the Cassidy, et al [43] study in assessing the association between visits to chiropractors and visit to primary care physicians in patients with vertebral artery-related stroke and healthy controls. They compared 1,829 patients with vertebral artery-related stroke with 4,633 age and gender matched controls. The data were obtained from two administrative databases, one from a commercial program and the other from a government program. They found no increased association between vertebral artery- related stroke and visits to chiropractors. They did find an increased association between patients with vertebral artery-related stroke and visits to primary care physicians.

Importantly, Kosloff, et al [47] also found that, among those patients who experienced vertebral artery-related stroke after seeing a chiropractor, in one-third of visits in the commercial population and half of visits in the government population *no CMT was applied at the time of these visits*. This means that, aside from the lack of increased statistical association between vertebral artery-related stroke and visits to chiropractors, even in those patients with stroke who had seen a chiropractor, only 1/2 to 2/3 had even received CMT.
In addition to these more recent case control studies, further biomechanical [48-52] and vascular [53-56] studies have been performed regarding the effects of CMT on the vertebral arteries. Taken collectively, these studies show that:

1. The mechanical strains on the vertebral artery during CMT are less than during normal range of motion movements and well below those required for mechanical failure of the artery and;

2. CMT does not have any deleterious effect on the flow of blood within the vertebrobasilar system.

Particularly interesting was the study by Wynd, et al [52]. In a canine model they used angioplasty to induce a lesion in the vertebral artery prior to the implementation of CMT. They found that, even in an already-compromised vertebral artery, no further damage to the artery occurred after CMT.

Therefore, based upon the current best evidence, the most plausible explanation for the statistical association between CMT and VADS is #2 discussed earlier. That is, individuals who are experiencing a vertebral artery dissection seek care from a chiropractic physician or other manual practitioner for relief of the neck pain and headache *that results from* the dissection. Sometime after the visit, the dissection proceeds along its natural course to produce arterial blockage, leading to stroke. This natural progression from dissection to stroke occurs independent of the application of CMT.

Do primary spine practitioners not have to worry about VADS?

The concern for the primary spine practitioner (PSP) has shifted. Previously the focus had been on trying to "screen" for a patient who is "at risk" of a rare "complication to CMT" [57-60]. However, multiple publications have pointed to the lack of reliability of screening in the clinic for risk of an episode of VADS that has not yet occurred [42, 58, 61, 62]. Also, as discussed here, current evidence indicates that VADS is not a "complication to CMT" *per se*. Therefore, issue for PSPs now is one of differential diagnosis. The responsibility of the practitioner is not to attempt to identify the patient who is at risk of "post-manipulative stroke", but to attempt to identify the patient who is having a dissection in progress so appropriate referral can be made.

Certainly, in many cases (perhaps most) there are no clear signs or symptoms that can serve to alert the PSP to the possibility of VADS. In addition, some of the early symptoms of VADS such as dizziness, vertigo, imbalance, nausea and tinnitus are common in patients without VADS who present to practitioners who use manipulation and other forms of manual therapy (as well as PCPs). However there likely are those cases in which history and examination may be useful in identifying the patient with true VADS.

See Chapter 1 for specifics on the diagnosis of cervical artery dissection.

Vertebral Artery Dissection and Stroke: The Public Health Message

Public health campaigns have been effectively used for decades to provide important health information to individuals on a wide scale [63-65]. Up to the present, most public discourse regarding the relationship between the chiropractic profession and VADS has revolved around, on the one side, publications [8] and advertising campaigns [66] regarding cervical manipulation being a "risky" treatment with the potential to cause stroke and, on the other side, the chiropractic profession defending the safety of this treatment [67]. However the chiropractic profession now has an opportunity to utilize all that is currently known about VADS to change the discussion from one of defensiveness to one of public health. That is, to engage in a public health campaign to educate the public about the warning signs and symptoms of this uncommon but potentially devastating disorder. While public education materials regarding stroke in general are widely available, these almost invariably focus on ischemic stroke secondary to arteriosclerosis or hemorrhagic stroke secondary to aneurism or arteriovenous malformation. They do not provide information regarding VADS. Thus, there is no widely available source of information for the public regarding this rare but potentially devastating disorder. Because the chiropractic profession has found itself linked to VADS and because of the paucity of information available to the lay person regarding VADS, it would appear to be beneficial to the profession and, more importantly, the pubic, for Chiropractic Medicine to take the lead on a public education campaign on this topic. A public education campaign specific to VADS would be beneficial on several levels:

- It would be of benefit to the public as it would provide information regarding a potentially serious disorder that can initially be mistaken for a common, benign condition. Such information is not readily available from other sources, even leading stroke societies.

- The chiropractic profession has historically taken a defensive approach to the issue of cervical manipulation and stroke. This is certainly understandable given the history of attacks on the profession in this area. However the current understanding of this issue allows the profession to move away from defensiveness toward a positive, proactive, patient-oriented approach. A public health campaign would allow the profession to do this.

- The chiropractic profession does not have a solid history of involvement in public health [68]. This is evidenced by the relatively small number of members of the Chiropractic Health Section of the American Public Health Association. Because the issue of cervical manipulation and stroke has caused such concern amongst chiropractic physicians over the years, taking a public health approach to this topic may provide the impetus for members of the chiropractic profession to recognize the importance of involvement in public health efforts in general.

There are a number of important points that can be included in a public health campaign regarding VADS:

- VADS is a rare but potentially serious disorder.

- Some of the initial symptoms of this disorder can mimic more common and relatively benign neck and headache problems.

- Because of this, diagnosis can be difficult, so some individuals and their health care providers are not aware that they are experiencing VADS.

- However there often can be subtle signs and symptoms that may alert a health provider to the possibility of the presence of VADS

- If you experience any of these signs and symptoms inform your health care provider immediately or call your local emergency service.

References

1. Thornton FV. Malpractice: death resulting from chiropractic treatment of headache (medicolegal abstract). JAMA. 1934;103:1260.

2. Lee KP, Carlini WG, McCormick GF, Albers GW. Neurologic complications following chiropractic manipulation: a survey of California neurologists. Neurology. 1995 Jun;45(6):1213-5. PubMed PMID: 7783892. eng.

3. Norris JW, Beletsky V, Nadareishvili ZG. Sudden neck movement and cervical artery dissection. CMAJ. 2000;163(1):38-40.

4. Dabbs V, Lauretti WJ. A risk assessment of cervical manipulation vs NSAIDs for the treatment of neck pain. J Manipulative Physiol Ther. 1995;18(8):530-6.

5. Haneline MT, Lewkovich G. Ongoing stroke dialogue: A response to the Smith, et al study on the association of spinal manipulation and vertebral artery dissection. JACA. 2003;40(10):24-7.

6. Haneline MT, Lewkovich G. Critique of the Canadian Stroke Consortium's spontaneous vs. traumatic arterial dissection. JACA. 2004;41(5):18-22.

7. Refshauge KM, Parry S, Shirley D, Larsen D, Rivett DA, Boland R. Professional responsibility in relation to cervical spine manipulation. Aust J Physiother. 2002;48(171-179).

8. Ernst E. Spinal manipulation: are the benefits worth the risks? Expert Rev Neurother. 2007 Nov;7(11):1451-2. PubMed PMID: 17997693. eng.

9. Schievink WI. Spontaneous dissection of the cartoid and vertebral arteries. N Engl J Med. 2001;344(12):898-906.

10. Horn SW, 2nd. The "Locked-In" syndrome following chiropractic manipulation of the cervical spine. Ann Emerg Med. 1983 Oct;12(10):648-50. PubMed PMID: 6625270. eng.

11. Schwarz GA, Geiger JK, Spano AV. Posterior inferior cerebellar artery syndrome of Wallenberg after chiropractic manipulation. AMA Arch Intern Med. 1956 Mar;97(3):352-4. PubMed PMID: 13291914. eng.

12. Schellhas KP, Latchaw RE, Wendling LR, Gold LH. Vertebrobasilar injuries following cervical manipulation. JAMA. 1980 Sep 26;244(13):1450-3. PubMed PMID: 7420633. eng.

13. Nadgir RN, Loevner LA, Ahmed T, Moonis G, Chalela J, Slawek K, et al. Simultaneous bilateral internal carotid and vertebral artery dissection following chiropractic manipulation: case report and review of the literature. Neuroradiology. 2003 May;45(5):311-4. PubMed PMID: 12692699. eng.

14. Quintana JG, Drew EC, Richtsmeier TE, Davis LE. Vertebral artery dissection and stroke following neck manipulation by native american healer. Neurology. 2002;58:1434-5.

15. Sedat J, Dib M, Mahagne MH, Lonjon M, Paquis P. Stroke after chiropractic manipulation as a result of extracranial postero-inferior cerebellar artery dissection. J Manipulative Physiol Ther. 2002;25(9):588-90.

16. Tinel D, Bliznakova E, Juhel C, Gallien P, Brissot R. Vertebrobasilar ischemia after cervical spine manipulation: a case report. Ann Readapt Med Phys. 2008 Jun;51(5):403-14. PubMed PMID: 18586346. eng fre.

17. Green D, Joynt RJ. Vascular accidents to the brain stem associated with neck manipulation. J Am Med Assoc. 1959 May 30;170(5):522-4. PubMed PMID: 13653990. eng.

18. Smith RA, Estridge MN. Neurologic complications of head and neck manipulations. JAMA. 1962 Nov 3;182:528-31. PubMed PMID: 13989552. eng.

19. Miller RG, Burton R. Stroke following chiropractic manipulation of the spine. JAMA. 1974 Jul 8;229(2):189-90.

20. Easton JD, Sherman DG. Cervical manipulation and stroke. Stroke. 1977 Sep-Oct;8(5):594-7. PubMed PMID: 906059. eng.

21. Sherman DG, Hart RG, Easton JD. Abrupt change in head position and cerebral infarction. Stroke. 1981 Jan-Feb;12(1):2-6. PubMed PMID: 7222154. eng.

22. Mas JL, Henin D, Bousser MG, Chain F, Hauw JJ. Dissecting aneurysm of the vertebral artery and cervical manipulation: a case report with autopsy. Neurology. 1989 Apr;39(4):512-5. PubMed PMID: 2927675. eng.

23. Terrett AGJ. Misuse of the literature by medical authors in discussing spinal manipulative therapy injury. J Manipulative Physiol Ther. 1995; 18(4):203-10.

24. Wynd S, Westaway M, Vohra S, Kawchuk G. The quality of reports on cervical arterial dissection following cervical spinal manipulation. PLoS One. 2013;8(3):e59170. PubMed PMID: 23527121. Pubmed Central PMCID: 3604043.

25. Haldeman S, Kohlbeck FJ, McGregor M. Risk factors and precipitating neck movements causing vertebrobasilar artery dissection after cervical trauma and spinal manipulation. Spine (Phila Pa 1976). 1999 Apr 15;24(8):785-94. PubMed PMID: 10222530. eng.

26. Dvorak J, Orelli FV. How dangerous is manipulation to the cervical spine? Case report and results of a survey. Man Med. 1985;2:1-4.

27. Klougart N, Leboeuf-Yde C, Rasmussen LR. Safety in chiropractic practice. Part II: Treatment to the upper neck and the rate of cerebrovascular incidents. J Manipulative Physiol Ther. 1996 Nov-Dec;19(9):563-9. PubMed PMID: 8976474. eng.

28. Symons BP, Leonard T, Herzog W. Internal forces sustained by the vertebral artery during spinal manipulative therapy. J Manipulative Physiol Ther. 2002 Oct;25(8):504-10. PubMed PMID: 12381972. eng.

29. Haldeman S, Carey P, Townsend M, Papadopoulos C. Clinical perceptions of the risk of vertebral artery dissection after cervical manipulation: the effect of referral bias. Spine J. 2002 Sep-Oct;2(5):334-42. PubMed PMID: 14589464. eng.

30. Haldeman S, Kohlbeck FJ, McGregor M. Unpredictability of cerebrovascular ischemia associated with cervical spine manipulation therapy: a review of sixty-four cases after cervical spine manipulation. Spine (Phila Pa 1976). 2002 Jan 1;27(1):49-55. PubMed PMID: 11805635. eng.

31. Carey TS, Boden SD. A critical guide to case series reports. Spine (Phila Pa 1976). 2003;28(15):1631-4.

32. Gordis L. Epidemiology. 2nd ed. Philadelphia: W.B. Saunders; 2000.

33. Hebel JR, McCarter RJ. Study Guide to Epidemiology and Biostatistics. 6th ed. Sudbury, MA: Jones and Bartlett; 2006.

34. Hiebert R, Nordin M. Methodological aspects of outcomes research. Eur Spine J. 2006;15:S4-S16.

35. Maclure M. The case-crossover design: a method for studying transient effects on the risk of acute events. Am J Epidemiol. 1991 Jan 15;133(2):144-53. PubMed PMID: 1985444. eng.

36. Horwitz RI, Feinstein AR. The problem of "protopathic bias" in case-control studies. Am J Med. 1980 Feb;68(2):255-8. PubMed PMID: 7355896.

37. Rothwell DM, Bondy SJ, Williams JI. Chiropractic manipulation and stroke: a population-based case-control study. Stroke. 2001 May;32(5):1054-60. PubMed PMID: 11340209. eng.

38. Smith WS, Johnston SC, Skalabrin EJ, Weaver M, Azari P, Albers GW, et al. Spinal manipulative therapy is an independent risk factor for vertebral artery dissection. Neurology. 2003 May 13;60(9):1424-8. PubMed PMID: 12743225. eng.

39. Dittrich R, Rohsbach D, Heidbreder A, Heuschmann P, Nassenstein I, Bachmann R, et al. Mild mechanical traumas are possible risk factors for cervical artery dissection. Cerebrovasc Dis. 2007;23(4):275-81. PubMed PMID: 17192705. eng.

40. Williams LS, Biller J. Vertebrobasilar dissection and cervical spine manipulation A complex pain in the neck. Neurology. 2003;60:1408-9.

41. Rubinstein SM, Haldeman S, van Tulder MW. An etiologic model to help explain the pathogenesis of cervical artery dissection: implications for cervical manipulation. J Manipulative Physiol Ther. 2006 May;29(4):336-8. PubMed PMID: 16690389.

42. Thiel H, Rix G. Is it time to stop functional pre-manipulation testing of the cervical spine? Man Ther. 2005;10:154-8.

43. Cassidy JD, Boyle E, Cote P, He Y, Hogg-Johnson S, Silver FL, et al. Risk of vertebrobasilar stroke and chiropractic care: results of a population-based case-control and case-crossover study. Spine (Phila Pa 1976). 2008 Feb 15;33(4 Suppl):S176-83. PubMed PMID: 18204390. eng.

44. Ernst E. Ophthalmological adverse effects of (chiropractic) upper spinal manipulation: evidence from case reports. Acta Ophthalmol Scand. 2005;83:581-5.

45. Ernst E. Adverse effects of spinal manipulation: a systematic review. J R Soc Med. 2007 Jul;100(7):330-8. PubMed PMID: 17606755. eng.

46. Engelter ST, Grond-Ginsbach C, Metso TM, Metso AJ, Kloss M, Debette S, et al. Cervical artery dissection: trauma and other potential mechanical trigger events. Neurology. 2013 May 21;80(21):1950-7. PubMed PMID: 23635964.

47. Kosloff TM, Elton D, Tao J, Bannister WM. Chiropractic care and the risk of vertebrobasilar stroke: results of a case-control study in U.S. commercial and Medicare Advantage populations. Chiropr Man Therap. 2015;23:19. PubMed PMID: 26085925. Pubmed Central PMCID: 4470078.

48. Herzog W, Leonard TR, Symons B, Tang C, Wuest S. Vertebral artery strains during high-speed, low amplitude cervical spinal manipulation. J Electromyogr Kinesiol. 2012 Oct;22(5):740-6. PubMed PMID: 22483611.

49. Wuest S, Symons B, Leonard T, Herzog W. Preliminary report: biomechanics of vertebral artery segments C1-C6 during cervical spinal manipulation. J Manipulative Physiol Ther. 2010 May;33(4):273-8. PubMed PMID: 20534313. eng.

50. Kawchuk G, Wynd S, Anderson T. Defining the effect of cervical manipulation on vertebral artery integrity: establishment of an animal model. J Manipulative Physiol Ther. 2004;27(9):539-46.

51. Kawchuk GN, Jhangri GS, Hurwitz EL, Wynd S, Haldeman S, Hill MD. The relation between the spatial distribution of vertebral artery compromise and exposure to cervical manipulation. J Neurol. 2008 Mar;255(3):371-7. PubMed PMID: 18185906. eng.

52. Wynd S, Anderson T, Kawchuk G. Effect of cervical spine manipulation on a pre-existing vascular lesion within the canine vertebral artery. Cerebrovasc Dis. 2008;26(3):304-9. PubMed PMID: 18667811. eng.

53. Erhardt JW, Windsor BA, Kerry R, Hoekstra C, Powell DW, Porter-Hoke A, et al. The immediate effect of atlanto-axial high velocity thrust techniques on blood flow in the vertebral artery: A randomized controlled trial. Man Ther. 2015 Aug;20(4):614-22. PubMed PMID: 25814193.

54. Quesnele JJ, Triano JJ, Noseworthy MD, Wells GD. Changes in vertebral artery blood flow following various head positions and cervical spine manipulation. J Manipulative Physiol Ther. 2014 Jan;37(1):22-31. PubMed PMID: 24239451.

55. Thomas LC, McLeod LR, Osmotherly PG, Rivett DA. The effect of end-range cervical rotation on vertebral and internal carotid arterial blood flow and cerebral inflow: A sub analysis of an MRI study. Man Ther. 2015 Jun;20(3):475-80. PubMed PMID: 25529191.

56. Thomas LC, Rivett DA, Bateman G, Stanwell P, Levi CR. Effect of selected manual therapy interventions for mechanical neck pain on vertebral and internal carotid arterial blood flow and cerebral inflow. Phys Ther. 2013 Nov;93(11):1563-74. PubMed PMID: 23813088. eng.

57. George PE, Silverstein HT, Wallace H, Marshall M. Identification of the high risk stroke patient. JACA. 1981;15(S-26):65-6.

58. Ivancii JJ, Bryce, D., Bolton PS. Use of provocational tests by clinician to predict vulnerability of patients to vertebrobasilar insufficiency. Chiro J Aust. 1993; 23(2):59-63.

59. Childs JD, Flynn TW, Fritz JM, Piva SR, Whitman JM, Wainner RS, Greenman PE. Screening for vertebrobasilar insufficiency in patients with neck pain: manual therapy decision-making in the presence of uncertainty. J Orthop Sports Phys Ther. 2005;35:300-6.

60. Barker S, Kesson M, Ashmore J, Turner G, Conway J, Stevens D. Guidance for pre-manipulative testing of the cervical spine. Man Ther. 2000;5(1):37-40.

61. Rivett DA, Milburn PD, Chapple C. Negative pre manipulative vertebral artery testing despite complete occlusion a case of false negativity? Man Ther. 1998;3(2):102-7.

62. Cote P, Kreitz BG, Cassidy JD, Thiel H. The validity of the extension-rotation test as a clinical screening procedure before neck manipulation: a secondary analysis. J Manipulative Physiol Ther. 1996 Mar-Apr;19(3):159-64. PubMed PMID: 8728458. eng.

63. Public health campaign: getting the message across: World Health Organization; 2009.

64. Burns EK, Levinson AH. Reaching Spanish-speaking smokers: state-level evidence of untapped potential for QuitLine utilization. Am J Public Health. 2010 Apr 1;100 Suppl 1:S165-710. PubMed PMID: 20147692. eng.

65. Buchbinder R, Jolley D, Wyatt M. Population based intervention to change back pain beliefs and disability: three part evaluation. BMJ. 2001 Jun 23;322(7301):1516-20. PubMed PMID: 11420272. eng.

66. Devitt M. Anti-Chiropractic campaign continues in Connecticut. Dynam Chiropr. 2006;24(13):1-2.

67. Feather K. Defending chiropractic in Connecticut. Dynam Chiropr. 2008;26(1):1-2.

68. Murphy DR, Schneider MJ, Seaman DR, Perle SM, Nelson CF. How can chiropractic become a respected mainstream profession? The example of podiatry. Chiropr Osteop. 2008;16:10.

•Chapter 7•

Treatment Approaches for Diagnostic Question #3

Introduction

Diagnostic question #3 in Clinical Reasoning in Spine Pain® (the CRISP® protocols) asks, "What has happened with this person as a whole that would cause the pain experience to develop and persist?" Another way of asking this question is, "what factors are present that are perpetuating the ongoing pain, disability and suffering experience or are causing recurrent episodes?" This question is most pertinent to the patient in the subacute or chronic stage, i.e., the patient who has not recovered from an acute episode. It is also important in the patient who has chronic, recurrent episodes of pain.

In the acute patient, potential perpetuating factors are often important from the standpoint of prevention, i.e., limiting the likelihood of the development of chronic pain. However, it is in the patient who has already transitioned to the subacute or chronic stage that the factors detected by diagnostic question #3 become a key part of the diagnostic and management strategy.

The perpetuating factors considered under diagnostic question #3 are:

Dynamic and passive instability
Oculomotor dysfunction
Nociceptive system sensitization
Psychological factors

It will be noted that in the section on the management of psychological factors, it is stressed that all communications should be carried out in a "CBT/ACT context". "CBT" stands for Cognitive-Behavioral Therapy" and ACT "Acceptance and Commitment Therapy."

In Volume I of this series that Cognitive-Behavioral Therapy was abbreviated "Cog-B". However, in this volume the more standard "CBT" abbreviation is used.

Dynamic and passive instability

Dynamic instability is believed to occur as a result of dysfunction in the motor control system in which the normal neuromuscular reactions to common perturbations to the spine do not function at optimum efficiency. It is critical to note that dynamic instability is induced by acute nociception and sustained by chronic nociception (see Nijs, et al in the Recommended Reading list). Thus, reducing nociception, through effectively addressing the factors related to diagnostic question #2 in the CRISP® protocols, is the essential first step in the treatment of dynamic instability. In fact, in many patients, the motor control dysfunction that leads to dynamic stability will normalize simply by effectively treating the primary pain generator. In these cases, extensive stabilization exercise is not necessary. However, in patients whose dynamic instability does not fully resolve despite effective management of the factors related to diagnostic question #2, cervical stabilization exercise is the management decision of choice.

Passive instability is far less common and results from failure of the passive holding elements of the spine. Patients with passive instability should generally be started on cervical stabilization exercise from the start. The notable exception is the small minority of patients whose passive instability is of sufficient magnitude to cause neurologic compromise (see Chapters 2 and 4). These patients should be referred for surgical consult.

Cervical stabilization exercise

The purpose of cervical stabilization exercise is to train the motor control system to more efficiently provide protective muscular responses to common perturbations that have the potential to cause irritation or injury to the cervical spine. The exercise approach presented here is designed to translate easily to a home exercise program. This maximizes efficiency and places the patient in charge of the process, which promotes self-efficacy and functional independence. Typically, an attempt should be made to have the patient perform two sets of 10-20 repetitions of each exercise twice per day in the beginning. Once adequate cervical stability is achieved, reduction to once per day is appropriate.

As discussed in Chapter 4 it appears that in patients who develop dynamic instability in the cervical spine the deep cervical flexors and lower cervical and upper thoracic extensors consistently become inhibited (see Falla, et al and Schomacher, et al in the Recommended Reading list). Therefore, cervical stabilization training starts with a co-contraction of these muscles.

Effective co-contraction may be aided by the patient establishing the resting tongue position.

Resting Tongue Position

The patient can establish normal resting position by placing the tongue in position to make a "cluck" sound. The position that the tongue takes against the hard palate just behind the upper incisors prior to making this sound is the normal resting position. Firm pressure of the tongue against the hard palate in this position can help facilitate co-contraction of the deep cervical flexors and lower cervical and upper thoracic extensors.

The Cervical Posture Exercise

This is a simple postural exercise for both co-contracting the deep cervical flexors and lower cervical and upper thoracic extensors as well as for training ideal craniocervical position (see Beer, et al in Recommended Reading list). The patient is sitting in an upright position with a natural lordosis. It is helpful to have the knees apart and the feet turned outward. The patient is asked to lift the base of the skull from the top of the neck as if to lengthen the cervical spine (Fig. 7-1a and b). Another command that is often useful is to have the patient imagine that there is a helium-filled balloon attached by a string to the posterior aspect of the top of the head. Once the patient has this image in mind, the patient is told to allow the head and neck to follow the pull of the helium-filled balloon.

Once this position is established the patient is asked to relax the shoulders. The patient holds this position for 10 seconds. The exercise should be repeated at least once per hour or close to this as possible.

Cervical Brace

The cervical brace further facilitates co-contraction of the deep cervical flexors and lower cervical and upper thoracic extensors by using the weight of the head.

The patient is in the quadruped position with the eyes looking straight at the floor. The patient is asked to protract the head by moving the chin straight toward the floor (Fig. 7-2). Then, in a smooth, scooping motion the patient is asked to flex the upper cervical spine (Fig. 7-3) and return the head the neutral position, with the upper cervical spine slightly flexed (Fig. 7-4). It is critically important that the maneuver is carried out in one fluid movement rather than in steps. A useful image is to have the patient imagine a small bucket of water on the floor just below his or her face and a scoop attached to the patient's chin. In carrying out the cervical brace the patient attempts to scoop water out of the bucket.

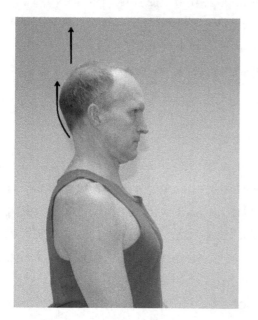 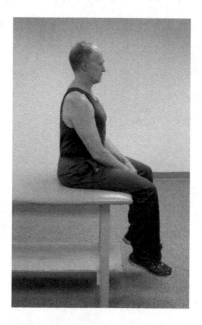

Figure 7-1a and b. The Cervical Posture Exercise.

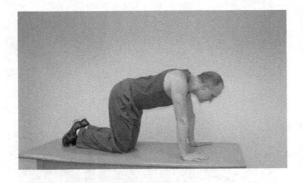

Figure 7-2. Protraction of the head at the start of the cervical brace exercise.

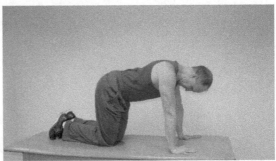

Figure 7-3. Flexion of the upper cervical spine during the cervical brace exercise.

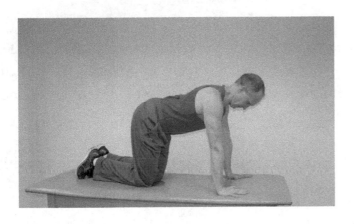

Figure 7-4. The cervical brace position. Note that the upper cervical spine is slightly flexed and the lower cervical spine is relatively neutral.

If the patient performs the movement correctly he or she should feel a slight tension just behind the throat and in the lower cervical and upper thoracic spine. If the patient does not feel this, the maneuver should be repeated with the proper form.

It is important for the practitioner to watch for incorrect form with the cervical brace. The most common mistakes are excessive flexion of the cervical spine (Fig. 7-5) or losing the upper cervical flexed position (Fig. 7-6).

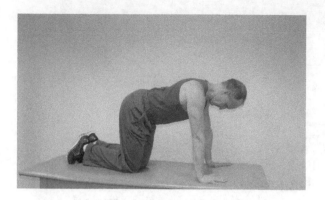

Figure 7-5. Incorrect form with the cervical brace: excessive flexion.

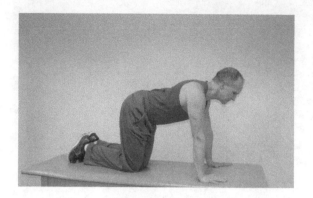

Figure 7-6. Incorrect form with the cervical brace: losing the upper cervical flexion.

It is also important for the practitioner to monitor scapular and lumbar positioning. The scapulae should be stable with no winging of the medial border or inferior angle. The lumbar spine should be positioned in a neutral lumbar lordosis. Good stability of these body parts should be maintained while establishing and maintaining the cervical brace.

In patients with passive instability it may be necessary to reduce the amplitude of the initial head protrusion.

Progression along the quadruped track

The patient can then be given a progression of exercises that challenge the motor control system by introducing load as well as driving the co-contraction to become unconscious and automatic through increasingly complex extremity movements. Typically, each exercise is performed for 10-20 repetitions with each extremity.

Quadruped single arm raise: The patient is in the quadruped position and establishes the resting tongue position and the cervical brace. While maintaining the cervical brace as well as scapular and lumbar position the patient raises one arm overhead without losing stability (Fig. 7-7). This arm is then lowered and the other is raised in the same manner.

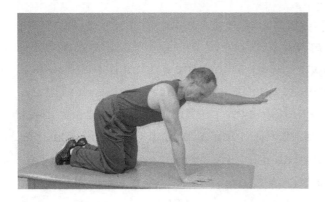

Figure 7-7. Quadruped single arm raise.

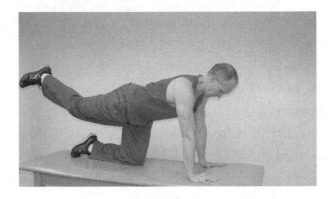

Figure 7-8. Quadruped single leg raise.

Quadruped single leg raise: The patient is in the quadruped position and establishes the resting tongue position and the cervical brace. While maintaining the cervical brace as well as scapular and lumbar position the patient raises one leg without losing stability (Fig. 8). This leg is then lowered and the other is raised in the same manner.

Quadruped single arm and leg raise: The patient is in the quadruped position and establishes the resting tongue position and the cervical brace. While maintaining the cervical brace as well as scapular and lumbar position the patient raises one arm and the opposite leg without losing stability (Fig. 7-9). This arm and leg is then lowered and the other arm and leg are raised in the same manner.

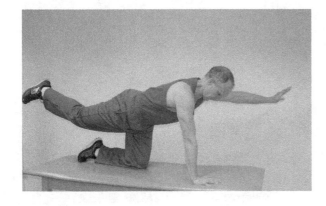

Figure 7-9. Quadruped single arm and leg raise.

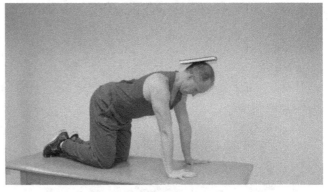

Figure 7-10. Balancing a book while holding the cervical brace.

Quadruped book balance: The patient is in the quadruped position and establishes the resting tongue position and the cervical brace. A small hardcover book (1-2 kilograms/ 2-4 pounds is ideal) is placed on the back of the patient's head so that the patient has to balance the book (Fig. 7-10). As with the previous exercises, the patient maintains the cervical brace as well as scapular and lumbar position. The patient holds the position until he or she loses stability and/or the book falls, or up to 30 seconds. At the point at which the patient is able to hold the position with good stability and without shaking for 30 seconds, the patient can then be progressed along the extremity movement track as described above, all while maintaining balance of the book.

Cervical strengthening exercises

There are a variety of exercises that can be performed that are designed to promote strength in the cervical muscles. Presented here is a simple approach that is easily performed at home and is applicable to the majority of patients with cervical disorders (CDs). It utilizes a rubber ball that can be purchased in any sporting goods store.

The exercises are performed in flexion, extension and lateral flexion to both sides. Each exercise is performed for 10-20 repetitions.

Flexion: The ball is placed on the wall and the patient places the forehead on the ball. The feet should be placed slightly farther away from the wall than the ball, so the patient is leaning slightly into the ball (Fig. 7-11). The patient applies pressure straight into the ball and, while maintaining this pressure, flexes the head in a nodding fashion (Fig. 7-12). The patient then returns to the starting position.

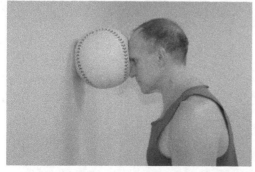

Figure 7-11. Starting position for cervical strengthening with a ball in flexion.

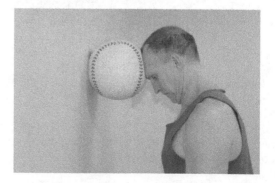

Figure 7-12. Flexion strengthening.

Extension: The ball is placed on the wall and the patient places the back of the head on the ball. The feet should be placed slightly farther away from the wall than the ball, so the patient is leaning slightly into the ball. The patient applies pressure straight into the ball and, while maintaining this pressure, extends the head (Fig. 7-13). The patient then returns to the starting position.

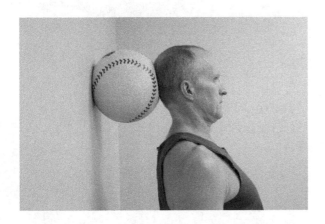

Figure 7-13. Starting position for extension strengthening.

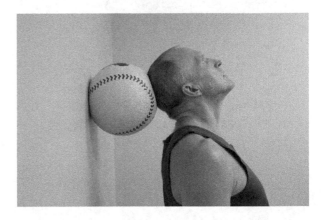

Figure 7-14. Extension strengthening.

Lateral flexion: The ball is placed on the wall and the patient places the side of the head on the ball (Fig. 7-15). The feet should be placed slightly farther away from the wall than the ball, so the patient is leaning slightly into the ball. The patient applies pressure straight into the ball and, while maintaining this pressure, laterally flexes the head (Fig. 7-16). The patient then returns to the starting position. This maneuver is repeated on the other side.

Some patients will have difficulty performing the lateral flexion movement. In these patients, an alternative is to perform the exercise statically rather than dynamically by applying pressure into the ball then maintaining the pressure for up to 30 seconds. To make this more challenging, the feet can be moved father from the wall.

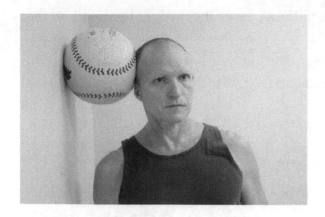

Figure 7-15. Starting position for lateral flexion strengthening.

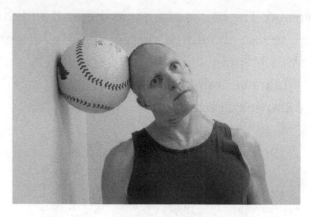

Figure 7-16. Lateral flexion strengthening.

Scapular stabilization exercise

As was discussed in Chapter 4, there is no consistent pattern of muscle dysfunction that occurs with scapular instability. Scapular stabilization exercise is designed to promote coordinated activity of the all the muscles involved in motor control of the scapula. These muscles include all three sections of the trapezius, the rhomboids, levator scapulae, pectoralis minor and serratus anterior.

The Brugger exercise

The purpose of this exercise is to train coordinated activity of the scapular muscles but it is also excellent for training proper lumbar and cervical posture. The patient should do it as a regular exercise in addition to using it as a "break" at work or home after sitting for a period of time.

The patient sits with his or her ischial tuberosities at the edge of a chair, with the pelvis positioned forward into an anterior tilt and the rest of the body upright (Fig. 7-17). The anterior tilt creates a natural lordosis in the lumbar spine and causes the cervical spine and head to automatically assume a neutral position. The patient should not be told to actively "tuck" the chin.

The patient is then instructed to open the fingers as wide as possible and externally rotate the arms as far as possible (Fig. 7-18). The patient should feel the middle and lower trapezii contracting, although at first the feeling of stretch in the arms and pectoral muscles may overpower the feeling of trapezius activation. The patient holds this position for up to 10 seconds. If the patient is unable to maintain the position for a full 10 seconds, a reduction in the holding time is appropriate, with gradual building to 10 second holds over time. The patient should progress up to 10 repetitions of the exercise, holding the position for 10 seconds on each repetition.

It is important when performing the Brugger exercise that the patient not try to pull the scapulae together, as this will decrease the effectiveness of the exercise. This is for two reasons. First, pulling the scapulae together will shorten the middle and lower trapezii and create active insufficiency of these muscles, in which the attachments of the muscles are so close together that full activation is compromised. Second, the purpose of providing this exercise is to promote coordinated activation of the scapular muscles, particularly the trapezii. By having the patient focus on opening the fingers and turning out the hands, rather than trying to activate the muscles consciously, the appropriate muscles will be indirectly, reflexively activated and a more natural recruitment of these muscles will occur.

Wall Angels

The patient places the buttocks, scapulae and back of the head against a wall, with the feet approximately two to three feet from the wall and slightly more than shoulder width apart.

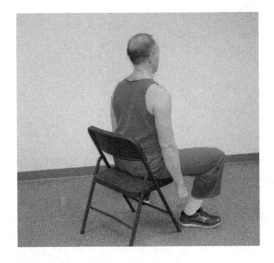
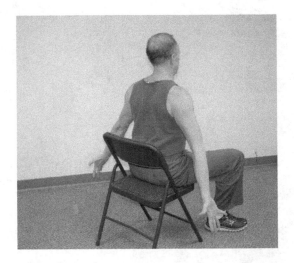

Figure 7-17. Starting position for the Brugger exercise.

Figure 7-18. The Brugger exercise.

The lumbar spine is positioned in lordosis. The upper extremities are placed against the wall with the shoulders and elbows abducted to 90 degrees. The hands are supinated and fingers open as wide as possible. The palms are facing each other (Fig. 7-19). The patient maintains pressure of the arms against the wall and slowly slides the arms downward (Fig. 7-20) then upward (Fig. 7-21).

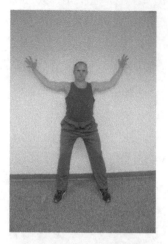

Figure 7-19. Starting position for wall angels.

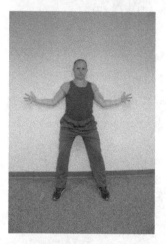

Figure 7-20. Downward movement of the arms while performing wall angels.

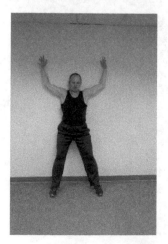

Figure 7-21. Upward movement of the arms while performing wall angels.

Push-up with a plus

This exercise is primarily designed to activate the serratus anterior. The patient is in the push-up position and performs a regular push-up but at the top adds a "plus" to the movement by pushing the shoulders into full protraction (Fig. 7-22). If the patient is not strong enough to perform this exercise in this manner, the exercise can be performed with the knees on the floor.

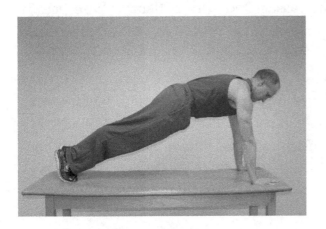

Figure 7-22. Push-up with a plus.

Readers who are interested in other scapular stabilization exercises, particularly in the context of rotator cuff training, are directed to:

https://www.shouldermadesimple.com/ [accessed 13 June 2016]

Presented here is a basic approach to cervical and scapular stabilization training that is applicable to the majority of patients with cervical disorders (CDs) and can easily be applied in a busy primary spine care environment. Some patients will require a more extensive and/or a more closely supervised exercise approach. With these patients, the primary spine practitioner (PSP) should consider referral for formal physical therapy or to a rehab facility that can provide such an approach. It is important in these cases for the PSP to follow up with the patient at regular intervals to monitor progress.

Some patients with passive instability will experience ongoing pain and activity intolerance despite intensive cervical stabilization training. In these cases, surgical consult should be considered.

See Chapter 12 of Volume I of this series for specifics regarding clinical decisions in patients who do not respond adequately to primary spine care.

Oculomotor dysfunction

Oculomotor dysfunction can occur in patients whose CD began after a traumatic event such as an automobile accident. It is particularly associated with patients whose pain is focused in the upper cervical spine. Oculomotor dysfunction is thought to result from disturbed afferent input from the cervical joint and muscle receptors (i.e., dysafferentation – see Chapter 2 in Volume I of this series). Therefore, as was discussed regarding cervical stabilization exercise, it is likely that many patients' oculomotor dysfunction will improve with effective treatment of the factors related to diagnostic question #2 in the CRISP® protocols. However, some patients will require exercises designed to restore normal oculomotor reflexes.

Phasic exercises

These exercises were developed by Fitz-Ritson (see the Recommended Reading list) for the purpose of training eye-head-neck-upper extremity coordination and eye-head-neck-trunk coordination. An elaborate progression was originally developed by Fitz-Ritson. Presented here is a streamlined version that is applicable to the majority of patients with CDs who have signs of oculomotor dysfunction.

Eye-head-neck-upper extremity exercise: The patient is standing. It is best to have an object in front upon which to fix the eyes. The patient abducts one arm with the thumb up and turns the eyes and head to look at that thumb (Fig. 7-23a). The patient then lowers the arm and returns the eyes to the starting point. The patient then abducts the opposite arm with the thumb up and turns to look at that thumb (Fig. 23b). This is followed by return to the starting position again. The movement is repeated for 20 repetitions. If, in the beginning, pain, dizziness or limited rotation range of motion do not allow full rotation, a shorter range of motion should be provided (Fig. 7-24). Also, if the patient is not able to perform a full 20 repetitions in the beginning, the patient should perform as many repetitions as is comfortable, and gradually build up to 20.

Figure 7-23a and b. Eye-head-neck-upper extremity phasic exercise. It is important that the patient stop and fix the gaze at a point directly in front between repetitions.

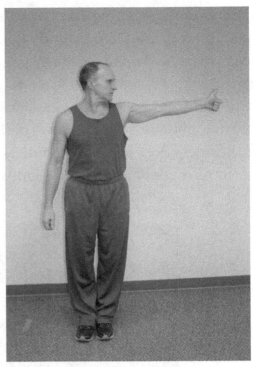

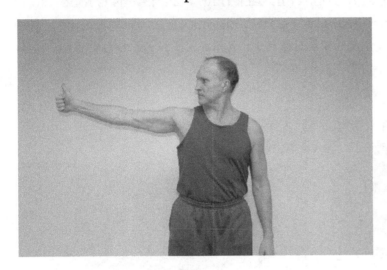

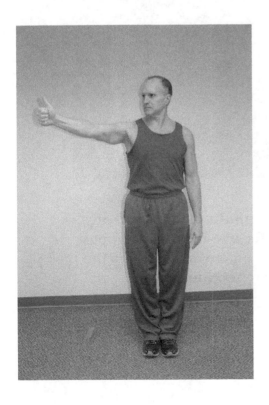

Figure 7-24. Reducing the range in a patient is not ready for full cervical rotation.

Eye-head-neck-trunk exercise: This exercise can only be performed if the patient has full rotation mobility of the head, neck and trunk. The patient is standing. It is best to have an object both in front and behind upon which to fix the eyes. The patient fixes the eyes on the object in front, then turns the eyes, head and trunk to the left and looks at the object in back (Fig. 7-25a). The patient returns to the starting position. The patient then turns the eyes, head and trunk to the right and looks at the object in back (Fig. 7-25b). This is followed by return to the starting position. This is repeated for 20 repetitions. If, in the beginning, pain or dizziness does not allow a full 20 repetitions, the patient should perform as many repetitions as is comfortable, and gradually build up to 20.

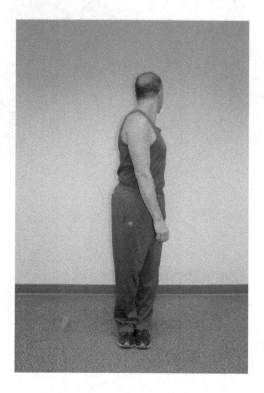 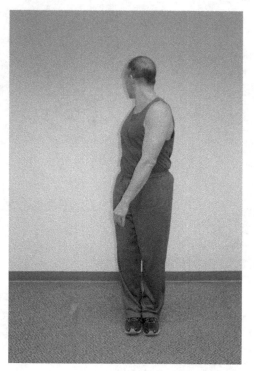

Figure 7-25a and b. Eye-head-neck-trunk phasic exercise rotating to the left (a) and the right (b). As with the eye-head-neck-upper extremity exercise, it is important that the patient stop and fix the gaze at a point directly in front between repetitions. .

Oculomotor reflex exercises

These exercises are designed to train oculomotor reflexes, specifically the vestibulo- and cervico-ocular reflex, smooth pursuit reflex (gaze stability) and saccade reflex. In the majority of patients the exercises can be patient-generated however, in some it might be necessary to start with practitioner-generated movements.

Vestibulo-ocular reflex (VOR) and cervico-ocular reflex (COR) (gaze stability): The patient can be seated or standing. The patient holds an object such as a pen at arm's length upon which he or she can fix the gaze. The patient rotates the head to the left while maintain eye fixation on the object (Fig. 7-26a). The patient returns to the starting position, and then rotates the head to the right, again maintain eye fixation on the object (Fig. 7-26b). This can be repeated for 20 repetitions. If in the beginning pain or dizziness does not allow a full 20 repetitions, the patient should perform as many repetitions as is comfortable, and gradually build up to 20.

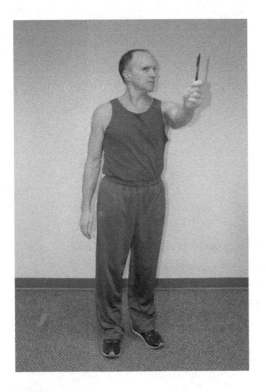 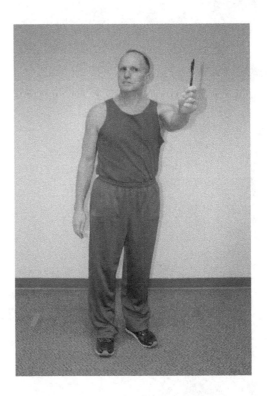

Figure 7-26a and b. Vestibulo-ocular and cervico-ocular reflex exercise

Smooth pursuit reflex (eye follow): The patient can be seated or standing. The patient holds an object such as a pen at arm's length upon which he or she can fix the gaze. The patient moves the object to the left while visually following the object (Fig. 7-27). The object should be moved as far to the left as the patient can follow. The patient should freely turn the head and eyes as in normal pursuit of an object moving across the visual field. The object is then moved back to neutral, with the patient visually following. The patient exchanges the object to the right hand (Fig. 7-28), and then moves it to the right in the same fashion (Fig. 7-29). After the patient learns to maintain stability while engaging in slow smooth pursuit movements, the speed can be increased by moving the object more quickly.

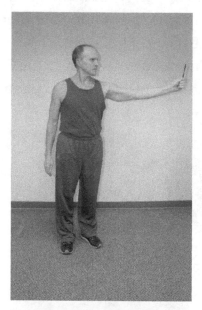

Figure 7-27. Smooth pursuit reflex exercise to the left.

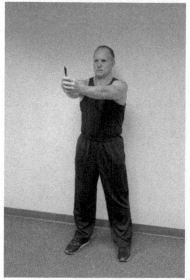

Figure 7-28. Switching the object that is being pursued from the left hand to the right hand in order to carry out movement to the right.

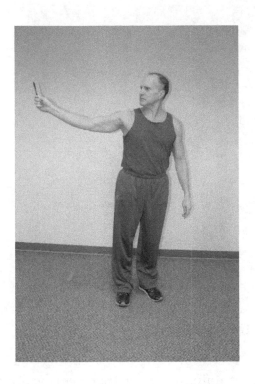

Figure 7-29. Smooth pursuit reflex exercise to the right.

Training smooth pursuit, with the inclusion of eye-head-neck-upper extremity coordination, can also be accomplished by having the patient throw a tennis ball into the air from one hand to the other, while following it with his or her eyes. As with the other smooth pursuit exercise, it is important that the head remain free to move along with the eyes.

Saccade reflex: The patient can be seated or standing. The patient holds an object such as a pen at arm's length upon which he or she can fix the gaze. The patient moves the object quickly in various directions while visually following the object, moving both the eyes and head in a natural fashion (Figs. 30 and 2319). These movements must be carried out quickly with the patient re-establishing eye fixation on the object as quickly as possible. This can be repeated for 20 repetitions. If in the beginning pain or dizziness does not allow a full 20 repetitions, the patient should perform as many repetitions as is comfortable, and gradually build up to 20.

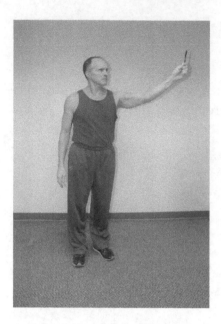 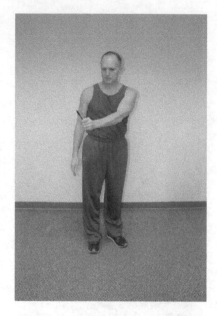

Figures 7-30 and 7-31. Training of the saccade reflex.

A convenient patient booklet has been created that contains most of these cervical and scapular stabilization, cervical strengthening and oculomotor exercises and many more. This booklet was created for the purpose of allowing the practitioner to provide the patient with take-home instructions and photographs of the exercises. The booklet is helpful for patient compliance and adherence to proper form. The booklets can be found at:

http://www.optp.com/ [accessed 13 June 2016]. Just search for the name "Murphy".

Nociceptive System Sensitization

The primary spine care management of nociceptive system sensitization (NSS) is covered in detail in Chapter 11 in Volume I of this series. The principles of management are the same for CD patients as with patients with low back disorders. So the reader is directed to that chapter for the application of education and graded exposure in patients with CDs in whom NSS is an important aspect of the diagnosis.

One important point that is critical for the spine practitioner is that, as was discussed above with regard to dynamic instability, the mechanism of NSS is initiated by acute nociception and sustained by chronic nociception (see Schneider, et al in the Recommended Reading list). Thus, as with cervical stabilization training, it is essential that the factors related to diagnostic question #2 in the CRISP® protocols are addressed prior to the institution of a detailed graded exposure process. In many patients in whom NSS is a prominent factor in diagnostic question #3, the NSS will substantially reduce or resolve with reduction or resolution of the primary pain generator. This will save both the practitioner and the patient a great deal of time and effort because the graded exposure process can be made far less demanding by dealing effectively with the source of nociception.

Psychological Factors

As with NSS, the primary management of the psychological perpetuating factors under diagnostic question #3 in the CRISP® protocols is largely the same in CD patients as in patients with low back disorders. In addition, as has been stated throughout this chapter, in many cases these factors will resolve with effective management of the pain generators related to diagnostic question #2 *as long as this management is provided in the CBT/ACT context, i.e., applying the principles of Cognitive Behavioral Therapy and Acceptance and Commitment Therapy, that is discussed throughout this book series*. Thus the reader is urged to be intimately familiar with the process of framing all management processes in a way that empowers the patient, improves self-efficacy and confers an accurate and realistic picture regarding what CDs *are* and what they *are not*. See Chapters 8, 9 and 11 in Volume I for specifics.

One psychological perpetuating factor that has particular relevance to the CD patient, and thus deserves detailed discussion here, is perceived injustice. Perceived injustice (also frequently referred to as "experience of injustice") is described in Chapter 2 of Volume I of this series as well as in Chapter 4 in this volume. Perceived injustice is frequently an important perpetuating factor in the patient with whiplash associated disorder, in which another driver has been determined, by the patient and/or the "system", as being "at fault".

Readers interested in learning more about perceived injustice and its impact on the pain, disability and suffering experience are directed to the work of Dr. Michael Sullivan which can be found at:

http://sullivan-painresearch.mcgill.ca/publications.php [accessed 23 April 2016]

The essence of perceived injustice is that the patient feels that his or her basic human rights have been unfairly violated, irreparable loss has occurred, people do not understand how severe the suffering is and, importantly, that this injustice is *someone else's fault*. Perceived injustice can cripple the patient's ability to recover, primarily because it creates a conflicting incentive for the patient (an example of the "ambivalence" that is addressed by Motivational Interviewing – see Chapter 9 of Volume I in this series). On the one hand, the patient wants to recover and get his or her life back. On the other hand, from a psychological perspective, the patient's suffering, and its related disability, is perceived to be *the only "power" the patient has over the other person who "did this to me"*.

This seems extremely illogical (and it is!) but the reader need only to think about the numerous times he or she has engaged in perceived injustice to realize that it is a universal human experience. This is one of the reasons that Volume I of this series emphasizes strongly the importance of the spine practitioner looking within, and being mindful during situations in which he or she engages in any of the various psychological perpetuating factors that are discussed throughout this book series. Doing this places the spine practitioner in the best position to truly understand and empathize with the patient, without judgement, and to be most helpful in guiding the patient toward recovery.

In the primary management of patients with CDs, helping the patient overcome perceived injustice and the impact it has on recovery involves two critically important things: validation and acceptance.

Validation means acknowledging and legitimizing the patient's *emotional experience*. This must be distinguished from validation of the *specific actions* that the patient perceives to be the cause of the suffering. In other words, communicating messages such as "boy, it seems like you have been through a lot with this whole ordeal" or "it is clear to me that you feel violated in this situation" communicate validation of the patient's *emotional experience*. Statements such as these will lead the patient in the direction of acceptance.

However, statements such as "yeah, that insurance company has really treated you unfairly", "that other driver should have been paying more attention or they wouldn't have hit you" and "those other doctors you saw obviously didn't believe you, nor did they care about helping you get better" are examples of validating *specific actions*. Statements like these can reinforce the patient's sense of perceived injustice, leading them further away from acceptance and further down the path of chronic pain, disability and suffering.

Thus, communicating validation of the emotional experience, but not the specific actions others have taken, is the most effective way to guide the patient toward *acceptance*.

Acceptance means being willing to place oneself in the present moment and to accept the situation as it is, without judgement. Further, acceptance entails the willingness to engage in activities that are most consistent with one's most deeply held values despite the presence or absence of pain at any given moment. Two processes that are helpful in promoting acceptance are *mindfulness* and *forgiveness*.

Mindfulness is discussed in Chapters 8, 9 and 11 in Volume I in this series and is the process of objectively observing one's experiences as well as one's reactions to those experiences. In the context of perceived injustice, this means helping the patient to:

- Recognize his or her sense of perceived injustice;

- Accept its presence *in this moment* allowing it to simply "be there;"

- Then to consider, in the context of his or her values, i.e., what is most important in the patient's life, whether the sense of perceived injustice enhances his or her ability to live a happy, productive life, or whether it interferes with this ability.

The patient is then free to make a choice as to whether to be guided by the sense of perceived injustice, or whether to make another choice. Helping the patient to this "choice point" allows him or her to decide what is best. This provides the patient the opportunity to forgive.

Forgiveness is often thought of as a purely religious concept, but it has great usefulness in helping patients overcome spine related disorders. As with validation, forgiveness is most effective when it does not focus on specific actions. That is, forgiveness does not mean "forgiving the bad thing that person did to me" or "pretending this never happened". Forgiveness, in the context of spine related disorders, is not about another person's *action*, it is about the patient's *reaction*. That is, once the patient is at the "choice point" he or she can make a choice. The choice is between, on the one hand, continued suffering and, on the other hand, living a "valuing" life, i.e., living a life that is consistent with what is most personally important. Thus, the patient forgives by simply choosing for recovery rather than for bitterness. Again, forgiveness is not about form (the *action*) but rather about content (the *reaction*).

Very useful in the process of overcoming the effects of perceived injustice, as well as the other important psychological factors that perpetuate the pain, disability and suffering experience, is helping promote *psychological flexibility* (see McCracken and Morley in the Recommended Reading list). Psychological flexibility is the capacity to objectively observe one's thoughts and feelings, consider them in light of a specific situation, and engage in behavior that is guided by one's goals and values, rather than being strictly tied to thoughts and feelings that may not be consistent with one's goals and values.

All human beings tend to create rules for themselves and their environment. This allows us to attempt to make sense of our lives. However, cognitive fusion (which is discussed in Chapter 2 of Volume I of this series) can often cause us to become rigidly attached to these rules, despite whether the rules serve us in living life to the fullest in a certain situation.

Psychological flexibility involves, in part, *cognitive defusion*, i.e., the capacity to detach from our thoughts and feelings (and rules) about a certain situation and to look at the situation objectively, independent of any preconceived notions that may or may not be useful. Cognitive defusion helps us understand that we are neither determined by nor harmed by our thoughts and feelings, but rather our thoughts and feelings are simply "things" that float around in our minds and that are available to us at any given moment. It is for us to determine, based on our goals and values, whether the thoughts and feelings we are experiencing are useful to us or not in a certain situation.

In the case of a patient with a spine related disorder, any thoughts that arise from fear, catastrophizing, passive coping, low self-efficacy, depression or any other of the psychological perpetuating factors discussed in this book series, are not *bad* or *wrong*. They should simply be looked at on the basis of whether they are *useful* or *not useful* in helping the patient return to a happy, healthy and productive life (obviously, in the vast majority of cases they are not useful). Looked at in this way, these factors are not enemies against which to wage battle, but simply benign thoughts that float around, to be used or not used, completely at the patient's choice and based on the patient's best interest.

As was discussed in Chapter 8 of Volume I in this series, it is important for all spine practitioners to actively apply the principles of Cognitive-Behavioral Therapy and Acceptance and Commitment Therapy and, ideally, to live by these principles themselves. In most cases, it is not necessary for the spine practitioner to practice psychotherapy with the patient (even if he or she were appropriately trained to do so). However, CBT/ACT principles should *inform everything the spine practitioner does*. In other words, these principles should permeate all interactions between the practitioner and the patient.

The reader is directed to the useful books by Hayes & Smith and Dahl & Lundgren that are found in the Recommended Reading list for practical self-application of Acceptance and Commitment Therapy. There are also a number of mindfulness apps that can be obtained through a simple online search.

As with the majority of factors related to diagnostic questions #2 and #3 in the CRISP® protocols, most patients can be managed quite well at the primary spine care level. Other patients require more extensive or invasive approaches. In the case of psychological factors, in patients who do not respond adequately to primary spine care, referral to a psychologist, preferably one who is trained in Cognitive Behavioral Therapy and/or Acceptance and Commitment Therapy, is indicated.

In some chronic pain patients, failure to respond to primary spine care relates to a combination of intense NSS and intense psychological factors. Often (but not always) there is an element of opioid-induced hyperalgesia (a form of NSS) and/or dependence. In these patients, a more extensive opioid management program and/or a chronic pain management program may be indicated.

As stated earlier, the reader is directed to Chapter 12 of Volume I of this series for specific recommendations in cases in which a patient does not respond to an adequate trial of primary spine care.

General Management Strategies

Chapter 9 in Volume I of this series covered general approaches that are applicable to all patients with low back disorders, regardless of diagnosis. These approaches included:

- Education regarding the nature of spine related disorders in general, with emphasis on dispelling many of the frightening myths that exist regarding these disorders

- Posture and lifting

- Limiting early morning flexion

- Anti-inflammatory nutrition

- Mindfulness, acceptance, commitment and values

- Motivational interviewing

All these topics apply equally to the patient with CDs and the reader is directed to that chapter for specifics. However, there are strategies related to posture and ergonomics that are particular to the patient with CDs. These will be presented here.

In Chapter 9 in Volume I of this series it was discussed that the key to proper posture and lifting technique for the lumbar spine is maintaining lumbar lordosis. For the cervical spine it is maintaining ideal craniocervical position. This applies to static postures as well as dynamic activities. Actually, maintaining lumbar lordosis is one of the keys to maintaining ideal craniocervical position.

The first step in training normal craniocervical position is the Cervical Posture Exercise (see Fig. 7-1a and b). By teaching the patient to get into the habit of imagining a helium balloon gently pulling on the posterosuperior aspect of the head, particularly when this is done with the lumbar spine in a natural lordosis, improved postural habits can be formed. This can then be translated into daily life such as sitting at a computer (Fig. 7-32) and lifting (Fig. 7-33).

Further training in posture can utilize the Brugger exercise (see Figs. 7-15 and 7-16). As discussed above, with this exercise, a natural lumbar lordosis is established as well as natural scapular positioning. In this position, the craniocervical area naturally falls into correct alignment as well.

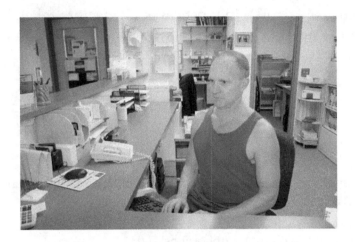

Figure 7-32. Sitting at a computer with proper craniocervical posture.

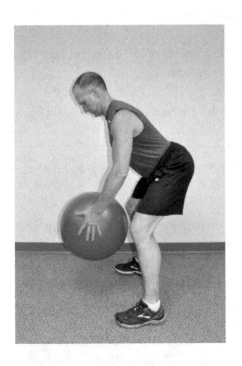

Figure 7-33. Lifting with proper craniocervical posture. Reprinted with permission from Murphy DR. Clinical Reasoning in Spine Pain Volume I: Primary Management of Low Back Disorders. Pawtucket, RI: CRISP Education and Research; 2013.

Further exercises to train proper posture can be found in the disc derangement section of Chapter 3.

Diagnostic question #3 in the CRISP® protocols primarily involves neurophysiological and psychological perpetuating factors. The treatment usually involves some type of reprogramming of central nervous system processes (in the case of dynamic instability, oculomotor system dysfunction and NSS) and reframing the situation so that the patient can make new choices (in the case of psychological factors). In most cases, the factors related to diagnostic question #3 can be managed at the primary spine care level. However, in a minority of cases, more intensive or invasive procedures may be helpful.

Recommended Reading:

Beer A, Treleaven J, Jull G. Can a functional postural exercise improve performance in the cranio-cervical flexion test?--a preliminary study. Man Ther 2012;17(3):219-24

Butler DS, Moseley GL. Explain Pain. Adelaide, Australia: Noigroup Publications, 2003.

Dahl J, Lundgren T. Living Beyond Your Pain. Oakland; New Harbinger Publications, 2006.

Falla D, Jull G, Dall'Alba P, Rainoldi A, Merletti R. An electromyographic analysis of the deep cervical flexor muscles in performance of craniocervical flexion. Phys Ther. 2003;83(10):899-906.

Fitz-Ritson D. Phasic exercises for cervical rehabilitation after "whiplash" trauma. J Manipulative Physiol Ther. 1995;18(1):21-4.

Fitz-Ritson D. Cervicogenic vertigo and disequilibrium. In: Murphy DR. Conservative Management of Cervical Spine Syndromes. New York: McGraw-Hill; 2000.

Hayes SC, Smith S. Get Out of Your Mind and Into Your Life. The New Acceptance and Commitment Therapy. Oakland; New Harbinger Publications, 2005.

McCracken LM, Morley S. The psychological flexibility model: a basis for integration and progress in psychological approaches to chronic pain management. J Pain. 2014 Mar;15(3):221-34.

Nijs J, Daenen L, Cras P, Struyf F, Roussel N, Oostendorp RA. Nociception affects motor output: a review on sensory-motor interaction with focus on clinical implications. Clin J Pain. 2012 Feb;28(2):175-81.

Pelletier R, Higgins J, Bourbonnais D. Is neuroplasticity in the central nervous system the missing link to our understanding of chronic musculoskeletal disorders? BMC Musculoskelet Disord. 2015;16:25.

Schneider GM, et al. Minimizing the source of nociception and its concurrent effect on sensory hypersensitivity: an exploratory study in chronic whiplash patients. BMC Musculoskelet Disord 2010;11:29

Schomacher J, Farina D, Lindstroem R, Falla D. Chronic trauma-induced neck pain impairs the neural control of the deep semispinalis cervicis muscle. Clin Neurophysiol. 2011 Dec 27.

Sullivan MJ, Adams H, Martel MO, Scott W, Wideman T. Catastrophizing and perceived injustice: risk factors for the transition to chronicity after whiplash injury. Spine (Phila Pa 1976) 2011;36(25 Suppl):S244-9.

Sullivan MJ, Scott W, Trost Z. Perceived injustice: a risk factor for problematic pain outcomes. Clin J Pain. 2012;28(6):484-8.

Treleaven J. Sensorimotor disturbances in neck disorders affecting postural stability, head and eye movement control. Man Ther 2008;13(1):2-11.

• Chapter 8 •

Diagnosis and Management of Patients with Thoracic Disorders Using the Clinical Reasoning in Spine Pain® Protocols

Introduction

Thoracic pain is sort of the poor stepchild in the family of spine related disorders. Very little research is focused on this area of the spine, yet spine practitioners regularly encounter patients with thoracic problems. This book series emphasizes taking an evidence-based approach to the primary management of SRDs. So the question as this relates to thoracic problems is: how do we take an evidence-based approach in the absence of a strong body of evidence?

The best way to do this is by applying the same general principles that apply to cervical and low back disorders. This includes sound, evidence-based clinical reasoning, minimalism ("less is more"), the promotion of patient empowerment and self-efficacy, and patient education. Clinical Reasoning in Spine Pain® (the CRISP® protocols) helps inform the approach. This means asking the Three Essential Questions of Diagnosis.

Diagnostic question #1: Do the presenting symptoms reflect a visceral disorder, or a serious or potentially life-threatening illness?

As was discussed in Chapter 2 of this volume, there is a great deal of overlap with regard to the disorders that fall under the first question of diagnosis. Much of what is presented in Chapter 4 in Volume I of this series applies to the cervical and thoracic spine. Therefore, it is recommended that the reader review that chapter prior to reading this chapter, as here the focus will be on information that is specific to patients with thoracic complaints.

The most important questions to ask on history in seeking the answer to diagnostic question #1 in thoracic pain patients are:

1. Do you have chest pain?

A "yes" answer suggests the possibility of heart, lung or esophageal disease. Heart disease should particularly be suspected if there is also accompanying sweating, pallor, heart palpitations and nausea. In addition, it is important to ask if the pain increases with exertion. Cardiac pain can refer to the thoracic spine as well as into the shoulder and medial aspect of the upper extremity. The pain can be experienced on the right side, although left-sided pain is far more common.

Pleurisy can cause pain to refer to the upper trapezius or lateral rib cage areas though not typically to the thoracic spine itself. The pain can be aggravated by coughing, sneezing or quick movements, making differentiation from somatic pain challenging. For this reason it is important to note that pleuritic pain is often accompanied by shortness of breath and/or pain when taking a deep breath (see below).

Esophageal pain is most commonly caused by gastroesophageal reflux disease. The pain is usually well localized to the sternum as well as in the mid thoracic spine. The patient may also have abdominal or throat pain and difficulty swallowing. In addition, the pain may be worse after a large meal, particularly when lying down.

2. Do you have shortness of breath?

A "yes" answer suggests the possibility of heart or pulmonary disease, particularly pulmonary embolus or pleurisy. Pulmonary embolus is of particular concern in a patient with a history of deep vein thrombosis.

3. Have you had a recent fall?

A "yes" answer suggests the possibility of thoracic vertebral fracture or rib fracture. This is particularly of concern in a patient who is potentially osteopenic or osteoporotic, whether age-related or related to other factors such as prolonged steroid use. Patients with acute thoracic compression fracture will often exhibit extreme pain behavior in response to movements. It is important to note that older patients with osteoporosis, or younger patients with risk factors for osteoporosis, such as those on long-term steroids, can develop rib fractures as a result of violent coughing.

4. Do you have pain when taking a deep breath?

A "yes" answer suggests the possibility of rib fracture, pleurisy or lung cancer.

5. Do you have abdominal pain? Do you have increased pain after eating?

A "yes" answer suggests the possibility of a gastrointestinal disorder, particularly gall bladder disease or ulcer (gastric or duodenal). Classically, gall bladder disease tends to cause referred pain to the right scapula and is exacerbated after a fatty meal.

6. Do you have lower extremity neurologic symptoms such as numbness, tingling, pins and needles, weakness or difficulty with walking or balance?

A "yes" answer suggests the possibility of thoracic myelopathy, which can be caused by spondylosis, disc herniation, syrinx, infection or tumor. See the discussion in Chapter 2 regarding cervical myelopathy. The examination to localize the lesion is the same as for the cervical spine. In patients with thoracic myelopathy the patient may have difficulty standing in Romberg's position with eyes closed, exhibit upgoing toes, and have hyperreflexia and spasticity in the lower extremities. However examination of the upper extremities will be normal. That is, the patient will not have hyperreflexia and spasticity in the upper extremities and Hoffman's and Tromner's signs as well as the scapulohumeral reflex will be absent. In addition, if there is a sensory level, it will be in the thoracic spine rather than the cervical spine.

DR. DONALD R. MURPHY

7. Do you have rash, itching or skin eruptions in the area of pain?

A "yes" answer suggests the possibility of herpes zoster (shingles). With herpes zoster the pain often develops spontaneously and is quite severe, although the initial symptom may be paresthesia rather than pain. The paresthesia and pain typically follow along a specific thoracic dermatome. Patients often feel generally ill, with myalgia, malaise, headache and, sometimes, fever. It is important to ask about and examine for erythema and grouped vesicles although these often develop sometime after the onset of pain.

8. Have you been having fever or chills?

A "yes" answer suggests the possibility of infection or cancer.

9. Have you been having constitutional symptoms such as malaise, fatigue or general feeling of being unwell?

A "yes" answer suggests the possibility of infection or cancer.

10. Have you had unexplained weight loss?

A "yes" answer suggests the possibility of cancer.

11. Do you have a history of cancer?

A "yes" answer suggests the possibility of metastasis, particularly if the primary cancer involved a tissue that has predilection for metastasis to the thoracic spine, such as breast or lung cancer.

12. Do you have localized or generalized stiffness in the morning lasting greater than 45 minutes?

A "yes" answer suggests the possibility of seronegative spondyloarthropathy or inflammatory arthritide. However, particularly in the case of seronegative spondyloarthropathy, it would be expected that the lumbopelvic area would be involved before the thoracic spine.

13. Have you had pain with urination, urinary urgency or frequency, unusual smelling urine or blood in your urine?

A "yes" answer suggests the possibility of kidney or ureter disease. The pain is typically felt in the lower rib cage area and often extends into the lower abdomen or groin.

Other important clinical factors to be aware of in seeking the answer to diagnostic question #1 in patients with thoracic pain are:

- Sudden onset of severe, unrelenting pain that is not relieved by rest raises the possibility of dissecting aortic aneurism.

- Factors that increase the risk of cardiovascular disease include history of smoking, hypertension, diabetes (particularly if poorly controlled) and age over 50.

- It is important in examining patients with upper thoracic pain to observe for unilateral Horner's syndrome (ptosis, cormiosis and anhydrosis of the forehead). This is because a Pancoast tumor in the superior sulcus of the lung apex can cause compression on the sympathetic chain and/or stellate ganglion.

Diagnostic question #2: Where is the pain coming from?

Disc derangement

While very little has been published in the area of detection of derangement as a possible cause of thoracic pain, end range loading protocols adapted from the McKenzie system, as discussed in Chapter 5 in Volume I of this series and in Chapter 3 in this volume, can be applied to the thoracic spine.

In many patients with pain in the upper thoracic spine and/or scapular area, if disc derangement is the source of pain it can be identified by applying the cervical protocols presented in Chapter 3. In many patients with pain in the lower thoracic spine, if derangement is the source of pain it can be identified by applying the lumbar protocols presented in Chapter 5 in Volume I of this series. However there is a small number of patients with midthoracic pain that arises from thoracic derangement in whom end range loading maneuvers may have to be applied to the thoracic spine itself.

As the mobility of the thoracic spine is more limited that the cervical or lumbar spine, in general sagittal plane movements are most important. The direction of movement that most commonly produces centralization, and thus most commonly serves as the Direction of Benefit, is extension.

Examination of extension can be performed with the use of a foam roller. Some examination tables allow the center of the table to "peak". This can be used in place of a foam roller provided the peak is narrow enough to create a focal extension of the thoracic spine.

Presented here is examination using a foam roller.

The patient sits on the examination table and the practitioner places the foam roller at the level of pain (Fig. 8-1). The practitioner holds the foam roller in place and guides the patient into the supine position while maintaining roller position (Fig. 8-2). The practitioner then moves to the head of the table and, supporting the head and upper thoracic spine, moves the patient to end range, or the point at which pain is elicited (Fig. 8-3). To examine the effect of repetition, the practitioner repetitively moves the patient away from the point of obstruction and returns to the point of obstruction, with the patient completely relaxed. The practitioner asks the patient to observe and report what happens to the pain, while at the same time the practitioner feels whether the mechanical obstruction lessens. If the pain centralizes or decreases in intensity as a result of repetition, and/or if the obstruction decreases, this suggests thoracic disc derangement with extension as the Direction of Benefit for exercise.

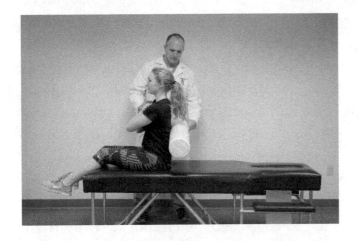

Figure 8-1. Placement of the foam roller in preparation for end range loading of the thoracic spine in extension.

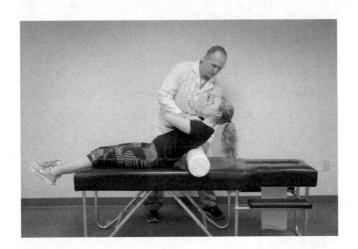

Figure 8-2. Moving the patient onto the foam roller.

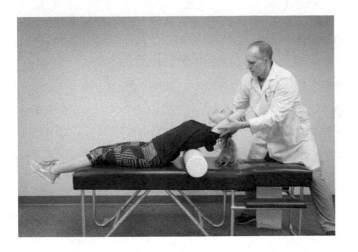

Figure 8-3. Extending the thoracic spine to end range or to the point of obstruction.

As with the cervical and lumbar spine, an alternative to repetition in the identification of centralization is sustained positioning. Sustained positioning is carried out in the same manner as repetition except instead of the practitioner repeatedly moving the spine to the point of obstruction and away from the point of obstruction, the practitioner holds the patient at the point of obstruction for 30-60 seconds. The practitioner then moves the patient away from that point, then back to the same position, asking the patient to observe and report on any pain that might be present. In patients with thoracic derangement, the pain will be located more centrally and/or be less severe in intensity upon return the point in the range of motion that had previously been obstructed. If this is the case, the patient should be moved farther into extension until an obstruction is again perceived and/or pain is elicited. The patient is held in this position for 30-60 seconds, then moved away from that point again. The effect of sustained positioning can again be determined by returning the patient the point that had previously been obstructed and/or painful, to determine whether the pain and obstruction centralizes further or further lessens in intensity.

If end range loading of the thoracic spine in extension reveals painful obstruction, and centralization and/or reduction in pain intensity is found as a result of repetitive or sustained loading in extension, the diagnosis of thoracic derangement is established. Further, extension is determined to be the Direction of Benefit for treatment.

For treatment of thoracic disc derangement in which extension is identified as the Direction of Benefit, the patient can self-treat with the use of a foam roller. Alternatively, a thick book with a pillow placed on top can be used.

The patient lies on the foam roller with the focus at the point of pain (Fig. 8-4). The patient then slowly extends, to the point of obstruction (Fig. 8-5). The patient tries to relax into this position and remain there for 30-60 seconds, after which the patient rolls out of the position to one side (Fig. 8-6). It is important that the patient does not try to get out of the position by flexing (Fig. 8-7). The patient then repeats the extension positioning for 30-60 seconds. Two sets of 30-60 second positioning should be performed 4-6 times per day.

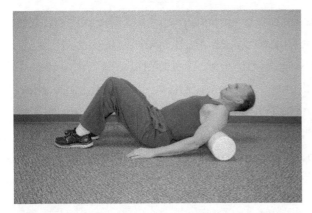

Figure 8-4. Initial positioning for end range loading self-treatment in extension.

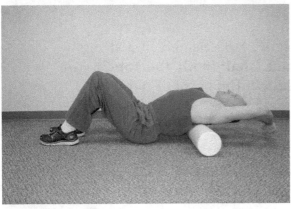

Figure 8-5. End range loading self-treatment in extension.

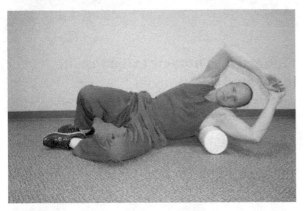

Figure 8-6. Rolling out of the end range extension position.

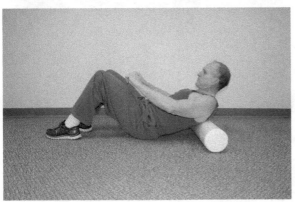

Figure 8-7. The patient should avoid flexing the thoracic spine when moving out of the end range extension position.

End range extension can also be performed in the seated position, provided the patient has a straight-back chair for which the back portion can be placed at the point of pain (Fig. 8-8). This allows the creation of a fulcrum around which the involved segment can extend. The patient clasps the hands behind the neck and extends backward to the point at which the obstructed end range prevents further movement (Fig. 8-9). This position is maintained for a moment and then the patient slowly backs away from that point just enough to decrease the pain. The exercise is performed up to 10 repetitions, the patient attempting to increase the range of extension with each repetition.

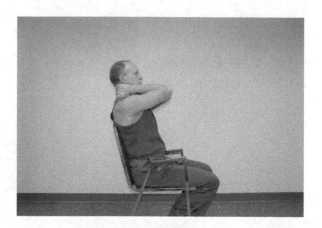

Figure 8-8. Seated in a straight-back chair with the top of the chair at the point of pain.

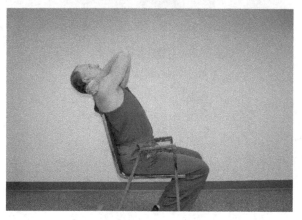

Figure 8-9. Thoracic extension in the seated position.

Joint Dysfunction

Unlike the lumbar spine, and more so than the cervical spine, the thoracic zygapophyseal joints are amenable to manual joint palpation. Thus it is reasonable to use manual joint palpation in detecting thoracic joint dysfunction. This is best done with the patient in the prone position.

The practitioner places the flat surface of one or both thumbs over the zygapophyseal joint just lateral to the spinous process. The practitioner applies gentle but firm pressure in much the same way as with manual joint palpation in the cervical spine (see Chapter 3) (Fig. 8-10). The practitioner perceives the amount of resistance to movement and asks the patient if the palpation is painful and, more importantly, whether the palpation reproduces the patient's chief complaint. As with the cervical spine, the patient's report of pain should be given more relevance than the practitioner's perception of resistance.

Also, as with the cervical spine, if a segment appears to be "positive" upon palpation, it is important to compare this segment to "control" segments, i.e., the same segment on the opposite side (in a patient whose pain is unilateral) and other thoracic levels. If palpation of a single thoracic joint exhibits increased resistance and reproduces the patient's pain, and the findings are distinctly different from "control" segments, the practitioner can be confident in the diagnosis of joint dysfunction. If all segments are equally painful, the practitioner should repeat the procedures, but apply less firm pressure. If after reducing the amount of pressure the patient continues to report equal amounts of pain at all segments, the practitioner should be less confident in the diagnosis of joint dysfunction (though this does not rule out this diagnosis) and should consider the possibility of nociceptive system sensitization (see below and Chapter 4).

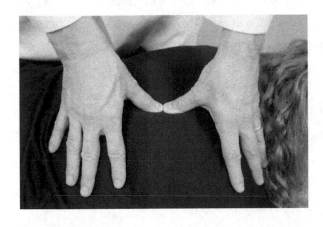

Figure 8-10. Manual joint palpation of a thoracic zygapophyseal joint.

Another potential source of thoracic pain is joint dysfunction involving the costotransverse joints. Costotransverse joint dysfunction can cause localized thoracic pain that is usually felt more laterally than with thoracic zygapophyseal joint dysfunction. Also, costotransverse joint dysfunction can at times cause referred pain around to the lateral rib cage. Costotransverse joint dysfunction can be identified with palpation in the same manner as the thoracic zygapophyseal joints, except that the palpation should be applied approximately two finger widths lateral to the spinous process.

Palpation is applied in exactly the same manner as described above for the thoracic zygapophyseal joints looking for reproduction of the patient's pain with gentle but firm pressure, and using "control" segments for confirmation.

As with the other areas of the spine, the treatment of choice for thoracic zygapophyseal or costotransverse joint dysfunction is manipulation. Also as with other areas of the spine, there are a variety of methods of manipulation for the thoracic spine, and it is beyond the scope of this book to present an exhaustive review of all available methods. It is incumbent upon the spine practitioner to be skilled in several different methods of providing this treatment, and manipulation should *not* be attempted in the absence of adequate training in this skill.

In addition, as with other areas of the spine, patients should always be instructed in self-mobilization strategies to complement the manipulative care and to promote self-efficacy. Presented here are some useful methods of thoracic manipulation and self-mobilization that are widely applicable. The methods presented here can be applied equally well to the thoracic zygapophyseal joints and the costotransverse joints. The only difference is that with the thoracic zygapophyseal joints the contact should be focused just lateral to the spinous process and with the costotransverse joints the contact should be focused approximately two finger widths lateral to the spinous process. Of course, it is unknown how precisely these contacts can be made, but the practitioner should attempt to be as precise as possible.

The same principles that apply to the cervical and lumbopelvic spine are applicable to the thoracic spine:

1. All manipulative movements should take place at the barrier.

2. High-velocity, low amplitude (HVLA) techniques can be used as well as low-velocity, low-amplitude techniques (LVLA).

3. LVLA techniques include muscle energy technique (MET) and oscillatory mobilization (OM).

4. The choice as to whether to use HVLA or LVLA maneuvers should be based on patient preference as well as clinical factors such as bone density, tissue sensitivity (actually, nociceptive system sensitivity) and other factors reviewed in Chapter 6.

For a more extensive examination of thoracic manipulation, the reader is directed to the book by Bergmann and Peterson in the Recommended Reading list.

Prone manipulation

The practitioner can stand on the side of involvement or on the opposite side. In patients with bilateral involvement, both sides can be manipulated at the same time. The patient lies prone and the practitioner applies a contact to the involved segment with the antero-medial aspect of the hand (in the vicinity of the pisiform bone). The other hand is placed on the opposite side to stabilize that side (Fig. 8-11). Gentle posterior-to-anterior pressure is applied until the barrier is engaged. From the point of the barrier a HVLA, ME or OM maneuver can be applied.

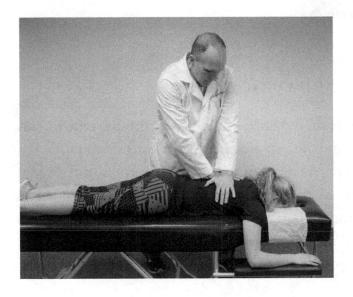

Figure 8-11. Prone manipulation directed to a segment in the mid thoracic spine.

DR. DONALD R. MURPHY

Supine manipulation

The practitioner can stand on the side of involvement or on the opposite side. The patient is seated and the practitioner makes a contact with the thenar eminence on the side of involvement and with the flexed fingers on the opposite side. The practitioner gently lays the patient supine so that the back of the practitioner's hand contacts the table, allowing pressure to be applied to the segment until the barrier is engaged (Fig. 8-12). From the point of the barrier a HVLA, ME or OM maneuver can be applied.

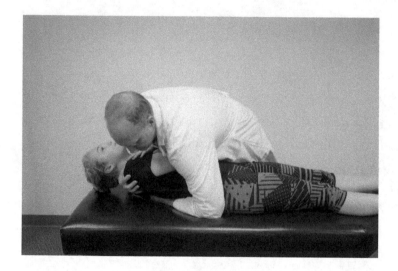

Figure 8-12. Supine manipulation directed to a segment in the mid thoracic spine. The same maneuver can be applied to lower thoracic segments.

Standing long axis manipulation - upper thoracic spine

The patient is standing and places both hands on the back of the head with the elbows out to the sides. The practitioner stands behind the patient and places each arm inside the triangle created by the patient's arms and makes a contact with the index and middle fingers inferior to the spinous process of the involved segment (as close as possible) (Fig. 8-13). The practitioner places his or her chest on the patient's mid thoracic area for support. The patient first inhales, then exhales. On exhalation the patient relaxes into the practitioner and moves the elbows forward (Fig. 8-14). From that point, a HVLA, ME or OM maneuver can be applied.

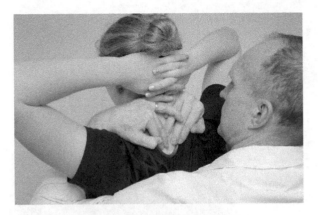

Figure 8-13. Practitioner finger placement for standing long axis manipulation in the upper thoracic spine.

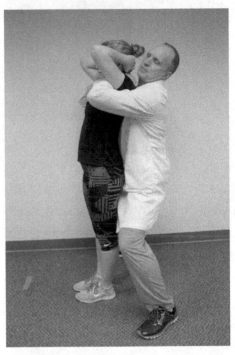

Figure 8-14. Final practitioner and patient positioning for standing long axis manipulation in the upper thoracic spine.

Standing long axis manipulation - mid thoracic spine

The patient is standing and places both hands over the eyes with the elbows together. The practitioner stands behind the patient and makes a contact with the chest as close to the involved segment as possible. The practitioner places one hand on each of the patient's elbows and applies pressure with both the hands and the chest until the barrier is engaged. The patient inhales, then exhales and relaxes into the practitioner (Fig. 8-15). From that point, a HVLA, ME or OM maneuver can be applied.

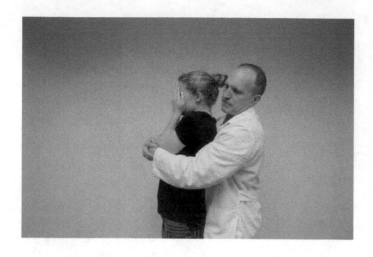

Figure 8-15. Practitioner and patient positioning for standing long axis manipulation in the mid thoracic spine.

Self-Mobilization Exercises

Thoracic long axis stretch

The patient is standing and places the hands behind the upper thoracic spine with the elbows pointing to the superior. The patient is instructed to push the elbows upward toward the ceiling, elevating the shoulders in the process (Fig. 8-16). This stretch is held for up to five seconds, and the patient returns to the starting position. This is repeated for five to ten repetitions.

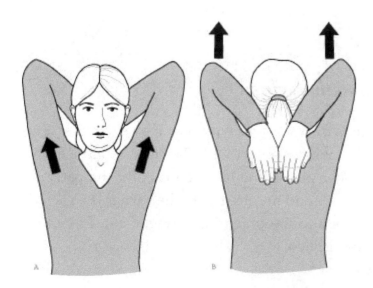

Figure 8-16. The thoracic long axis stretch exercise. Reprinted with permission from Murphy DR, ed. Conservative Management of Cervical Spine Syndromes. New York: McGraw-Hill, 2000.

Thoracic flexion and extension self-mobilization

The patient is seated and clasps the hands behind the back of the neck with the elbows facing forward. The patient flexes the thoracic spine (Fig. 8-17) then extends the thoracic spine (Fig. 8-18). The movement in each direction is carried out as far as possible, or to the point of initial discomfort. This is repeated for 10 to 20 repetitions. Depending on the situation, the practitioner may choose to provide only the flexion phase or only the extension phase.

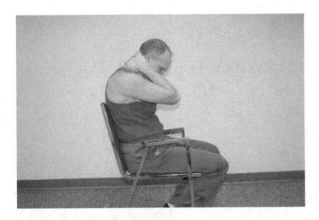

Figure 8-17. Thoracic flexion self-mobilization.

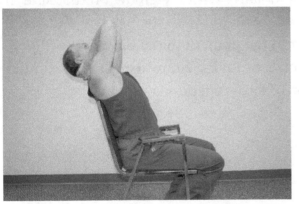

Figure 8-18. Thoracic extension self-mobilization.

Thoracic breathing self-mobilization

The patient is seated with the knees approximately four to six inches from a wall. The patient crosses the arms and places the forearms against the wall, with the forehead resting on the forearms (Fig. 8-19). The patient inhales, attempting to focus the breath to the painful thoracic segment, them exhales fully, allowing the thoracic spine to drop into extension on exhalation. This is repeated for 10 to 20 repetitions.

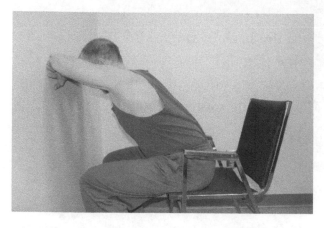

Figure 8-19. Patient positioning for thoracic breathing self-mobilization.

The "Cat and Camel" was presented in Chapter 10 of Volume I of this series for general mobilization of the lumbar spine. This exercise can also be used for general mobilization of the thoracic spine.

Thoracic rotation self-mobilization

The patient is on the knees and one forearm, sitting back in the "lumbar lock" position. The patient places one hand on the side of the head and starts with the elbow on that side in contact with the opposite elbow (Fig. 8-20). The patient then rotates the thoracic and cervical spine, raising the elbow as high as possible, or to the point of initial discomfort (Fig. 8-21). It is helpful to tell the patient to keep the eyes on the moving elbow to ensure maximum cervical and thoracic rotation. This is repeated for 10 to 20 repetitions.

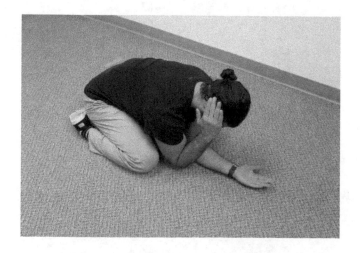

Figure 8-20. Starting position for the thoracic rotation self-mobilization exercise.

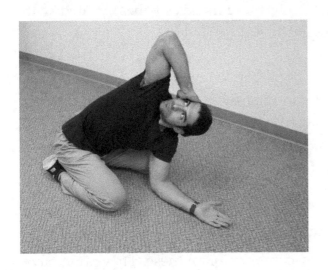

Figure 8-21. End point of thoracic rotation self-mobilization exercise.

Radiculopathy

Thoracic radiculopathy is very uncommon, however the busy spine practitioner will occasionally encounter patients with this condition. In the majority of cases the cause is disc herniation (except those whose pain is related to herpes zoster – see the earlier discussion of this). However, it must be noted that disc herniation is a very common incidental finding on thoracic MRI; the vast majority of these are asymptomatic.

Patients with thoracic disc herniation with radiculopathy will typically complain of severe pain in the thoracic spine that radiates around the rib cage. They will often report paresthesia or numbness along the involved thoracic dermatome. Sensory loss may be detected on pin prick examination. Motor loss, if it occurs, cannot be reliably detected on examination.

Acute thoracic radiculopathy can be expected to self-limit and the most important factor in management is reassurance and pain management.

Myofascial pain

Myofascial pain in the thoracic area is fairly common but, as is the case with myofascial pain in the cervical and lumbar spine, is usually secondary to one of the other pain generators. Myofascial trigger points (TrPs) commonly occur in the rhomboid, middle and lower trapezius and thoracic erector spinae muscles. TrPs in these muscles is best treated with manual or instrumented pressure release techniques.

One less common but important myofascial cause of pain in the thoracic area is that of the diaphragm. Very little published work can be found regarding myofascial pain from the diaphragm and this author credits the late Karel Lewit, MD (personal communication, 1999 and see recommended reading list) for the approach to diagnosis and treatment presented here which, anecdotally, has been very successful but for which systematic investigation is needed.

The patient with diaphragm TrPs will typically present with pain in the rib cage area – the location can be posterior, lateral or anterior, or any combination of these. They often have been worked up for GI disease, with this investigation obviously being unrevealing. If they have not been worked up for GI disease, it is important for the spine practitioner to consider GI disease, as discussed earlier with regard to diagnostic question #1, in patients with pain in the area of the posterior, lateral or anterior rib cage.

The pain can be constant, although many patients will describe increased pain with exercise or any physical activity that increases respiration. Palpation of the diaphragm will often reveal exquisite tenderness on the side of pain. It is important to note that because only the anterior and anterolateral attachment of the diaphragm can be palpated, in many patients the causative TrPs cannot be examined directly. Therefore, in most cases palpation will not exactly reproduce the pain. However if palpation of the diaphragm reveals pain on the involved side that is distinctly more intense than on the uninvolved side, the diagnosis should be suspected.

To palpate the diaphragm, the patient is seated, with the practitioner standing behind the patient. It is important that the practitioner fully explains the procedure prior to commencing. The patient leans back against the practitioner and completely relaxes. This ensures that the rectus abdominis is relaxed and does not obstruct palpation. The practitioner places the hands on the lower edge of the anterolateral aspect of the rib cage. The patient inhales, then exhales. As the patient is exhaling, the practitioner reaches the fingers under the ribcage and applies pressure anteriorward against the posterior aspect of the ribs, attempting to apply direct pressure on the diaphragm (Fig. 8-22). The practitioner asks the patient if this is painful, and if there is a distinct difference in pain between sides.

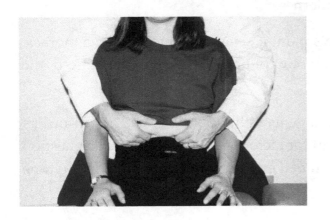

Figure 8-22. Palpation of the diaphragm. Reprinted with permission from Murphy DR, ed. Conservative Management of Cervical Spine Syndromes. New York: McGraw-Hill, 2000.

Diagnostic question #3. What is happening with this person as a whole that would cause the pain experience to develop and persist?

Dynamic and Passive Instability

The thoracic spine is a very stable part of the spine and as such it is very unlikely that it would be affected by dynamic or passive instability, at least in the absence of severe trauma. However, it is reasonable that pain in the upper thoracic spine could be perpetuated by dynamic instability in the cervical spine and that pain in the lower thoracic spine and thoracolumbar junction could be perpetuated by dynamic instability in the lumbopelvic spine. Therefore, in subacute, chronic or chronic-recurrent patients it is reasonable to asses for dynamic instability in these areas (see Chapter 4 in this volume and Chapter 6 in Volume I of this series).

Nociceptive System Sensitization

The Smart criteria for NSS apply equally to patients with cervical, thoracic or low back disorders. To reiterate these criteria:

- Pain disproportionate to the tissue injury or pathology.

- Strong association with psychological factors.

- Disproportionate, non-mechanical and unpredictable exacerbating and remitting factors in the history.

- Diffuse, nonanatomic areas of pain/ tenderness

As stated earlier, if segmental palpation reveals pain at several segments in the thoracic spine, particularly if it persists even when the amount of applied pressure is reduced, the practitioner should suspect the presence of NSS.

The management of NSS is the same as that in patients with neck and low back disorders – the reduction of nociception through treatment for factors related to diagnostic question #2, education regarding pain mechanisms and graded exposure (see Chapter 11 in Volume I of this series).

Psychological Factors

As with NSS, the identification and management of significant psychological perpetuating factors is the same in patients with thoracic disorders as for patients with neck and low back disorders. See Chapters 8, 9 and 11 in Volume I and Chapter 7 of this volume for specifics.

While there is little published research regarding the diagnosis and management of patients with thoracic disorders, the CRISP® protocols allow the spine practitioner to apply sound clinical reasoning in attempting to help these patients overcome the problem. The principles that apply to patients with neck and low back disorders apply equally well to these patients.

Recommended Reading

Bergmann T, Peterson D. Chiropractic Technique Principles and Procedures; 3rd Ed. St. Louis: Elsevier, Mosby, 2011.

Postacchini R, Paolino M, Faraglia S, Cinotti G, Postacchini F. Assessment of patient's pain-related behavior at physical examination may allow diagnosis of recent osteoporotic vertebral fracture. Spine J. 2013 Sep;13(9):1126-33.

Roman M, Brown C, Richardson W, Isaacs R, Howes C, Cook C. The development of a clinical decision making algorithm for detection of osteoporotic vertebral compression fracture or wedge deformity. J Man Manip Ther. 2010 Mar;18(1):44-9.

Klineberg E, Mazanec D, Orr D, Demicco R, Bell G, McLain R. Masquerade: medical causes of back pain. Cleve Clin J Med. 2007 Dec;74(12):905-13.

Pateder DB, Brems J, Lieberman I, Bell GR, McLain RF. Masquerade: Nonspinal musculoskeletal disorders that mimic spinal conditions. Cleve Clin J Med. 2008;75(1).

Blumenfeld H. Neuroanatomy Through Clinical Cases. 2nd ed. Sunderland, MA: Sinaouer Associates, 2010.

Papagoras C, Drosos AA. Seronegative Spondyloarthropathies: Evolving Concepts Regarding Diagnosis and Treatment. J Spine 2011;1(1).

• Chapter 9 •

Case Studies in Primary Spine Care – Part I

Introduction

The purpose of these chapters is to present clinical scenarios of patients managed in a primary spine care setting. The emphasis will be on diagnosis and management decisions, utilizing Clinical Reasoning in Spine Pain® (the CRISP® protocols), as well as case management. This includes primary spine care treatment as well as triage and case coordination, in those cases in which this are necessary. Thus, an important aspect of these chapters is that they illustrate one of the key roles of the primary spine practitioner (PSP), which is *managing the situation across the full cycle* (see Chapter 1 for a discussion of the concept of management across the full cycle). In other words, the PSP's purpose is to guide the patient along the path from the point of having a pain, disability and suffering experience for which he or she seeks help, to resolution. "Resolution" can mean different things to different patients at different times. The course that the case takes along the path to resolution will also be different in different situations. It is the PSP's job to make evidence-based, relationship-centered decisions along that path that will most rapidly and expeditiously lead the patient to resolution.

Review of the CRISP® Protocols

Recall that the CRISP® protocols involve three questions of diagnosis:

Diagnostic question #1: Do the presenting symptoms reflect a visceral disorder, or a serious or potentially life-threatening illness?

Diagnostic question #2: Where is the pain coming from?

    a. Disc derangement

    b. Joint dysfunction

    c. Radiculopathy

    d. Myofascial pain

Diagnostic question #3: What is happening with this person as a whole that would cause the pain experience to develop and persist?

    a. Dynamic or passive instability

    b. Nociceptive system sensitization

    c. Oculomotor dysfunction (in cervical patients)

    d. Psychological factors

The answers to these three questions form the diagnosis. In most cases, the diagnosis is multifactorial, as this is the nature of spine related disorders. Management decisions are then made based on the answers to the three questions, i.e., based on the diagnosis:

1. Do the presenting symptoms reflect a visceral disorder, or a serious or potentially life-threatening illness?

    a. Investigate or refer

2. Where is the pain coming from?

    a. Disc derangement – end range loading maneuvers in the Direction of Benefit, distraction manipulation (for lumbar patients)

    b. Joint dysfunction – joint manipulation, self-mobilization maneuvers

c. Radiculopathy – anti-inflammatory measures if acute, neural mobilization if subacute or chronic, possible surgical consult

d. Myofascial pain – myofascial therapies and self-treatment

3. What is happening with this person as a whole that would cause the pain experience to develop and persist?

a. Dynamic or passive instability – stabilization exercise, possible surgical consult (for passive instability that does not respond to exercise)

b. Nociceptive system sensitization – treatment of the pain source, education, graded exposure

c. Oculomotor dysfunction – oculomotor exercise

d. Psychological factors – education, appropriate communication, possible behavioral health referral

The Structure of the Case Presentations

Each case presentation is formatted to simulate a real-world case of a patient consulting a PSP. As in the normal course of clinical practice, the history is presented, including the History of Present Illness, Past Medical History, Review of Systems, Social History, Family History, and Questionnaire Data. The reader is then asked to stop and think about impressions of possible diagnostic factors based on the three questions of diagnosis.

Following this, examination findings are presented. After the examination, the reader is again asked about impressions regarding the diagnosis based on the three questions of diagnosis. The reader is also asked to think about whether further investigation is indicated in the form of imaging, lab tests or specialist consult.

The diagnosis is presented and the reader is again asked to stop and think about how the PSP can apply the CRISP® protocols is devising the most appropriate management strategy, based on the diagnosis. The case is then followed through the course of primary spine care, illustrating how the PSP manages the case *across the full cycle*. Periodically along the way, the reader will be asked to stop and ponder questions for thought. The patient's case is followed throughout the entire clinical management cycle, with the reader being asked to make decisions at key points. This helps reinforce the clinical reasoning process that is the essence of this book series.

Of course, every patient is unique, and these cases cannot be absolutely generalized. Therefore, in many cases there are "gray areas" regarding clinical decision making, rather than a single absolute correct response. However, the purpose of these cases is to illustrate how the principles of primary spine care and the CRISP® protocols are applied in a real-world clinical setting and to challenge the reader to apply clinical decision skills to each case.

The cases presented are based on actual patients managed in a primary spine care environment. However, none of the presentations reproduce all the clinical information regarding any particular patient. Nearly all cases are based on a compendium of patients seen by the author (DRM) over the years that illustrate implementation of the CRISP® protocols and primary spine care. For those cases that are based more closely on a particular patient, certain facts have been changed to protect the identity of the individual. Any close resemblance of a case to an actual person is unintentional.

Because these cases are not "real" patients, when references are made to imagining findings, the actual images are, naturally, not presented. In clinical practice the PSP is encouraged to obtain and read the radiographs, CT and MRI images that he or she orders or that other practitioners may have ordered prior to seeing the the patient. This also extends to EMG studies and relevant hematology studies. However as the purpose of this chapter is training in clinical reasoning and case management, the absence of actual images should not detract from the learning experience. Education in reading imaging studies and interpreting electrodiagnostic tests can be obtained through other sources such as the formal training for primary spine practitioners. Information can be obtained at **www.primaryspineprovider.com** [accessed 30 March 2016].

It will be seen that in certain cases the patient is described as having had "physical therapy" or "chiropractic care". In these cases, the terms "physical therapy" and "chiropractic care" are presented in quotes. The rationale for this is that these terms are often used as if "physical therapy" and "chiropractic care" were specific treatments. However, it is important to be aware that physical therapy and chiropractic are professions, not treatments. Because it is so common for these terms to be (mis)used as if one were referring to a specific intervention, the terms are put in quotes at appropriate places in this chapter.

It will also be noted that in each case it is made clear that "all communications during these sessions are carried out in a CBT/ACT context". "CBT" is the abbreviation for Cognitive-Behavioral Therapy" and ACT for "Acceptance and Commitment Therapy". It will be remembered from Volume I of this series that Cognitive-Behavioral Therapy was abbreviated "Cog-B". However, in this volume the more standard "CBT" abbreviation is used.

Finally, the reader will recall that in Chapter 4 a 2-question screen was presented for the purpose of measuring self-efficacy. The cases presented here were written prior to the introduction of this screen. Therefore, in these case presentations, the single-tem self-efficacy screen, which is also presented in Chapter 4, is used.

Case 1

History of the Present Illness:

The patient is a 56-year-old man who complains of low back pain and right lower extremity pain. This began during the course of his work as a registered nurse. He was helping a patient sit up when the patient suddenly grabbed him and pulled him forward and slightly to the left. He felt immediate pain at the time and it became quite severe that night. He was seen at his hospital's Employee Health clinic and was referred for "physical therapy". He states that this consisted "mostly of stretching exercises". He was out of work for approximately six weeks. He eventually returned to work and his pain improved somewhat but persisted, particularly in the right lower leg. He followed up with the occupational medicine physician at Employee Health who referred him for a lumbar spine MRI as well as for primary spine care.

The pain is located in the right lumbosacral and sacroiliac area with referral in the right posterolateral thigh and leg into the anterior foot. The pain frequently comes on unexpectedly but flexing while performing patient transfers and standing after prolonged sitting particularly aggravate the pain. He has relief with ibuprofen and hydrocodone combined with acetaminophen, but is concerned about ongoing medication use particularly as it might affect his work.

He denies numbness, paresthesia or motor loss in the extremities. He denies saddle anesthesia. He denies bowel or bladder difficulties as well as any other gastrointestinal (GI), genitourinary (GU) or chest symptoms related to the pain. He also denies fever, chills, rigors, constitutional symptoms and unexplained weight loss.

Past Medical History:

Remarkable for hypertension for which he takes a beta blocker and diuretic, type II diabetes for which he takes a biguanidine medication and hypercholesterolemia for which he takes a statin medication. He sees his primary care physician regularly and has regular cancer screenings.

Review of Systems:

Remarkable for symptoms related to a recent sinus infection.

Social History:

He is married with two grown children. He quit smoking two years ago, drinks alcohol occasionally and does not exercise regularly.

Family History:

Remarkable for hypertension, heart disease and type II diabetes in his mother.

Questionnaire data:

Bournemouth Back Disability Questionnaire – 51
Average pain intensity over the past week - 8/10

Anxiety item on the Bournemouth Back Disability Questionnaire – 7/10
Depression item on the Bournemouth Back Disability Questionnaire – 7/10
Coping Strategies Screening Questionnaire - 6/12
Tampa Scale for Kinesiophobia - 24/44.

What are your impressions based on the history?

Diagnostic question #1:

Diagnostic question #2:

Diagnostic question #3:

Physical Examination:

Reveals a well-nourished, pleasant man who appeared in no acute distress. Blood pressure is 150/100 on the left. Temperature is 98.8 degrees Fahrenheit. Pulse is 104 per minute. Respirations are 20 per minute.

End range loading examination reveals painful obstruction upon extension in the prone position that reproduces the patient's low back and leg pain. The obstruction reduces and the pain gradually centralizes with both repetition and overpressure. Specifically, the leg pain gradually reduces and the low back pain gradually increases with repetition of the prone extension maneuver; the low back pain then reduces in intensity with the application of overpressure. Straight Leg Raise is positive on the right for exact reproduction of the patient's leg pain. There is no change in this pain with ankle dorsiflexion or ankle plantar flexion. Well Leg Raise is negative. Active Straight Leg Raise Test is positive. Hip Extension Test and Prone Instability Test are both negative.

The patient is oriented to person, place and time. Heel, toe and tandem walking are within normal limits. Romberg's position is held with eyes closed without difficulty. Sensory examination to pinprick in the lower extremities reveals no abnormalities. Motor strength is 5/5 bilaterally in the lower extremities. Muscle stretch reflexes are 1+ and symmetric in the knees and ankles. Plantar responses are downgoing bilaterally.

The lower extremity peripheral pulses are intact bilaterally.

Diagnostic Imaging:

Both the MRI report and the images are reviewed and they are essentially unremarkable, only revealing normal age-related degenerative changes.

What are your diagnostic impressions based on the history and examination?

Diagnostic question #1:

Diagnostic question #2:

Diagnostic question #3:

Diagnosis:

The diagnosis is lumbar disc derangement with extension as the direction of benefit for exercise (diagnostic question #2) along with dynamic instability of the lumbopelvic spine (diagnostic question #3). There is some concern about anxiety and depression as perpetuating factors as well (diagnostic question #3). No findings on history and examination are significant with regard to diagnostic question #1.

What is your initial management strategy?

The patient is instructed in end range loading exercises in extension ("press up" – see Chapter 5 in Volume I of this series). He is to perform 10 repetitions 4-6 times per day. He is told to stop the exercise if his pain should steadily increase or peripheralize during a set or over the next few days. It is made clear to him that this is not expected, but that it is the guideline provided to all patients.

He is scheduled for four additional visits, which consist of distraction manipulation (aka Cox Technique – see Recommended Reading list) and stabilization exercises. These sessions also include instruction on maintaining lumbar lordosis during active movements, particularly patient transfers (see Chapter 9 in Volume I of this series). The PSP and patient agree that he should remain at his full-duty work status.

He is given information on anti-inflammatory nutrition [**http://www.deflame.com/** accessed 16 March 2016]. All communications during the sessions are carried out in a CBT/ACT context.

At re-examination on the fourth visit the patient rates himself to be 70% improved. He states that he occasionally has episodes of pain with patient transfers but these are less frequent and less severe. He states that patient transfers are much easier and less painful when he remembers to maintain lordosis.

Questionnaire data at re-exam:

Bournemouth Disability Questionnaire – 24
Average pain intensity over the past week - 4/10
Anxiety item on the Bournemouth Back Disability Questionnaire – 2/10
Depression item on the Bournemouth Back Disability Questionnaire – 3/10
Coping Strategies Screening Questionnaire - 9/12
Tampa Scale for Kinesiophobia - 21/44

End range loading examination is pain-free and unobstructed in all directions. Active Straight Leg Raise Test remains positive. Hip Extension Test and Prone Instability test remain negative.

What is the best course of action now?

The patient has experienced marked improvement in pain and functional ability. The disc derangement is resolved. His anxiety and depression have markedly improved. He does still appear to have residual dynamic instability (positive ASLR test).

It is explained to the patient that he has improved as expected, largely due to his diligence with sticking to his exercises and self-care strategies. Because of the residual instability it is recommended that he and the PSP continue working together on expanding his home stabilization exercise program.

The patient is followed once per week for three weeks for the purpose of advancing him on his lumbar stabilization program and to monitor his pain and functional progress.

At the next re-examination the patient reports 85% improvement. He states that he still occasionally has pain with patient transfers but these have continued to become less frequent and severe.

Questionnaire data at re-exam:

Bournemouth Disability Questionnaire – 15
Average pain intensity over the past week - 2/10
Anxiety item on the Bournemouth Back Disability Questionnaire – 2/10
Depression item on the Bournemouth Back Disability Questionnaire – 2/10
Coping Strategies Screening Questionnaire - 10/12
Tampa Scale for Kinesiophobia - 21/44.

End range loading examination remains unremarkable and Active Straight Leg Raise is negative. The patient demonstrates a good ability to perform his exercises properly and to bend forward and mimic patient transfers while maintaining lumbar lordosis.

What is the best course of action now? Is the patient ready to be released from the active care plan? Is this alright to do even though he remains mildly symptomatic? What should the patient be told at this point?

It is determined that in all likelihood the patient is at a point at which he can continue his improvement with the home exercises and self-care strategies he has been taught. It is explained to him that it is likely that he will continue to experience occasional flare-ups of pain but that these are expected to happen less frequently and to be less severe over time. It is also explained that this is simply the natural fluctuation of pain and not typically reflective of "re-injury". The patient is asked if he understands this and he acknowledges that he does.

It is recommended to the patient that he monitor these fluctuations and if he should have pain he should utilize the "press up" exercise for self-treatment. If the finds that pain is starting to occur more frequently and/or is becoming more severe he is advised return to the PSP. Otherwise there is no need for him to schedule any follow-ups.

Case 2

History of the Present Illness:

The patient is a 35-year-old woman who complains of neck pain and "numbness" in her right arm and the right side of her trunk. The pain began insidiously approximately one month ago, with the numbness in her arm and trunk developing sometime later. She saw her primary care physician who ordered cervical radiographs, prescribed nonsteroidal anti-inflammatory and muscle relaxant medications and referred her for PSP consultation.

She states that she had an episode of neck pain approximately six years ago and saw a chiropractor. She was treated with high-velocity, low amplitude manipulation which "helped a lot".

The pain is located in the right anterolateral and lateral cervical spine. There is no radiation of pain down her right arm but she does have what she describes as "numbness" starting in her hand and extending into her entire arm and into the right side of her trunk. Upon further questioning she states that the "numbness" is not true sensory loss but "a feeling of numbness – like when your foot falls asleep". She denies sensory symptoms on the left as well as weakness in either upper extremity. She states that laterally bending her head to the left provokes the right-sided pain somewhat. Lateral bending to the right is not painful.

She denies rashes, itching or skin eruptions in the area of numbness. She denies ataxia or balance problems. She denies blurred vision, double vision, dysarthria, dysphasia, vertigo or other bulbar symptoms related to the pain. She denies numbness, paresthesia or motor loss in the lower extremities. She denies GI or chest symptoms related to the pain. She also denies fever, chills, rigors, constitutional symptoms and unexplained weight loss.

The patient notes that in the past couple of months she has had two episodes of "pins and needles" extending down her spine provoked by flexion of the cervical spine. These episodes were short-lived and she never gave them much thought.

Past Medical History:

Remarkable for occasional migraine headaches that she self-treats with over-the-counter non-steroidal anti-inflammatory medications (NSAIDs). She sees her primary care practitioner regularly.

Review of Systems:

Remarkable for fatigue that she has had for approximately six months and that she has not reported to her primary care physician.

Social History:

She lives with a partner and has no children. She does not smoke, drinks wine occasionally and runs and weight trains for exercise.

Family History:

Unknown, as she was adopted.

Questionnaire data:

Neck Pain Screening Tool - long form - 18
Neck Disability Index - 28%
Average pain intensity over the past week - 4/10

Coping Strategies Screening Questionnaire - 3/12
Self-efficacy scale - 2/10
Problem-specific depression scale - 4/10

What are your impressions based on the history?

Diagnostic question #1:

Diagnostic question #2:

Diagnostic question #3:

Physical Examination:

Reveals a well-nourished, pleasant woman who appears in no acute distress. Blood pressure is 117/70 on the left. Temperature is 98.0 degrees Fahrenheit. Pulse is 68 per minute. Respirations are 12 per minute.

End range loading examination is unremarkable in rotation and lateral flexion to either side, however extension in the supine position causes neck pain without obstruction. The neck pain does not change with repetition or sustained loading. Flexion of the head in the seated position with firm pressure into flexion elicits what the patient describes as "those pins and needles down my back".

The Brachial Plexus Tension Test is painful on the right but this is equal to that on the left. Structural differentiation (see Chapter 3) reveals the elicited pain to be of neural origin on each side. Palpation for segmental tenderness and manual joint palpation reveal resistance to motion and severe pain at approximately C2-3 and C5-6 on the right that exactly reproduces the patient's neck pain. There is no pain or resistance to motion upon examination of the same segments on the left. The Extension-Rotation Test is positive on the right for reproduction of the patient's neck pain. Foraminal Compression Test, Cervical Distraction Test and Cervical Rotation Test to the right are all unremarkable. Cervical Stability Test is negative.

The patient is oriented to person, place and time. Heel, toe and tandem walking are within normal limits. Romberg's position is held with eyes closed without difficulty. Examination of cranial nerves II through XII is within normal limits. Pupils are equal, round and reactive to light and accommodation. Funduscopic examination is unremarkable. Sensory examination to pinprick in the upper and lower extremities and trunk reveals no abnormalities. Motor strength is 5/5 bilaterally throughout. Muscle stretch reflexes are 3+ and symmetric throughout. Plantar responses are downgoing bilaterally. The umbilical reflexes are present and Hoffman's and Tromner's signs are absent bilaterally. The jaw jerk reflex is normal. Rapid alternating movements, heel to shin movements and finger to nose movements are carried out without dysmetria or tremor. There is no evidence of pronator drift.

What are your impressions based on the history and examination? Is there any indication for imaging, specials tests or specialist consult? Why or why not?

Diagnostic question #1:

Diagnostic question #2:

Diagnostic question #3:

Diagnosis:

The impression is that the patient has right-sided mid-and lower cervical joint dysfunction with the possibility, but not a strong likelihood, of cervical radiculopathy (diagnostic question #2).

However, there are concerns related to diagnostic question #1. Because of the trunk sensory symptoms and the presence of Lhermitte's sign*, both on history and examination, combined with the hyperreflexia on examination, it is decided that a central nervous system (CNS) process should be ruled out. There are no clear signs on examination that allow for definitive localization of the lesion, but cranial nerve examination and jaw jerk are normal (see Chapter 2), so it is determined that cervical MRI would be the study with the highest potential for positive findings. A cervical MRI is ordered to rule out CNS infection, spinal cord compression or multiple sclerosis. As this is a screening MRI, it is ordered without contrast.

The MRI report states, "There is abnormal signal within the spinal cord at the C2-C4 level. Differential considerations include demyelinating disease, neoplastic considerations and cord infarction."

What is the best course of action now?

It is decided that neurologic consult is necessary. A cervical MRI with contrast along with a brain MRI with contrast is ordered as well so this information is available for the neurologist.

Is the PSP's job done at this point? What about the patient's neck pain?

It is decided that the most important thing is to get a definitive diagnosis for the neurologic findings. It is suspected that these findings relate to multiple sclerosis (MS). If that is the case, the neck pain likely is caused by joint dysfunction, and is unrelated to MS. However,

---

* Lhermitte's sign is a phenomenon in which a patient reports sensory symptoms, usually a feeling of "electricity", that runs down the spine and often into the extremities. It is typically provoked by cervical flexion. It often occurs in patients with a spinal cord lesion. It can be found in patients with MS although it is not specific to this particular disease.

it is decided that the best course of action is to get confirmation of the MS diagnosis prior to addressing the neck pain.

The post-contrast cervical MRI and brain MRI further support the diagnosis of MS. The patient sees the neurologist, who confirms the diagnosis of MS, and starts treatment for the MS. She returns to the PSP with continued neck pain.

What is the best course of action now?

It is decided that management strategy should involve manipulation at approximately the C2-3 and C5-6 segments on the right along with exercises to self-mobilize these segments. The patient is also given information on anti-inflammatory nutrition [http://www.deflame.com/ accessed 16 March 2016]. All communications are carried out in a CBT/ACT context.

Are there any special precautions or procedures that need to be considered given the patient's diagnosis of MS? Should HVLA manipulation be considered contra-indicated?

Discussion takes place between the PSP and patient and, given the patient's prior positive experience with HVLA manipulation, this method is used. There is no reason to think manipulation of any kind, including HVLA manipulation, should be avoided in this patient. The patient is given cervical retraction and self-mobilization exercises (see Chapter 6).

The patient is treated three times, with re-examination on the fourth session. At that time the patient reports that her neck pain is resolved and she is engaging in all activities of daily living.

Questionnaire data at re-examination:

Neck Pain Screening Tool - long form - 5
Neck Disability Index - 0%
Average pain intensity over the past week - 2/10
Coping Strategies Screening Questionnaire - 12/12
Self-efficacy scale - /10
Problem-specific depression scale - 4/10

The patient is followed up two weeks later and remains symptom-free with regard to her neck pain complaint. It is recommended that she continue the cervical retraction exercises regularly and use the self-mobilization exercises to self-treat any recurrences that may arise. She is welcomed to return to the PSP if she has recurrence of pain that she is not able to resolve with the self-treatment strategies she has been taught.

Case 3

History of the Present Illness:

The patient is a 16-year-old girl, accompanied by her mother, who complains of chronic neck pain. She has had this for "at least three years". She saw a chiropractor initially who treated her with manipulation and electrical stimulation. She states that the manipulation "felt great" but the improvement was short-lived. She later had three months of "physical therapy" that consisted of heat, ultrasound and stretching exercises. There was no improvement with this treatment regimen. She saw her pediatrician for a regular checkup and mentioned the neck pain to her, after which the pediatrician referred her to the PSP.

The pain is located in the posterior cervical spine bilaterally without radiation or referral. She states that "the pain is constant" and especially bothers her when she is in school and when she is studying with books or the computer. She plays soccer, basketball and softball and the pain does not interfere with those activities. Her only source of relief is self-manipulation. Upon questioning, she states that "I crack my neck constantly all day". When asked to estimate how many times per day on average she self-manipulates, she states "probably 20 or 30".

She denies numbness, paresthesia or motor loss in the extremities. She denies problems with gait or balance. She denies chest or abdominal pain as well as bowel or bladder difficulties. She denies fever, chills, rigors, constitutional symptoms and unexplained weight loss.

Past Medical History:

Otherwise unremarkable. She sees her pediatrician regularly.

Review of Systems:

Remarkable for occasional abdominal pains for which she has seen her pediatrician with no definitive diagnosis.

Social History:

She lives with her family and plays soccer, basketball and softball.

Family History:

Unremarkable.

Questionnaire data:

Neck Pain Screening Tool Long Form - 14
Neck Disability Index - 22%
Average pain intensity over the past week - 8/10
Coping Strategies Screening Questionnaire - 8/12
Problem-specific self-efficacy scale - 6/10
Problem-specific depression scale - 4/10

What are your impressions based on the history?

Diagnostic question #1:

Diagnostic question #2:

Diagnostic question #3:

Physical Examination:

Reveals a well-nourished, pleasant girl who appears in no acute distress. Blood pressure is 110/70 on the left. Temperature is 97.4 degrees Fahrenheit. Pulse is 68 per minute. Respirations are 16 per minute.

End range loading examination is pain-free and within normal limits in all directions. The Extension-Rotation Test is negative bilaterally. Palpation for segmental tenderness and manual joint palpation are painful without perceived resistance to motion at all segments. The intensity of the pain on examination is equal at all segments and is present even with light palpation. Palpation of the posterior cervical muscles reveals diffuse myofascial trigger points that reproduces the patient's neck pain. Cervical Stability Test is positive.

The patient is oriented to person, place and time. Heel, toe and tandem walking are within normal limits. Romberg's position is held with eyes closed without difficulty. Sensory examination to pinprick in the upper and lower extremities is unremarkable. Motor strength is 5/5 bilaterally in the upper and lower extremities. Muscle stretch reflexes are 2+ and symmetric throughout. Plantar responses are downgoing bilaterally.

What are your impressions based on the history and examination? Is there any indication for imaging, specials tests or specialist consult? Why or why not?

Diagnostic question #1:

Diagnostic question #2:

Diagnostic question 3#:

Diagnosis:

The diagnosis is self-manipulation induced hyperalgesia (nociceptive system sensitization) and dynamic instability (diagnostic question #3). Myofascial trigger points are the pain source (diagnostic question #2) however these are seen as secondary to the nociceptive system sensitization and dynamic instability.

What is your initial management strategy?

Self-manipulation induced hyperalgesia is explained to the patient. Included in this explanation is the fact that the most important aspect of the management strategy is for her to stop self-manipulation of her neck. The patient is placed on a weaning schedule designed to gradually reduce the frequency of self-manipulation. The following schedule is agreed to between the PSP and the patient:

Week one: Six self-manipulations per day, spaced throughout the day at the patient's discretion.
Week two: Four self-manipulations per day, spaced throughout the day at the patient's discretion.
Week three: Two self-manipulations per day, one first thing in the morning and the other at a time of the patient's choosing.
Week four: One self-manipulation first thing in the morning.
Week five: No self-manipulations.

During this time, the patient is educated not to worry if her neck "cracks" when she moves her neck during the course of a normal activity, but to strictly adhere to the schedule with regard to deliberate self-manipulation.

The patient is also placed on a program of cervical stabilization exercise, with the Cervical Brace exercise (see Chapter 7). The patient is scheduled twice per week for three weeks for the purpose of cervical stabilization exercise and ischemic compression to the trigger points in the posterior cervical muscles and for monitoring of the self-manipulation schedule. She is also given information on anti-inflammatory nutrition [**http://www.deflame.com/** accessed 16 March 2016]. All communications during the sessions are carried out in a CBT/ACT context.

At the sixth session a formal re-examination is undertaken. The patient is again accompanied by her mother. At that time the patient reports 20% improvement. She states that on the one hand she feels she is making overall progress but her pain has increased since starting the weaning schedule. She states that she finds it very difficult to stick to the schedule but that she has largely been successful. Her mother reinforces the fact that she has kept to the schedule for the most part although she has "cheated" at times.

Questionnaire data at re-examination:

Neck Pain Screening Tool Long Form– 10
Neck Disability Index - 18%
Average pain intensity over the past week - 9/10
Coping Strategies Screening Questionnaire - 8/12
Problem-specific self-efficacy scale - 8/10
Problem-specific depression scale - 2/10

On examination myofascial trigger points are again noted in the posterior cervical muscles. The Cervical Stability Test is mildly positive.

What is the best course of action now?

A detailed discussion takes place between the PSP, patient and mother. There is concern that the patient may not have a great deal of confidence in her ability to carry on the management strategy on her own. This concern was reflected in the problem-specific self-efficacy scale as well as the conversation during the visit. Therefore, although the patient likely has the skills to self-manage her condition, a decision is made for the PSP to continue to see her once per week to have her do her cervical stabilization exercises under supervision at each session. In addition, it is thought that weekly visits would allow the PSP to provide guidance and encouragement in following the weaning schedule, particularly when she reaches the "no self-manipulation" stage. She is scheduled once per week for four weeks, with another formal re-examination on the fourth week.

At the next re-examination the patient reports 70% improvement. She states that her pain is much less intense and that she has been able to complete the weaning schedule. This is again reinforced by her mother. The patient states that she is functioning normally and is engaging in all normal activities.

Questionnaire data at re-examination:

Neck Pain Screening Tool Long Form– 8
Neck Disability Index - 10%
Average pain intensity over the past week - 2/10
Coping Strategies Screening Questionnaire - 10/12
Problem-specific self-efficacy scale - 2/10
Problem-specific depression scale - 2/10

On examination there are mild myofascial trigger points in the posterior cervical muscles. The Cervical Stability Test is negative.

What is the best course of action now?

Based on discussion between the PSP, the patient and the patient's mother, it is decided at this point that the patient is ready to be released to self-care. It is impressed upon her that she should continue with her 10-15 minute cervical stabilization exercise routine and avoid any self-manipulation. She is instructed to return as needed.

For consideration: Manipulation-induced hyperalgesia is unfortunately not well represented in the literature but the busy PSP will encounter it frequently. It is a phenomenon in which repetitive exposure to the *hypo*analgesic effects of manipulation lead to the paradoxical induction of nociceptive system sensitization (NSS). It is not unlike the phenomenon of rebound headache or opioid-induced hyperalgesia. In fact, the mechanisms, while not well understood, are likely very similar. When the nervous system is repeatedly exposed to pain-relieving chemicals, this can lead to a plastic change in the peripheral and central portions of the nociceptive system in which the system as a whole becomes more sensitive to subsequent nociceptive stimuli (i.e., NSS develops). As the pain becomes more frequent and/or severe, the patient naturally will do what has always worked – take additional analgesic medication or self-manipulate. However, this becomes a downward spiral in that the more *hypo*algesia the patient seeks, the more pronounced the induced *hyper*algesia becomes. This then leads to even more frequent pursuit of pain relief, worsening the condition.

The weaning process discussed above is one that this author has used with a number of patients. While it requires a firm commitment on the part of the patient, empirically, the approach is often successful.

Case 4

History of the Present Illness:

The patient is a 57-year-old woman who complains of low back pain, left lower extremity pain and "numbness" in both feet. She had developed "soreness" in her lower back while exercising in the gym approximately six months ago. Approximately two months ago the pain markedly worsened. This is about the time that she developed the numbness in her feet. The pain is located in the lumbosacral area with radiation into the left posterior thigh and calf.

Flexion activities, sitting, lifting, coughing and sneezing aggravate the pain. She has relief with heat, massage and sitting with a pillow supporting her lower back. She generally feels better when she is upright compared to when she is sitting, although she does develop pain after a prolonged period of being upright. There is no particular time of day at which the pain is better or worse although she reports that she occasionally has severe pain at night. Upon questioning, she is not sure whether this pain relates to turning in bed or whether it develops spontaneously.

She describes "numbness" in her left leg in the same location as the pain as well as in both feet. Upon questioning, she states that she thinks that the numbness covers the entire foot on each side although she is not sure. Also upon questioning, she states that this is a "feeling of numbness" rather than actual loss of sensation. She denies numbness or paresthesia in her groin area, motor loss, bowel or bladder difficulties and abdominal or pelvic symptoms. She denies fever, chills, rigors, constitutional symptoms and unexplained weight loss.

Past Medical History:

Remarkable for anxiety for which she does not currently take medication.

Review of Systems:

Remarkable for occasional constipation.

Social History:

She is married with three children, all of whom live with her. She quit smoking 10 years ago, drinks approximately two glasses of wine per week and, goes to the gym to do weight training and to use cardio machines 2-3 times per week. She works full-time as a receptionist for a law firm.

Family History:

Remarkable for heart disease and hypertension in her mother and lung cancer in her father.

Questionnaire data:

STarT Back 9-Item Clinical Tool – 51
Fear item on the STarT Back 9-Item Clinical Tool – 7/10
Catastrophizing item of the STarT Back 9-Item Clinical Tool – 6/10
Problem-Specific Depression scale – 6/10
Self-Efficacy scale – 6/10
Average pain intensity over the past week - 8/10
Patient-Specific Functional Scale - deficits of working (which involves sitting for long periods) rated 8/10 and putting on boots rated 8/10

What are your impressions based on the history?

Diagnostic question #1

Diagnostic question #2

Diagnostic question #3

Physical Examination:

Reveals a well-nourished, pleasant women who appears in mild distress. Blood pressure is 158/102 on the left. Temperature is 98.6 degrees Fahrenheit. Pulse is 100 per minute. Respirations are 16 per minute.

Toe and tandem walking are within normal limits. She has trouble with heel walking on the left, with difficulty fully dorsiflexing her foot. Romberg's position is held with eyes closed without difficulty. Sensory examination in the lower extremities reveals decreased sensation to light touch and pinprick in the lateral feet bilaterally. Lower extremity motor strength is 5/5 bilaterally throughout with exception of the left extensor hallucis longus (EHL), which is 4/5. Muscle stretch reflexes are 3+ and symmetric in the knees and absent bilaterally in the ankles. Plantar responses are downgoing bilaterally. Upper extremity muscle stretch reflexes are 2+ and symmetric. Hoffman's and Tromner's signs are absent bilaterally. No ankle clonus or lower extremity spasticity is noted. Rapid alternating movements, heel-to-shin movements, and finger-to-nose movements are carried out without dysmetria or tremor. There is no evidence of pronator drift.

End range loading examination of the lumbar spine reveals painful obstruction upon extension in the prone position which does not change with repetition or overpressure. Right side gliding also reveals painful obstruction that reproduces her low back pain but not her leg pain. The pain and obstruction both improve with repetition of right side gliding. Left side gliding is unremarkable.

Straight Leg Raise with ankle dorsiflexion is positive on the left for reproduction of the low back and lower extremity pain. The intensity of this pain is decreased by ankle plantar flexion. Femoral Nerve Stretch Test produces low back pain but no lower extremity symptoms. Structural differentiation using the Femoral Nerve Slump Test reveals the low back pain produced on the initial test not to be of neural origin. Hip Extension Test is positive bilaterally for deviation of the lumbar spine. Prone Instability Test is also positive. Active Straight Leg Raise Test is negative.

What are your impressions based on the history and examination? Is there any indication for imaging, specials tests or specialist consult? Why or why not?

Diagnostic question #1:

Diagnostic question #2:

Diagnostic question 3#:

Diagnosis:

The initial diagnosis is lumbar radiculopathy, most likely involving the left L5 nerve root and most likely secondary to herniated disc (diagnostic question #2). Right side gliding is deemed the direction of benefit for exercise. Important perpetuating factors are dynamic instability of the lumbar spine as evidenced by the positive Hip Extension Test and Prone Instability Test and possible psychological perpetuating factors based on moderately high scores on the psychological data from the questionnaires (diagnostic question #3).

There is some concern related to diagnostic question #1 because of the motor loss that appears to be reflective of L5 radiculopathy. Also of concern is the hyperreflexia in the knees, however this does not require immediate investigation given the downgoing toes, normal upper extremity reflexes, absence of clonus or spasticity and absent Hoffman's and Tromner's signs.

An additional concern is the sensory loss in the lateral feet and the absent ankle jerks, which could reflect bilateral S1 radiculopathy. However, as there was no motor loss involving the S1 nerve roots, it is decided that this can be monitored.

The diagnosis and clinical concerns are discussed with the patient and a shared decision is made to undergo a trial of treatment. It is decided that no imaging is indicated at this time but that clinical progress will be monitored carefully.

What is your initial management strategy?

The patient is instructed in end range loading exercises in right side gliding. She is told to perform 10 repetitions of this exercise four times per day. She is told to stop the exercise if her pain should progressively increase in intensity or peripheralize during a set or over the duration of time until the next visit. The treatment plan is to also include distraction manipulation targeting the lumbosacral spine, with a plan to progress to lumbar stabilization exercise. The patient is told to plan for a treatment schedule of two sessions per week for three weeks with a formal re-examination planned for the sixth session, or sooner if progress occurs more quickly than expected. She is also given information on anti-inflammatory nutrition [**http://www.deflame.com/** accessed 16 March 2016]. All communications during the sessions are carried out in a CBT/ACT context.

It is also planned that neurologic findings, particularly motor strength, will be carefully monitored on each treatment session.

The patient tolerates both the home exercises and the treatments well although over the first three sessions she does not experience a significant change in her symptoms. Neurologic examination findings remain unchanged.

On the fourth visit the patient reports that over the past two days her leg pain has decreased somewhat. The numbness and tingling have not changed but she notices her left foot "dragging a bit" when she walks. She also reports that she occasionally experiences an "electrifying jolt" when she rises from a lying position. She has continued the side gliding exercise without difficulty or peripheralization of symptoms.

On examination during the fourth visit she is unable to rise on her left toe and she is unable to heel walk because of inability to maintain dorsiflexion of her left ankle. She is able to tandem walk and stand in Romberg's position with eyes closed. Muscle stretch reflexes remain 3+ bilaterally in the knees and absent bilaterally in the ankles. Plantar response is downgoing bilaterally. There is decreased sensation to light touch and pinprick over the dorsum of the left foot and the lateral aspects of both feet. Motor strength is now 3/5 in the left EHL and 4/5 in the left peroneus.

What is the best course of action now?

Because of the fairly rapid progression of motor loss, a lumbar spine MRI is ordered. A discussion takes place with the patient during which the PSP suggests that consultation with a spine surgeon will likely be necessary.

The MRI reveals complete marrow replacement of the S1 vertebral body with extension into the S2 vertebral body and the central canal causing severe central canal stenosis. The lesion fully enhances with the introduction of contrast medium.

What is the best course of action now?

The patient is seen for follow up and the findings of the MRI are discussed. It is explained to her that she has a tumor in her sacrum that will require further evaluation. A stat neurosurgical consult is set up. After the visit a phone call is placed to the patient's primary care practitioner to apprise her of the situation.

According to the neurosurgeon's report, he does not feel immediate decompression is necessary. CT scan of the chest, abdomen and pelvis are ordered to assess for the extent of the pathology. This reveals diffuse involvement of the bone marrow. Oncology is called in for biopsy which reveals plasma cell neoplasm and further evaluation determines this to be stage II multiple myeloma.

Further PSP follow-up is not deemed necessary other than periodic phone calls to check on the patient.

For consideration: On the initial visit a shared decision was made that MRI was not indicated and a trial of treatment was carried out. Did the delay in obtaining the MRI negatively impact the outcome of this case?

Among the important principles of primary spine care are minimalism and judicious use of special tests such as MRI. In this case, at the outset there were no red flags that would indicate the need for immediate investigation. There were a few findings that were of sufficient concern to warrant careful monitoring (motor loss of 4/5, hyper-reflexia in the knees, bilateral sensory loss) but none of these findings in any way suggested a medical emergency.

Had there been certain other findings, such as profound motor loss on exam (3/5 or greater), fever, rigors or other indications of infection, or saddle anesthesia, difficulty with urination or other indication of cauda equina syndrome, immediate action would have been indicated. However these were all ruled out through careful history and exam.

As it turned out, with careful monitoring, signs and symptoms were detected that changed the decision-making process and immediate action was taken by the PSP. As a result, the diagnosis was made and the patient was started on the appropriate path for her condition.

The two week delay in making the diagnosis did not in any way negatively impact the course of the case.

Case 5

History of the Present Illness:

The patient is a 45-year-old man who complains of neck pain and right upper extremity pain. This began approximately six months previously when he was at work, attempting to open the cover of a circuit breaker that was stuck. He saw his primary care physician initially who prescribed hydrocodone/ acetaminophen and muscle relaxant. His internist instructed him to stay out of work and referred him to a neurologist. It took four weeks to get an appointment with the neurologist. The neurologist ordered an MRI and scheduled the patient for an EMG.

The MRI was scheduled for one week after and the EMG two weeks after the neurologist visit. The patient followed up with the neurologist after these studies were completed (a total of three weeks). The patient indicates that the studies had revealed "disc injury" at C5-6 that resulted in "nerve damage" to the C6 nerve root. The neurologist reinforced the internist's instruction to remain out of work and referred the patient to a pain management physician for injections.

It took three weeks to get an appointment with the pain management physician. The pain management physician scheduled the patient for a "series of three" epidural steroid injections that were provided over a two month period. There was mild improvement for approximately three days after the first injection, but no improvement, even temporarily, after the second and third injections.

The patient later saw a neurosurgeon. It took five weeks to get an appointment with the neurosurgeon. The neurosurgeon recommended surgery. The patient wanted to avoid surgery if possible and therefore sought the advice of a PSP.

The pain is located in the right lower cervical spine and scapula with referral into the right lateral upper arm and dorsal forearm. Right cervical rotation and movements of the right arm increase his pain. He remains out of work. His daily activities include working around the house and he states that doing household chores that require the use of his right arm give him some discomfort. As a result he tries to avoid these activities for fear of "making the disc injury and nerve damage worse". He does not usually have pain at rest although there are times when leaving his arm in one position for a long time gives him pain and he has to change positions. He continues to take the hydrocodone/ acetaminophen and muscle relaxant although he states that "I'm not sure whether they help or not."

He describes "numbness" in his right thumb and index finger although on questioning he indicates that this is not true sensory loss but "a feeling of numbness". He denies focal motor loss although he states that his right arm (dominant) arm generally feels "weaker" than the left. He denies neurologic symptoms in the lower extremities as well as bowel or bladder difficulties. He denies GI or chest symptoms. He denies fever, chills, rigors, constitutional symptoms and unexplained weight loss.

Past Medical History:

Unremarkable. He does not take any medications other than those noted above. He sees his primary care physician regularly.

Review of Systems:

Remarkable for occasional heartburn when he eats spicy foods and constipation since he started taking the medications.

Social History:

He is married with one child. He does not smoke, drinks "a few beers on the weekend" and usually golfs regularly for exercise although he has not done so since the onset of his pain.

Family History:

Remarkable for hypertension and type II diabetes in his mother and prostate cancer in his father.

Questionnaire data:

Neck Pain Screening Tool Long Form - 50
Neck Disability Index - 62%
Average pain intensity over the past week - 7/10.
Fear item on the Neck Pain Screening Tool Long Form – 9/10
Catastrophizing item of the Neck Pain Screening Tool Long Form – 9/10
Problem-Specific Depression scale – 8/10
Self-Efficacy scale – 7/10
Coping Strategies Screening Questionnaire – 3/12

What are your impressions based on the history?

Diagnostic question #1

Diagnostic question #2

Diagnostic question #3

What is the significance of scores on the fear and catastrophizing items of the Neck Pain Screening Tool - long form as well as the depression, self-efficacy and coping scales?

The Neck Pain Screening Tool - long form was adapted from the STarT Back 9-Item Clinical Tool. These tools can be used both to identify the presence of important psychological factors at baseline. They can also be used to track progress in both function and psychological factors. Questions 5-9 on these tools include the fear and catastrophizing items. These items, along with the condition-specific depression scale, the self-efficacy scale and the coping strategies scale, allow the PSP to develop a clear impression regarding the "Big 5" psychological factors that can often be clinically relevant in perpetuating the ongoing pain, disability and suffering experience. Patients with high scores on these scales may require more intensive intervention and monitoring of psychological factors.

In this case, the scores on these items are quite high, suggesting the presence of significant fear, catastrophizing, passive coping, low self-efficacy and depression. These factors may be contributing to the perpetuation of the problem.

Physical Examination:

Reveals a well-nourished, pleasant man who appeared in no acute distress. End range loading examination of the cervical spine in the seated and supine positions reveals painful obstruction in extension in the seated position and this movement reproduces the patient's neck and scapular pain, but not his upper extremity pain. There is no change in range of motion, pain intensity or pain location with repeated movements into extension. Right lateral flexion is unobstructed and reproduces the patient's upper extremity pain. The intensity of the upper extremity pain increases after four repetitions, so the maneuver is stopped. Right rotation also reproduces the patient's upper extremity pain and repetition is not pursued. The Brachial Plexus Tension Test in the median bias position is positive on the right for reproduction of the patient's right upper extremity pain. Structural differentiation reveals this pain to be of neural origin. Palpation for segmental tenderness and manual joint examination reveal increased resistance to motion to manual pressure and reproduction of the patient's neck pain at approximately the C5-6 level on the right. Examination of other segmental levels on the involved side reveals only mild pain. No pain is noted upon examination of individual segments on the left. The Extension-Rotation Test is positive bilaterally for reproduction of the patient's neck pain. The Cervical Stability Test is positive.

The patient is oriented to person, place and time. Heel, toe and tandem walking are within normal limits. Romberg's position is held with eyes closed without difficulty. Sensory examination to pinprick in the upper and lower extremities reveals no abnormalities. Motor strength is 5/5 bilaterally throughout. Muscle stretch reflexes are 2+ and symmetric throughout. Plantar responses are downgoing bilaterally.

The MRI and EMG reports are reviewed and the MRI images are obtained online. The MRI reveals right-sided disc herniation at C5-6 with encroachment on the right C6 nerve root. No other significant findings are noted. The electrodiagnostic report indicates needle EMG findings of increased insertional activity, fibrillation potentials and positive sharp waves in the cervical paraspinal muscles at the C6 level on the right as well as in the right biceps and brachioradialis. The nerve conduction study was normal.

What are your impressions based on the history, examination and imaging? Is further diagnostic testing necessary? Why or why not?

Diagnostic question #1:

Diagnostic question #2:

Diagnostic question #3:

Diagnosis:

The diagnosis is right-sided C6 radiculopathy secondary to C5-6 disc herniation and joint dysfunction at approximately the right C5-6 facet joint (diagnostic question #2) with dynamic instability, fear, catastrophizing, depression, poor coping and low self-efficacy (diagnostic question #3). No findings on history and examination are significant with regard to diagnostic question #1. A further clinical concern is the prolonged work disability and the resultant risk of continued disability.

Further diagnostic testing is not deemed necessary as there are no lingering questions regarding the diagnosis following history and examination.

Are there any factors in the history that might explain the chronicity as well as the significant fear, catastrophizing, depression, poor coping and low self-efficacy?

While it is not possible to determine for certain how the case "would have gone" if it had been managed differently, there are strong indications that the patient's present pain, disability and suffering experience has been greatly influenced by how the situation was handled from the beginning by his primary care physician and subsequent specialists. Several factors support this contention:

1. The patient was prescribed narcotic and muscle relaxant medications despite the fact that these medications are not recommended as a first-line treatment, except in isolated circumstances, by most evidence-based guidelines.

2. The early referral to the neurologist subsequently led to a total of a six-month delay in the institution of an active care plan, given the delay in seeing the neurologist and all the unnecessary testing and referrals that followed the neurologist visit.

3. All of the practitioners who saw the patient employed non-evidence-based treatment recommendations, further delaying the institution of an active, evidence-based, patient-centered management strategy.

4. An MRI was ordered early in the process in spite of the fact that, in all likelihood, there were no clinical indications suggesting the need for this study. It is known that early MRI increases the likelihood of the development of prolonged disability (as well as increased costs – see Webster, et al in the Recommended Reading list). In addition to the unnecessary MRI, an unnecessary EMG was performed despite the fact that the diagnosis of radiculopathy was obvious and there was no need for further confirmation.

5. While it is not possible in this case to know how the findings of the MRI and EMG were communicated to the patient, discussion made it clear that he perceived himself as having "an injured disc" that resulted in "nerve damage". These terms suggest that the patient perceived that he had a serious spinal injury. It is certainly understandable that this, coupled with the fact that he was told that he should avoid work, would lead the patient to assume that a fearsome catastrophe had happened to him (i.e., fear and catastrophizing). It is natural that this would lead to feelings of despair, negative affect and a pessimistic outlook (i.e., depression). And since nothing had been done to help him overcome the problem, it is of no surprise that he has little confidence (i.e., self-efficacy) in his ability to get better and return to normal activities.

6. The patient remained out of work for an entire six months, and none of the practitioners who saw the patient engaged in a targeted return-to-work strategy. On the contrary, all practitioners told the patient to remain out of work. It is well known that the longer a worker remains out of work (either on a light-duty or a full-duty basis) the greater the likelihood of prolonged or even permanent work disability. Thus, it is critical that a clear strategy and discussion for getting back to meaningful work activities should begin right away with all patients. It is common for practitioners to give patients the impression that returning to normal activities, including and especially work, is somehow "dangerous" and increases the likelihood for "reinjury". In fact, the opposite is true – delayed return to normal activities puts patients at risk of chronic pain, disability and suffering.

This case, as with many of the cases presented in this chapter, provides an excellent example for the need to implement primary spine care services, provided by specially trained PSPs, throughout the health care system.

What is your initial management strategy?

The diagnosis is explained to the patient and a treatment plan is begun consisting of manipulation to the C5-6 segment along with neural mobilization in the median bias position. Before the introduction of practitioner-generated treatments the patient is instructed in self-mobilization maneuvers for both the joint and the nerve root (see Chapter 6). Because of the significant psychological findings and the prolonged work disability, the patient is referred to a work hardening (WH) program to immediately start the process of preparation for return to work. He is also given information on anti-inflammatory nutrition [**http://www.deflame.com/** accessed 16 March 2016]. All communications are carried out in a CBT/ACT context.

Manipulation/ neural mobilization/ self-treatment is instituted by the PSP over the course of four sessions in two weeks. WH takes place for four sessions per week. The patient is scheduled to follow up with the PSP two to three weeks after the 4th PSP session.

On the initial visit to the WH facility, functional capacity evaluation (FCE) reveals the patient to be functioning at a Light physical demand level (PDL). Specifically, the FCE report indicated a maximum lifting capacity of 20 pounds and frequent lifting capacity of 10 pounds. It is determined that his full-duty job requires a Heavy PDL. Specifically, the job requires a maximum lifting capacity of 100 pounds and frequent lifting capacity of 50 pounds.

For consideration: Why was self-treatment provided before practitioner-generated treatment?

In the majority of patients, particularly in those with low self-efficacy, it is important to provide patient-generated treatment prior to the institution of practitioner-generated treatment. This delivers a clear message to the patient that the key to recovery is self-care. In addition, it helps to build self-efficacy because in most cases the patient's first experience of benefit from the management strategy will come as a result of something *the patient did by him- or herself*, rather than something that was *done to* the patient.

On re-examination, after four sessions of primary spine care and four weeks of WH, the PSP reviews the most recent FCE report. It indicates that the patient is now functioning at a Medium PDL (maximum lifting capacity of 50 pounds and frequently lifting capacity of 25 pounds). The patient reports 50% improvement.

Questionnaire data at re-examination:

Neck Pain Screening Tool Long Form - 30
Neck Disability Index - 40%
Average pain intensity over the past week - 4/10
Fear item on the Neck Pain Screening Tool Long Form – 4/10
Catastrophizing item of the Neck Pain Screening Tool Long Form – 3/10
Problem-Specific Depression scale – 4/10
Self-Efficacy scale – 3/10
Coping Strategies Screening Questionnaire – 7/12

On examination, sensory examination to pinprick in the upper and lower extremities reveals no abnormalities. Motor strength is 5/5 bilaterally throughout. Muscle stretch reflexes are 2+ and symmetric throughout. Plantar responses are downgoing bilaterally.

For consideration: Why was the Brachial Plexus Tension Test, palpation for segmental tenderness, manual joint examination, Extension-Rotation Test and Cervical Stability Test not repeated on re-examination?

The reason for this is that the patient is feeling better and, most important, gaining confidence (i.e., self-efficacy) in his ability to recover and return to normal activities. Given the duration of his symptoms and the initial significant psychological factors, there is a good likelihood that a certain degree of nociceptive system sensitization is present. While this has likely improved somewhat there is still a chance that some residual hypersensitivity remains. Given this possibility, there is reason to expect that pain provocation tests will remain "positive". In other words, it is highly likely that the Brachial Plexus Tension Test, palpation for segmental tenderness, manual joint examination and Extension-Rotation Test will still be pain provoking. There is also a good chance that the Cervical Stability Test will still be difficult for the patient.

Repeating these tests has the potential to negatively impact the patient's perception of his improvement, causing him to think that he still has "significant damage" in his neck. So it is important for the PSP to consider the potential consequences of repeating the pain provocation tests at re-examination in light of the possibility that these may impair the gains in self-efficacy that have been made during the management strategy. The purpose of pain provocation tests is to establish the diagnosis. In this case, the diagnosis has already been established. Thus, there is no reason to repeat these tests.

What is the best course of action now?

The PSP reviews the report from the WH program with the patient and congratulates him on the great job he is doing. The PSP and patient discuss the importance of continuing the program and the patient is scheduled to return to the PSP in three weeks.

On the next re-examination the PSP reviews the most recent FCE report, which indicates that the patient is now functioning at his required Heavy PDL, specifically a maximum lifting capacity of 100 pounds and frequent lifting capacity of 50 pounds. The patient reports 90% improvement. He states that most of the time he is relatively pain-free although "it has its moments", meaning that there are times in which, for no apparent reason, he has fairly significant pain in his neck and scapula area. This usually does not last a long time. He states that he occasionally has a vague feeling of "numbness" in his right index finger but this does not trouble him.

Questionnaire data at re-examination:

Neck Pain Screening Tool Long Form - 10
Neck Disability Index - 20%
Average pain intensity over the past week - 2/10
Fear item on the Neck Pain Screening Tool Long Form – 2/10
Catastrophizing item of the Neck Pain Screening Tool Long Form – 1/10
Problem-Specific Depression scale – 3/10
Self-Efficacy scale – 2/10
Coping Strategies Screening Questionnaire – 10/12

On examination, sensory examination to pinprick in the upper and lower extremities reveals no abnormalities. Motor strength is 5/5 bilaterally throughout. Muscle stretch reflexes are 2+ and symmetric throughout. Plantar responses are downgoing bilaterally.

What is the best course of action now?

For consideration: Should the PSP explore why the patient has intermittent neck and scapular pain, i.e. look into whether there are residual pain generators, or things he is doing that are aggravating the condition, so these can be corrected?

This may be considered but caution is warranted. In all likelihood the intermittent pain is a normal manifestation of resolving nociceptive system sensitization and will gradually fade over time. If this is the case, there is no need to "explore" anything. The best thing the patient can do to facilitate normalization of his nociceptive system is to engage in normal activities, to "live life" and not worry about the residual pain.

By going through an investigation of lifestyle or tissue-related factors that might be producing the intermittent pain, the PSP runs the risk of giving the patient the impression that "something is still wrong". This can put the thought in the patient's mind that some mysterious pain generator is still lurking below the surface, ready to pounce. Or the patient can be given the impression that there is some activity in which he is engaging that is inconspicuously causing "damage". This has the potential to negatively influence his self-efficacy and his willingness to return to normal activities.

The PSP discusses with the patient that he is fully recovered and is ready to resume all normal activities, including work. It is explained that some residual pain is normal. It is explained that, in general, occasional pain that comes and goes is a normal part of life. The important thing is that he has regained the ability to "get his life back" and there is every indication that he will do well over the long term.

The patient is cleared to return to work on a full-duty basis. It is explained to him that he should initially expect some degree of pain, discomfort or just fatigue. This is normal when returning to work activities and in all likelihood will fade over time as his system adapts to work activities. Pain upon initial return to work does not usually indicate "re-injury" but is a normal result of "pain memory" (which is part of nociceptive system sensitization). When the tissues that had previously been painful return to rigorous activity, it is normal for "pain memory" in the CNS to be stimulated. However, as with any memory, "pain memory" fades over time. This fading occurs more rapidly when it is replaced by "movement memory". "Movement memory" comes from exercise and return to normal activities. Thus, as work activities continue, the CNS adapts and the pain gradually fades.

However, it is explained to the patient that if this adaptation does not occur over the period of a few weeks, returning to the PSP is in order so it can be addressed. The patient understands this and returns to work. It is recommended that the patient continue with his home exercise program. No further visits are scheduled but the patient is welcomed to return if there are future problems.

Case 6

History of the Present Illness:

The patient is a 38-year-old man who complains of low back pain. The pain began insidiously approximately six months previously. He had not sought medical care because for the first few months the pain was intermittent and not severe but as time has passed the pain has become more intense and persistent. It also has begun to disturb his sleep. This leads him to consult his PSP.

The pain is located in the sacroiliac and buttock areas bilaterally without radiation or referral. The pain is often present at night, particularly toward the early morning when it awakens him from sleep and he frequently has difficulty falling back to sleep. Nonsteroidal anti-inflammatory medication reduces the intensity of the pain. When he gets up in the morning his pain is at its worst and he is very stiff in the morning. Once he gets up and starts moving he gradually loosens up, but this can take "quite a bit of time". The PSP asks him specifically how long it takes for him to "loosen up" and he states "at least a couple of hours". He generally has pain after prolonged immobility such as when he is sitting at his desk at work. He goes to the gym regularly and feels fine when he is exercising. In fact, this is when he feels best.

He denies numbness, paresthesia or motor loss in the lower extremities. He denies GI or GU symptoms. He denies bowel or bladder symptoms as well as fever, chills, rigors, constitutional symptoms or unexplained weight loss.

Past Medical History:

Otherwise unremarkable. He is not currently taking any medications. He sees his primary care physician regularly.

Review of Systems:

Remarkable for frequent abdominal pain and diarrhea which he has had for "a few years" and which he never thought was severe enough to seek medical attention; right knee pain that he attributes to prior sports injuries and occasional severe headaches over the past several years that are not accompanied by neurologic symptoms.

Social History:

He is married with one child. He does not smoke, drinks alcohol occasionally and lifts weights and uses cardio machines several times per week for exercise.

Family History:

Remarkable for hypertension in both parents and "some kind of arthritis" in his mother.

Questionnaire data:

STarT Back 9-Item Clinical Tool – 28
Oswestry Low Back Pain and Disability Questionnaire - 32%
Average pain intensity over the past week - 7/10
Fear item on the STarT Back 9-Item Clinical Tool – 3/10

Catastrophizing item of the STarT Back 9-Item Clinical Tool – 7/10
Problem-Specific Depression scale – 4/10
Self-Efficacy scale – 6/10
Coping Strategies Screening Questionnaire – 3/12

What are your impressions based on the history?

Diagnostic question #1

Diagnostic question #2

Diagnostic question #3

Physical Examination:

Reveals a well-nourished, pleasant man who appears in no acute distress. End range loading examination is somewhat restricted and painful (though there is no abrupt obstruction to movement) in extension in the prone position and side gliding to either side. There is no change in range of motion, pain intensity or pain location with repetition or overpressure. Three out of five sacroiliac provocation maneuvers (thigh thrust, sacral thrust, Gaenslen's – see Chapter 5 in Volume I of this series) are positive for reproduction of his pain. Straight Leg Raise is negative bilaterally. Prone Instability Test and Hip Extension Test are both negative. Active Straight Leg Raise Test is positive bilaterally.

The patient is oriented to person, place and time. Heel, toe and tandem walking are within normal limits. Romberg's position is held with eyes closed without difficulty. Sensory examination to pinprick in the lower extremities reveals no abnormalities. Motor strength is 5/5 bilaterally in the lower extremities. Muscle stretch reflexes are 1+ and symmetric in the knees and ankles. Plantar responses are downgoing bilaterally.

What are your impressions based on the history and examination? Is there any indication for imaging, specials tests or specialist consult? Why or why not?

Diagnostic question #1:

Diagnostic question #2:

Diagnostic question 3#:

There is significant concern related to diagnostic question #1. Specifically, the location of the pain, age and gender of the patient, prolonged morning stiffness, relief with NSAID, relief with exercise and the presence of symptoms that might reflect colitis (frequent abdominal pain and diarrhea) raise the concern for the possibility of seronegative spondyloarthropathy.

Plain film radiographs and blood tests are ordered to rule out ankylosing spondylitis (AS). The radiographs include an A-P pelvis as well as a lumbosacral A-P and lateral. The blood work includes CBC with differential, C-reactive protein (CRP), sedimentation rate (sed rate), RA factor, antinuclear antibodies (ANA) and HLA-B27.

The plain film radiographs are normal. The blood work reveals elevated CRP (50mg/L) and sed rate (60mm/h) with normal RA factor and ANA. HLA-B27 is present.

What are your impressions now and what is the best course of action?

A call is placed to the patient's primary care practitioner and the findings are discussed. It is agreed that ankylosing spondylitis is the most likely diagnosis and referral for rheumatologic consult is the best course of action. The rheumatologist confirms the diagnosis and recommends ibuprofen for pain relief.

The patient returns to the PSP and it is decided that a trial of treatment focusing on gentle self-mobilization and exercise is reasonable to see if this produces symptomatic relief and to help the patient on a self-management strategy to maintain mobility and symptom control. The patient is referred for four sessions with a physical therapist who has experience with AS patients.

Because the patient is apparently in an inflammatory phase of the disorder (given the elevated CRP and sed rate) manipulation is not provided at this time. The patient is given information on anti-inflammatory nutrition [**http://www.deflame.com/** accessed 16 March 2016]. All communications are carried out in a CBT/ACT context.

The patient follows up with the PSP after the four sessions with the physical therapist. He states that he is upset about having an incurable disease but is relieved to have a diagnosis. He also states that the therapist was very helpful in giving him strategies to increase and maintain mobility and cope with the disorder. He is thrilled that the therapist and all of the doctors he has seen (including the PSP) have recommended that he continue going to the gym regularly.

Questionnaire data at re-examination:

STarT Back 9-Item Clinical Tool – 21
Oswestry Low Back Pain and Disability Questionnaire - 20%

Average pain intensity over the past week - 5/10
Fear item on the STarT Back 9-Item Clinical Tool – 0/10
Catastrophizing item of the STarT Back 9-Item Clinical Tool – 5/10
Problem-Specific Depression scale – 6/10
Self-Efficacy scale – 3/10
Coping Strategies Screening Questionnaire – 6/12

The PSP recommends the patient continue with the home exercise program and to return if should have an increase in pain or stiffness that he is not able to control himself.

Case 7

History of the Present Illness:

The patient is a 45-year-old man who complains of low back pain and left leg pain. This began approximately eight months previously when he was getting into his car and felt sudden severe pain. He saw a chiropractor and then later saw a spine surgeon who ordered an MRI. The spine surgeon discussed the options of epidural steroid injection (ESI) and surgery but the patient did not pursue treatment at that time. However because the pain persisted over the following several months and there developed greater interference with important activities he decided to pursue primary spine care. He tells the PSP that he regrets the decision to forgo the ESI, specifically stating, "If only I had gotten that shot, I wouldn't be in this situation".

The pain is located in the left lumbosacral area with referral into the left buttock and posterolateral thigh and leg into the lateral foot. Flexion activities particularly aggravate the pain. He has not tried exercise because he is afraid this will make the pain worse although he would like to get back to the gym as well as to running. He generally feels best when he is up and moving as long as he avoids flexion.

He has some "pins and needles" down the left leg but otherwise denies numbness, paresthesia and motor loss in the extremities. He denies numbness or paresthesia in his groin area. He denies bowel or bladder difficulties as well as any other GI, GU or chest symptoms related to the pain. He also denies fever, chills, rigors, constitutional symptoms and unexplained weight loss.

Past Medical History:

Otherwise unremarkable. He is not currently taking any medications.

Review of Systems:

Unremarkable.

Social History:

He is married with three children. He does not smoke, drinks alcohol occasionally and does not currently exercise regularly.

Family History:

Unremarkable.

Questionnaire data:

STarT Back 9-Item Clinical Tool – 33
Oswestry Low Back Pain and Disability Questionnaire - 38%
Average pain intensity over the past week - 8/10
Fear item on the STarT Back 9-Item Clinical Tool – 10/10
Catastrophizing item of the STarT Back 9-Item Clinical Tool – 1/10
Problem-Specific Depression scale – 6/10
Self-Efficacy scale – 5/10
Coping Strategies Screening Questionnaire – 6/12

What are your impressions based on the history?

Diagnostic question #1:

Diagnostic question #2:

Diagnostic question 3#:

Physical Examination:

Reveals a well-nourished, pleasant man who appears in no acute distress. Blood pressure is 138/72 on the left. Temperature is 97.6 degrees Fahrenheit. Pulse is 84 per minute. Respirations are 20 per minute.

End range loading examination is unremarkable in extension and left side gliding. Right side gliding is painfully obstructed and reproduces his low back pain and part, but not all, of his leg pain. Specifically, this maneuver causes pain in the lumbosacral area extending into the buttock and posterolateral thigh but does not extend below the knee. With repetition of right side gliding movements, the pain gradually centralizes out of the posterolateral thigh, into the buttock, and eventually to the lumbosacral area. Of note, the patient reports that as this centralization is occurring the lumbosacral pain steadily increases in intensity. Also, during the repetitive right side gliding movements the painful obstruction gradually lessens with repetition. Straight Leg Raise is positive on the left for reproduction of the patient's leg pain. Structural differentiation determines this pain to be of neural origin. That is, the pain that is produced during Straight Leg Raise is increased by ankle dorsiflexion and decreased by ankle plantar flexion. Well Leg Raise is negative. Prone Instability Test, Hip Extension Test and Active Straight Leg Raise Test are all negative.

The patient is oriented to person, place and time. Heel, toe and tandem walking are within normal limits. Romberg's position is held with eyes closed without difficulty. Sensory examination to pinprick in the lower extremities reveals no abnormalities. Motor strength is 5/5 bilaterally in the lower extremities. Muscle stretch reflexes are 2+ and symmetric in the knees and ankles. Plantar responses are downgoing bilaterally.

Diagnostic Imaging:

The lumbar MRI report and images that had been ordered by the spine surgeon are reviewed online. The study had been conducted approximately three weeks after the onset of pain. The study revealed a large left-sided disc herniation at L5-S1. Incidentally noted is a far lateral disc herniation at L4-5 to the right. No additional imaging is considered necessary at this time.

What are your impressions based on the history, examination and imaging findings?

Diagnostic question #1:

Diagnostic question #2:

Diagnostic question 3#:

Diagnosis:

The diagnosis is left-sided lumbosacral radiculopathy secondary to disc herniation (diagnostic questions #2). A portion of the pain centralized with end range loading examination in right side gliding. Thus right side gliding is the direction of benefit for exercise. An important perpetuating factor is high fear beliefs (diagnostic question #3). No findings on history and examination are significant with regard to diagnostic question #1.

Question for thought: The MRI was ordered by another practitioner, prior to presentation to the PSP. Was this MRI necessary?

Consider: As the MRI was ordered well before the patient saw the PSP, it is not possible to know for sure what the specific clinical findings were at that time. However, based on the history and examination findings at the time of the visit to the PSP there would have been no reason to order an MRI. All clinical indicators were that the patient had radiculopathy. There were no red flags for benign or malignant neoplasm, infection or any other possible cause of radiculopathy. Therefore, there were no clinical indicators that would suggest that the radiculopathy was due to anything other than herniated disc or spinal stenosis.

Given the fact that part of the patient's pain centralized with end range loading examination, the most likely cause of the radiculopathy in this case is herniated disc. This conclusion is based on the fact that the patient exhibited signs of both disc pain and nerve root pain. Either way, the primary-level treatment in this case does not necessitate knowing with absolute certainty the cause of the radiculopathy. Thus, MRI could have been deferred and treatment instituted, with consideration for MRI at a later time if the patient did not respond to primary spine care in a reasonable amount of time, or if the clinical findings changed in such a way as to suggest a factor related to Diagnostic Question #1.

Question for thought: What is an evidence-based response to the patient's statement "If only I had gotten that shot, I wouldn't be in this situation"?

The patient can be told that he should not get down on himself for this decision. While an ESI can often bring about substantial relief of acute pain, it generally does not, in and of itself, affect long-term prognosis. So with no treatment other than the ESI, it is unlikely that his condition would be any different eight months after onset, whether or not he had received the injection.

What is your initial management strategy?

The patient is set up with a home routine of end range loading exercises in right side gliding that he is to perform 10 repetitions 4-6 times per day. He is told to stop the exercise if the pain should steadily increase in intensity or peripheralize during a set or over the next few days of doing the exercise. However, he is assured that this is not expected to happen.

He is treated with distraction manipulation focused at the L5-S1 disc and with neural mobilization of the involved nerve root. He is given information on anti-inflammatory nutrition [**http://www.deflame.com/** accessed 16 March 2016]. All communications are carried out in a CBT/ACT context.

He is seen four times over a two week period followed by re-examination.

At re-examination the patient reports 60% improvement. He states that he tried running for the first time and was able to run for 40 minutes without difficulty. He states that he was "sore" in his lower back the next morning upon awakening but this markedly improved after doing his right side gliding exercise.

Questionnaire data at re-examination:

STarT Back 9-Item Clinical Tool score – 13
Oswestry Low Back Pain and Disability Questionnaire - 22%
Average pain intensity over the past week - 2/10
Fear item on the STarT Back 9-Item Clinical Tool – 4/10
Catastrophizing item of the STarT Back 9-Item Clinical Tool – 1/10
Problem-Specific Depression scale – 3/10
Self-Efficacy scale – 2/10
Coping Strategies Screening Questionnaire – 10/12

On examination, end range loading in right side gliding is pain-free and within normal limits. Extension in the prone position "feels tight" at end range but the patient states that with repetition it "seems to loosen up". Straight Leg Raise is positive on the left for "pulling" but not pain. Sensory examination to pinprick in the lower extremities is unremarkable. Motor strength is 5/5 bilaterally in the lower extremities. Muscle stretch reflexes are 2+ and symmetric in the knees and ankles. Prone Instability Test, Hip Extension Test and Active Straight Leg Raise Test are all negative.

Does the patient require continued treatment sessions with the PSP or another professional? If so, what should this consist of? If not, what it the best course of action now?

The patient is told that it is likely that he will be able to continue his progress on his own with exercise and self-management. He is given three additional exercises - the co-contraction maneuver (see Chapter 11 in Volume I of this series), the press up (see Chapter 5 in Volume I of this series) and the "Good Morning" exercise (see Chapter 9 in Volume I of this series). He is taught to use the "Good Morning" exercise to facilitate proper lifting technique by flexing at the hips and maintaining lumbar lordosis. He is told to gradually increase his running distance and to return to his weight training routine, starting with light weights and gradually increasing over time. It is recommended that he follow up in three weeks.

Question for thought: Why was the patient not put on a more extensive lumbar stabilization exercise program?

There were no signs of dynamic instability, as the Prone Instability Test, Hip Extension Test and Active Straight Leg Raise Test were all negative. In addition, the patient practiced good physical fitness habits prior to the onset of his pain, it was felt that the most efficient way to promote self-efficacy was to provide the patient with a basic, evidence-based program to limit the likelihood of frequent recurrence and to monitor the result of this basic program.

At three-week follow-up the patient reports that he is essentially pain-free although there are occasions when he experiences mild back and/or leg pain. He is functioning normally in all his usual activities of daily living and is back to his usual running and weight training regimen. He has continued with his home exercise program.

It is explained to the patient that he is fully recovered. He is told that some level of occasional pain is a normal part of life. There may continue to be occasions in which he may experience pain in his back and/or leg, sometimes for no apparent reason. Again, it is emphasized that this is normal. He is told that if he should experience back and or leg pain that is significant enough to be bothersome or to interfere with activities, he should return to the side gliding exercise that he had initially been given. It is reasonable to expect the pain to markedly improve within a day or so. If the pain does not improve, or if it peripheralizes while doing the side gliding exercise, he should return to the PSP.

Case 8

History of the Present Illness:

The patient is an 80-year-old woman who complains of lower thoracic pain. This began two days previously when she was cooking and tripped over an object that was on the floor behind her, causing her to fall onto her back. She had the immediate onset of pain. The pain is well localized to the lower thoracic area without radiation or referral. She states that "all movements are excruciating". When lying down she is gradually able to get comfortable in the supine or side lying position but it takes some time to get into the position and relax. She rates the pain intensity as 10/10. She denies rash or skin eruptions in the area. She denies recent illness or fever. She denies numbness, paresthesia or motor loss in the lower extremities as well as ataxia of gait. She denies bowel or bladder difficulty.

Past Medical History:

Remarkable for hypertension for which she takes a beta blocker, hypercholesterolemia for which she takes a statin and left breast cancer at age 62 which was treated with lumpectomy and radiation. She sees her primary care practitioner regularly and has regular cancer screenings.

Review of Systems:

Remarkable for occasional constipation and bilateral tinnitus that she has had "for years".

Social History:

She is married with four grown children. She does not smoke, drinks one glass of wine each night with dinner and approximately two weeks prior had started a "Strengthening for Seniors" exercise program that consists of strength exercises using dumbbells done in a group setting. She states that she was excited about this program because she had not exercised regularly for "decades". She very much wants to get back to the program as soon as possible. She also normally goes for walks in her neighborhood for exercise though she has not done so since the onset of her pain.

Family History:

Remarkable for heart disease in her father and two of her brothers and type 2 diabetes in her sister.

Questionnaire data:

STarT Back 9-Item Clinical Tool – 56
Oswestry Low Back Pain and Disability Questionnaire - 84%
Average pain intensity - 10/10
Fear item on the STarT Back 9-Item Clinical Tool – 8/10
Catastrophizing item of the STarT Back 9-Item Clinical Tool – 6/10
Problem-Specific Depression scale – 7/10
Self-Efficacy scale – 4/10
Coping Strategies Screening Questionnaire – 0/12

What are your impressions based on the history?

Diagnostic question #1:

Diagnostic question #2:

Diagnostic question 3#:

Physical Examination:

Reveals a well-nourished, pleasant woman who appears in acute pain. Blood pressure is 142/88. Temperature is 98.6 degrees Fahrenheit. Pulse is 92 per minute. Respirations are 20 per minute.

She does not appear to have an accentuated thoracic kyphosis on visual inspection.

The examination is difficult because of the intensity of the pain and difficulty with movement. The patient displays intense pain behavior when attempting to lie on the examining table. Once she is lying down and at rest, the pain is less intense. Segmental palpation at the level of pain is quite painful and percussion of the spinous processes is not attempted. The patient again exhibits intense pain behavior when arising from the table.

The patient is oriented to person, place and time. Heel, toe and tandem walking are within normal limits although they are somewhat painful. Romberg's position is held with eyes closed without difficulty. Sensory examination to pinprick in the lower extremities and trunk reveals no abnormalities. Motor strength is 5/5 bilaterally in the lower extremities. Muscle stretch reflexes are 1+ and symmetric in the knees and absent bilaterally in the ankles. Plantar responses are downgoing bilaterally.

What are your impressions based on the history and examination? Is there any indication for imaging, specials tests or specialist consult? Why or why not?

Diagnostic question #1:

Diagnostic question #2:

Diagnostic question #3:

Diagnosis:

There is significant concern related to diagnostic question #1. The PSP tells the patient that she likely has a fracture and that radiographs are needed to clarify the diagnosis. A stat thoracic spine radiographic study is ordered. The PSP receives the report on the same day and views the images online. They reveal a compression fracture of the vertebral body at T10 with approximately 15% loss of vertebral body height. There is no retropulsion noted and the posterior elements appear intact. Bone density appears normal.

A discussion takes place between the PSP and patient regarding options, which include surgical referral for consideration of kyphoplasty, bracing or watchful waiting. A shared decision is made to apply a brace for use when she is weightbearing, with specific instructions to gradually decrease the time in the brace as the intensity of the pain subsides and her functional abilities improve. She is instructed to rest completely for the next two days. After two days she is to get up and start walking around, as pain allows, while wearing the brace. Gradually she is to start normal activities such as housework, again while wearing the brace. She is also given information on anti-inflammatory nutrition [**http://www.deflame.com/** accessed 16 March 2016]. All communications are carried out in a CBT/ACT context.

At the same time a call is placed to her primary care practitioner so that she can be apprised of the situation and order a bone density study if she feels it is appropriate.

The patient follows up one week later and reports continued severe pain, although the overall intensity has decreased somewhat. She states that she was able to get up and start walking around after two days of complete rest, as instructed, and has increased the frequency from three times initially to five to six times for the past couple of days. The PSP recommends the patient continue this process and return in two weeks for follow up, although she can come in sooner if she feels the need.

The patient follows up two weeks later and reports 50% improvement. She states that her pain is substantially improved and that she is able to do most normal household chores without severe pain, though she continues to wear the brace for most of these activities. Simply moving around the house does not necessitate the use of the brace. She has gone out to take a short walk a couple of times but she is nervous about falling again so she has limited this activity.

Questionnaire data at re-examination:

STarT Back 9-Item Clinical Tool score – 29
Oswestry Low Back Pain and Disability Questionnaire - 38%
Average pain intensity over the past week - 5/10
Fear item on the STarT Back 9-Item Clinical Tool – 6/10
Catastrophizing item of the STarT Back 9-Item Clinical Tool – 3/10
Problem-Specific Depression scale – 3/10
Self-Efficacy scale – 2/10
Coping Strategies Screening Questionnaire – 5/12

No excessive kyphosis is noted on standing inspection.

What is the best course of action now?

The patient is instructed to start taking more walks outside but to move slowly and wear her brace. She is instructed to start gradually reducing the amount of time she spends in the brace during household activities, with the specific instruction to only wear it during activities that require heavy lifting, such as when doing laundry.

The patient follows up again three weeks later and reports 70% improvement. She is now doing all usual household chores and only wears the brace when lifting heavy objects. She has taken four or five walks outside although she is still somewhat nervous about this activity for fear of falling.

Questionnaire data:

STarT Back 9-Item Clinical Tool score – 22
Oswestry Low Back Pain and Disability Questionnaire - 22%
Average pain intensity over the past week – 3/10
Fear item on the STarT Back 9-Item Clinical Tool – 5/10
Catastrophizing item of the STarT Back 9-Item Clinical Tool – 2/10
Problem-Specific Depression scale – 2/10
Self-Efficacy scale – 2/10
Coping Strategies Screening Questionnaire – 7/12

No excessive kyphosis is noted on standing inspection.

What is the best course of action now?

The patient is instructed to continue wearing the brace for heavy lifting activities but not to wear it at other times. She is educated as to the fact that compression fractures can take up to three months to fully heal, so care must be taken during that time, even if she is relatively pain-free. It is recommended that the patient return in one month unless she has increased pain or other problems.

The patient follows up again one month later and reports 90% improvement. She is now doing all usual household chores and wears the brace only occasionally when lifting heavy objects. She has been taking her usual daily walks although she walks more slowly than usual to limit the likelihood of falling.

Questionnaire data:

STarT Back 9-Item Clinical Tool score – 10
Oswestry Low Back Pain and Disability Questionnaire - 16%
Average pain intensity over the past week – 1/10
Fear item on the STarT Back 9-Item Clinical Tool – 2/10
Catastrophizing item of the STarT Back 9-Item Clinical Tool – 1/10

Problem-Specific Depression scale – 1/10
Self-Efficacy scale – 1/10
Coping Strategies Screening Questionnaire – 10/12

On examination no excessive kyphosis is noted on standing inspection. Palpation and percussion in the middle and lower thoracic spine are both pain-free.

What is the best course of action now?

The PSP recommends that the patient wait three full months before returning to the "Strengthening for Seniors" class, and only to do so if she is able to carry out all activities of daily living without pain. She is told to return to the PSP if she develops any pain.

For consideration: Depending on the PSP's experience, comfort level and local professional regulations, an alternate and appropriate course of action from the beginning could have been early referral to an orthopedist or physiatrist for management and monitoring.

Case 9

History of the Present Illness:

The patient is a 68-year-old woman who is referred to the PSP by her primary care physician with a diagnosis of "spinal stenosis". She complains of left lower extremity pain that particularly bothers her when she is walking. Because of the lower extremity pain she has had to limit her exercise walks, which has been her primary form of exercise. The pain started insidiously approximately eight months previously and has been steadily worsening since that time. She finally reported it to her primary care practitioner who ordered an MRI. According to the report, the MRI revealed central and left lateral stenosis at L4-5.

The pain is located in the left buttock and lateral hip with referral into the left lateral thigh, extending just below the knee. She states the pain is very severe when she is walking and goes away almost immediately when she sits down. Upon questioning, she states that the pain starts right away when she first begins to walk and that it increases in intensity as she continues to walk. She has no pain when sitting but after she has been sitting for a long time she has trouble standing up due to the pain.

She denies numbness, paresthesia or motor loss in the lower extremities. She denies swelling, coldness or discoloration in the lower extremities. She denies bowel or bladder difficulties as well as any other GI or GU symptoms related to the pain. She also denies fever, chills, rigors, constitutional symptoms and unexplained weight loss.

Past Medical History:

Remarkable for hypertension for which she takes a beta blocker, hysterectomy at age 50 due to uterine fibroids, depression for which she takes a selective serotonin reuptake inhibitor and asthma for which she uses an inhaler. She also takes a statin medication to control her blood cholesterol. She sees her primary care physician regularly and has regular cancer screenings.

Review of Systems:

Remarkable for right-sided tinnitus which she has had for several years, occasional heart palpitations, particularly on days when she has a second cup of coffee, occasional heartburn for which she takes an other-the-counter medication and emotional distress due to her inability to take her regular walks.

Social History:

She is married with two grown children. She does not smoke, drinks alcohol occasionally and tries to walk as much as she can for exercise.

Family History:

Remarkable for hypertension and type II diabetes in both parents and lung cancer in her brother.

Questionnaire data:

STarT Back 9-Item Clinical Tool – 25
Oswestry Low Back Pain and Disability Questionnaire - 42%
Average pain intensity over the past week - 7/10
Fear item on the STarT Back 9-Item Clinical Tool – 6/10
Catastrophizing item of the STarT Back 9-Item Clinical Tool – 3/10
Problem-Specific Depression scale – 6/10
Self-Efficacy scale – 5/10
Coping Strategies Screening Questionnaire – 3/12

What are your impressions based on the history?

Diagnostic question #1:

Diagnostic question #2:

Diagnostic question #3:

Physical Examination:

Reveals a well-nourished, pleasant woman who appears in no acute distress. Blood pressure is 130/84 on the left. Temperature is 98.4 degrees Fahrenheit. Pulse is 80 per minute. Respirations are 16 per minute.

End range loading examination is somewhat restricted but not painful in extension and side gliding to either side. Straight Leg Raise on the left reveals "painful tightness" in the left posterior thigh and calf at approximately 60 degrees. Structural differentiation determines this to be of neural origin. Straight Leg Raise on the right reveals an identical finding - "painful tightness" in the posterior thigh and calf at approximately 60 degrees that increases with ankle dorsiflexion and decreases with ankle plantar flexion (i.e., the "painful tightness" is determined to be of neural origin). Sacroiliac provocation maneuvers are unremarkable. Placing the involved lower extremity in the "Figure 4" position and gently but firmly pressing downward on the knee (Patrick's Test) reproduces the patient's lateral hip and lateral thigh pain. Resisted abduction of the left lower extremity reproduces the patient's lateral hip pain. Palpation of the left greater trochanteric area also reproduces the patient's lateral hip pain. Palpation of the left piriformis muscle is unremarkable. Hip Extension Test, Prone Instability Test and Active Straight Leg Raise Test are all negative.

The patient is oriented to person, place and time. Heel, toe and tandem walking are within normal limits. Romberg's position is held with eyes closed without difficulty. Sensory examination to pinprick in the lower extremities reveals no abnormalities. Motor strength is 5/5 bilaterally in the lower extremities. Muscle stretch reflexes are 2+ and symmetric in the knees and absent bilaterally in the ankles. Plantar responses are downgoing bilaterally. The lower extremity peripheral pulses are intact bilaterally.

Diagnostic Imaging:

Both the MRI report and the images are reviewed and they confirm the finding of central and left lateral stenosis at L4-5.

What is your diagnostic impression based on history, examination and imaging?

Diagnostic question #1:

Diagnostic question #2:

Diagnostic question #3:

Diagnosis:

The diagnosis is greater trochanteric pain syndrome, which is sometimes referred to as "trochanteric bursitis". High fear and condition-specific depression are potential perpetuating factors however the score on these items is only 6/10 so this is not a strong concern.

What is your initial management strategy?

The patient is set up with a home routine of self-stretching exercises for the greater trochanteric area and is gradually transitioned to basic pelvic stabilization exercises. As the management strategy is provided in a CBT/ ACT context and involves primarily self-treatment, it is expected that the fear and condition-specific depression, as well as self-efficacy, will rapidly improve without specific intervention or discussion. She is given information on anti-inflammatory nutrition [**http://www.deflame.com/** accessed 16 March 2016].

This case presentation is not followed through the entire management process because it is presented for an important and specific reason. It is used as an example of a common occurrence in primary spine care. This is a patient who is suspected to have spinal stenosis but who actually has lower extremity pain and difficulty walking as a result of greater trochanteric pain syndrome.

In this case the diagnosis of spinal stenosis was based on the fact she complained of lower extremity pain that worsened with walking. In addition, she is at an age at which symptoms from spinal stenosis commonly begin. Finally, the MRI actually appeared to confirm the diagnosis of spinal stenosis.

However, upon further detailed history and examination by the PSP it became clear that greater trochanteric pain syndrome was the correct diagnosis. The finding of central and lateral stenosis on the MRI was actually a red herring – it was an asymptomatic finding that was not clinically relevant. This illustrates the important point that it is important to "treat the patient, not the image". Specifically in this case, it was the clinical findings that were informative in establishing the diagnosis, not the imaging findings.

It is common for patients with greater trochanteric pain syndrome to be mistakenly diagnosed with spinal stenosis (see Tortolani, et al in the Recommended Reading list at the end of the next chapter). Therefore, the PSP can expect to see a large number of patients with this disorder.

It should be noted that the current accepted terms for this disorder is "greater trochanteric pain syndrome" rather than the previous term, "trochanteric bursitis". The reason for this is that there a number of tissues in the greater trochanteric area that can become painful, including bursae, tendons and muscular structures. It is usually not possible in the vast majority of patients to distinguish the precise structure that is involved, but it is also usually not necessary to do so, because effective treatment can still be instituted. For more information see Williams and Cohen in the Recommended Reading list at the end of the next chapter.

•Chapter 10 •
Case Studies in Primary Spine Care - Part II

Introduction

This is a continuation of the case presentation format of the previous chapter. Presented here are additional patient scenarios encountered by the primary spine practitioner (PSP). Their purpose, as in the previous chapter, is to illustrate the diagnostic and treatment process, using Clinical Reasoning in Spine Pain® (the CRISP® protocols) as well as the role of the PSP in *managing the patient across the full cycle*. That is, guiding the patient and helping him- or her navigate through the process from the point of having the spine-related disorder to the point of resolution. See Chapter 1 for a more detailed discussion of this important concept.

As a reminder, the three questions of diagnosis within the CRISP® protocols are:

Diagnostic question #1: Do the presenting symptoms reflect a visceral disorder, or a serious or potentially life-threatening illness?

Diagnostic question #2: Where is the pain coming from?

      a. Disc derangement

      b. Joint dysfunction

      c. Radiculopathy

      d. Myofascial pain

Diagnostic question #3: What is happening with this person as a whole that would cause the pain experience to develop and persist?

a. Dynamic or passive instability

b. Nociceptive system sensitization

c. Oculomotor dysfunction (in cervical patients)

d. Psychological factors

Case 10

History of the Present Illness:

The patient is a 53-year-old man who complains of right-sided low back pain. This began insidiously approximately four months prior. He did not seek medical attention because "I kept waiting for it to go away" but the pain gradually increased in intensity so he decided to consult a PSP.

The pain is well localized to the right lumbosacral area without radiation or referral. The pain particularly bothers him when he is working overhead, which he frequently does during the course of his job doing taping and spackling of new houses. He has trouble finding a comfortable position when going to sleep but is eventually able to fall asleep. However, the pain often wakes him up at night when he turns in bed. Because of this, he has been very tired. He has no pain when walking, sitting or standing from a sitting position.

He denies numbness, paresthesia or motor loss in the extremities or groin. He denies bowel or bladder difficulties as well as any other GI or GU symptoms related to the pain. He also denies fever, chills, rigors, constitutional symptoms and unexplained weight loss.

Past Medical History:

Remarkable for hypertension for which he takes a beta blocker. He sees his primary care practitioner regularly and has regular cancer screenings.

Review of Systems:

Remarkable for occasional left foot pain, stemming from an injury he had a number of years ago, as well as occasional heart palpations after drinking coffee.

Social History:

He is divorced with two children, both of whom live with him part-time. He does not smoke, drinks alcohol occasionally and does not exercise regularly.

Family History:

Remarkable for prostate cancer and hypertension in his father and stroke in his mother.

Questionnaire data:

STarT Back 9-Item Clinical Tool - 30
Oswestry Low Back Pain and Disability Questionnaire - 40%
Average pain intensity over the past week - 7/10
Fear item on the STarT Back 9-Item Clinical Tool – 6/10
Catastrophizing item of the STarT Back 9-Item Clinical Tool – 7/10
Problem-Specific Depression scale – 5/10
Self-Efficacy scale – 6/10
Coping Strategies Screening Questionnaire – 6/12

What are your impressions based on the history?

Diagnostic question #1

Diagnostic question #2

Diagnostic question #3

Physical Examination:

Reveals a well-nourished, pleasant man who appears in no acute distress. Blood pressure is 118/68 on the left. Temperature is 98.6 degrees Fahrenheit. Pulse is 68 per minute. Respirations are 12 per minute.

End range loading examination in extension reveals reproduction of pain without obstruction. The pain increases in intensity with repetition and with overpressure but there is no peripheralization of pain. Flexion and side gliding to either side are mildly uncomfortable and unobstructed. Sacroiliac provocation maneuvers are all negative. The Extension-Rotation test is positive bilaterally for reproduction of the patient's pain. Hip Extension Test is positive on the right for deviation of the lumbar spine. Prone Instability Test and Active Straight Leg Raise Test are both negative.

The patient is oriented to person, place and time. Heel, toe and tandem walking are within normal limits. Romberg's position is held with eyes closed without difficulty. Sensory examination to pinprick in the lower extremities reveals no abnormalities. Motor strength is 5/5 bilaterally in the lower extremities. Muscle stretch reflexes are 2+ and symmetric in the knees and ankles. Plantar responses are downgoing bilaterally.

What are your impressions based on the history and examination? Is there any indication for diagnostic imaging, specials tests or specialist consult? Why or why not?

Diagnostic question #1:

Diagnostic question #2:

Diagnostic question #3:

Diagnosis:

The diagnosis is lumbosacral facet joint dysfunction (diagnostic question #2) with dynamic instability and moderate psychological factors (diagnostic question #3). There are no immediate concerns regarding diagnostic question #1, thus there is no indication for diagnostic imaging, special tests or specialist consult.

What is your initial management strategy?

The patient is set up with a home routine of self-mobilization exercises. Initially these consist of the Cat and Camel exercise (see Chapter 10 in Volume I of this series), and after one week bilateral side gliding (see Chapter 5 of Volume I of this series). In addition, manipulation is directed toward the lumbosacral facet joints on the right. He is given information on anti-inflammatory nutrition. All communications are carried out in a Cognitive-Behavioral Therapy/ Acceptance and Commitment Therapy (CBT/ACT) context.

The patient is seen four times over a two-week period after which re-examination takes place.

At re-examination the patient reports 10% improvement. He states that he "feels great after the manipulations" but the pain returns within a few hours. He has been compliant with the home exercises and while these "hurt a little", there is no lasting pain afterward.

Questionnaire data at re-examination:

STarT Back 9-Item Clinical Tool – 28
Oswestry Low Back Pain and Disability Questionnaire - 36%
Average pain intensity over the past week - 7/10
Fear item on the STarT Back 9-Item Clinical Tool – 5/10
Catastrophizing item of the STarT Back 9-Item Clinical Tool – 6/10
Problem-Specific Depression scale – 5/10
Self-Efficacy scale – 7/10
Coping Strategies Screening Questionnaire – 6/12

End range loading examination is repeated and reveals essentially the same findings as at initial examination – extension is painful but unobstructed; upon repetition there is increased pain without peripheralization. Flexion and side gliding to either side remain unremarkable. Sacroiliac provocation maneuvers are all negative. The Extension-Rotation test remains positive bilaterally for reproduction of the patient's pain. Neurodynamic examination is negative. Palpation of the lumbosacral multifidus muscle in the right lumbosacral area reveals myofascial trigger points that exactly reproduce the patient's pain. Hip Extension Test remains positive on the right for deviation of the lumbar spine. Prone Instability Test and Active Straight Leg Raise Test both remain negative.

What is the best course of action now?

Despite the initial trial of treatment the patient has not experienced clinically meaningful improvement in pain or function. Chapter 12 of Volume I in this series includes a discussion of strategies that can be applied to situations in which the patient does not respond as expected to an initial trial of treatment. Possibilities to consider are:

1. The diagnosis is not correct.

2. The diagnosis is partly correct but there are factors contributing to the patient's pain, disability and suffering experience that had not previously been detected or addressed.

3. The diagnosis is correct but the treatment being applied is not the best one in that particular case.

4. The diagnosis and treatment are appropriate but there are perpetuating factors, including activities of daily living, ergonomics, "stress" or other issues that are interfering with recovery.

5. The patient has not been compliant with exercise and self-care recommendations.

Therefore, the re-examination process should focus on investigating these possibilities and making alterations accordingly. This involves:

1. Re-applying the CRISP® protocols by repeating the history and examination to confirm or revise the diagnosis.

2. If the diagnosis appears to be correct, considering alternate treatments designed to address that diagnosis.

3. Discussing with the patient work, home and recreational behavior (or beliefs) to determine whether potential perpetuating factors can be uncovered.

4. Reviewing the exercise and self-care strategies to determine the patient's level of compliance or whether they are being performed as directed.

5. Asking the patient if he or she has any ideas as to why improvement has not occurred.

The PSP asks the patient what kinds of activities he has been engaging in and he states that he has not changed anything other than reducing the amount of time he spends with overhead activities at work since these provoke the pain. He states that his coworkers have been able to do most of the overhead work and he has taken over much of the work that involves sitting or kneeling, as these positions do not bother him. He states that "other than that, my everyday life has not changed much." He states that he has been consistent with his exercises and that these only bother him a little bit. The patient denies any new symptoms. Upon questioning he specifically denies GI or GU symptoms, fever, chills, rigors, constitutional symptoms or unexplained weight loss.

Because an additional diagnostic factor has been found, i.e., multifidus trigger points (diagnostic question #2) and the dynamic instability has persisted (diagnostic question #3) it is decided that treatment will continue with the addition of pressure release and muscle lengthening procedures targeting the multifidus muscles (see Chapter 10 in Volume I of this series) and spinal stabilization exercises (see Chapter 11 in Volume I of this series), that are taught and performed in the clinic with an emphasis on performing these daily at home. So that additional time can be spent on the stabilization exercise, the PSP arranges to have this phase of care take place in the physical therapy department. Sessions are scheduled twice per week for three weeks, after which the PSP follows up with the patient.

At the next re-examination the patient reports 40% improvement. He states that his pain has improved somewhat and he only occasionally has pain at night when turning in bed. However, he has tried gradually increasing the time he spends performing overhead activities and is still only able to tolerate these a few minutes at a time before the pain becomes severe.

The report from the physical therapist indicates that he has progressed well with his stabilization exercise program and has been performing exercise both on the floor and using an exercise ball (see Chapter 11 in Volume I of this series). The therapist reports that the patient has been compliant with his home exercise program and bought himself an exercise ball to use at home. The therapist has tried a graded exposure approach to increasing the amount of time spend with overhead activities (see Chapter 11 in Volume I of this series), but the patient continues to report pain after only a few minutes.

Questionnaire data at re-examination:

STarT Back 9-Item Clinical Tool score – 26
Oswestry Low Back Pain and Disability Questionnaire - 34%
Average pain intensity over the past week - 7/10
Fear item on the STarT Back 9-Item Clinical Tool – 6/10
Catastrophizing item of the STarT Back 9-Item Clinical Tool – 6/10
Problem-Specific Depression scale – 5/10
Self-Efficacy scale – 7/10
Coping Strategies Screening Questionnaire – 6/12

On examination the Extension-Rotation test remains positive bilaterally for reproduction of the patient's pain. Palpation of the right lumbosacral multifidus muscle also remains positive for reproduction of the patient's pain. Hip Extension Test is now negative bilaterally.

The patient has continued pain that is consistent with lumbosacral facet pain and multifidus myofascial pain. The dynamic instability has resolved, at least based on examination findings. Although the patient does not have any hard "red flags" for serious illness, because he has continued pain despite six weeks of targeted, evidence-based management, an MRI is ordered. It is recommended that the patient continue with his home exercise program.

The MRI is negative. It only reveals some normal age-related "degenerative" changes. The PSP follows up with the patient and explains the MRI findings ("completely normal for your age"). The PSP and patient discuss options. The PSP explains that facet joint dysfunction still appears to be the pain generator and recommends the patient see a physical medicine specialist (physiatrist) who might be able to help clarify this. The PSP explains that the physical medicine specialist might recommend facet injections to determine whether these provide reduction in pain intensity. If substantial reduction in pain intensity does occur, this increases the likelihood that the facet joint is the source of pain. Typically, the pain reduction is temporary but there are some individuals in whom it is longer lasting. In addition, the PSP recommends a trial of manipulation after joint analgesia, which would involve the patient seeing the PSP within two days of injection to take advantage of the analgesic effect of the injection. This might promote longer-lasting benefit. If it does not, the patient, PSP and physical medicine specialist can then discuss the possibility of further procedures such as medial branch block and radiofrequency ablation. However, the first step is to meet with the specialist to get further input.

For consideration: Specialists who utilize injections are most commonly physiatrists or anesthesiologists. Some orthopedic spine surgeons or neurosurgeons perform these procedures as well. The important thing for the PSP is to identify a practitioner in his or her community who has a solid reputation for judicious use of these procedures based on sound clinical reasoning.

The patient sees the physiatrist who agrees with the clinical diagnosis of facet pain and applies a facet block. The patient sees the PSP two days later and reports substantial improvement in pain intensity, rating his current pain as 2/10. The PSP applies manipulation targeting the lumbosacral facet joints and the patient is scheduled to follow up again in two weeks.

At two-week follow up the patient reports that the pain returned to an intensity of 7/10 within one or two days of the prior visit. Thus, no lasting benefit was seen as a result of the injection. However, the substantial short-term improvement supports the diagnosis of facet pain.

The patient sees the physiatrist again who recommends a medical branch block to further confirm the diagnosis, with a consideration, if this procedure provides substantial decrease in pain intensity, for the possibility of radiofrequency ablation (see Chapter 12 in Volume I of this series).

The PSP receives a report from the physiatrist that states that a diagnostic medial branch block had been performed with the short-acting local anesthetic agent lidocaine. The patient reported substantial decrease in pain intensity (a reduction to 2/10) for approximately six hours following the procedure. The pain then returned to the baseline 7/10 intensity. The patient followed up with the physiatrist three days later and together they decided that, as the patient experienced substantial temporary improvement in pain intensity after both facet block and a single medial branch block, confidence in the diagnosis of facet pain was great enough to warrant a radiofrequency neurotomy procedure. The procedure was performed and the patient follows up with the PSP two weeks later.

For consideration: Guidelines often recommend confirmation of facet-mediated pain with double medial branch blocks before consideration of radiofrequency ablation. With double medial branch blocks, an initial block is performed using short-acting local anesthetic agent such as lidocaine, followed by a second block being using a long-acting local anesthetic such as bupivacaine. It is determined whether there is substantial (50-80%) improvement in pain after each block that lasts for a period of time that would be consistent with each medication that is injected (i.e., approximately six hours after injection with lidocaine and approximately 12 hours after injection with bupivacaine). However, there are times in which it is deemed clinically prudent to make the decision based on clearly documented substantial decrease in pain intensity (as determined by pre- and post-injection pain scales) after a joint block and a single medial branch block, such as occurred in this case.

At follow up with the PSP the patient reports minimal pain since the radiofrequency ablation. He states that he is now able to work overhead with occasional discomfort, which he is able to relieve by briefly stretching into flexion. He has no pain that interferes with his work. He has been sleeping without pain as well.

Questionnaire data at re-examination:

STarT Back 9-Item Clinical Tool score – 4
Oswestry Low Back Pain and Disability Questionnaire - 4%
Average pain intensity over the past week - 1/10
Fear item on the STarT Back 9-Item Clinical Tool – 0/10
Catastrophizing item of the STarT Back 9-Item Clinical Tool – 0/10
Problem-Specific Depression scale – 0/10
Self-Efficacy scale – 2/10
Coping Strategies Screening Questionnaire – 10/12

The PSP discusses with the patient that the radiofrequency procedure has been successful. The PSP states that the duration of pain improvement with this procedure is highly variable but can last for eight months to a year, and sometimes longer. However occasional back pain is a normal part of life so the presence of some pain in the back at any given time does not necessarily indicate that "the problem has returned". The PSP recommends that the patient continue with the home lumbar stabilization exercise program and to start a fitness regimen, as these will decrease the likelihood and impact of any future low back pain. It is recommended that the patient return if he should develop pain that interferes with activity and lasts for more than a couple of days.

Case 11

History of the Present Illness:

The patient is a 45-year-old woman who complains of mid back pain. This began insidiously approximately eight months ago. She states that approximately four months ago she had "chiropractic care" which consisted of manipulation to the cervical, thoracic and lumbar spine as well as hot packs. She states that she had "about a dozen" sessions and that this treatment provided some temporary relief but the benefit did not last. She heard that her local hospital provided primary spine care services and so called to make an appointment.

The pain is well localized to the mid thoracic area, spreading bilaterally a few inches from the spine. She states that "sometimes it feels like it goes through to my chest." She denies chest pain with exertion as well as heart palpitations, shortness of breath or nausea. Prolonged standing and reaching overhead particularly aggravate the pain. She works as a librarian and frequently has to reach books that are on high shelves. She finds this difficult because of the pain. She also has pain when she spends a lot of time at the computer. She does not have pain when lying down. She sometimes takes over-the-counter anti-inflammatory medications when her pain is particularly severe and these seem to help.
She denies rash, itching or skin eruptions in the area. She denies abdominal pain or change in her pain with certain foods. She denies neurologic symptoms in the lower extremities as well as fever, chills, rigors, constitutional and unexplained weight loss.

Past Medical History:

Otherwise unremarkable. She is not taking any medications other than the occasional anti-inflammatories. She sees her primary care practitioner regularly.

Review of Systems:

Unremarkable.

Social History:

She is single with no children. She does not smoke, drinks alcohol occasionally and does not exercise regularly.

Family History:

Remarkable for breast cancer in her mother and hypertension in her father.

Questionnaire data:

STarT Back 9-Item Clinical Tool (applied to the thoracic pain) – 26
Oswestry Low Back Pain and Disability Questionnaire (applied to the thoracic pain) - 48%
Average pain intensity over the past week - 7/10
Fear item on the STarT Back 9-Item Clinical Tool – 5/10
Catastrophizing item of the STarT Back 9-Item Clinical Tool – 5/10
Problem-Specific Depression scale – 5/10

Self-Efficacy scale – 2/10
Coping Strategies Screening Questionnaire – 6/12

What are your impressions based on the history?

Diagnostic question #1

Diagnostic question #2

Diagnostic question #3

Physical Examination:

Reveals a well-nourished, pleasant woman who appears in no acute distress. Blood pressure is 120/80 on the left. Temperature is 98.2 degrees Fahrenheit. Pulse is 72 per minute. Respirations are 16 per minute.

End range loading examination in the cervical spine is unremarkable in all directions in the seated and supine positions. End range loading of the thoracic spine in extension (see Chapter 8) causes pain without significant obstruction. There is no change with repetition. Segmental palpation reveals restriction of motion and pain at approximately the T5-6 level that exactly reproduces the patient's pain. Palpation of the segments immediately above and below this segment reveals tenderness with less restriction and with no exact reproduction of pain. There is no tenderness or restriction at any other thoracic segment. Palpation of the thoracic erector spinae muscles reveals mild tenderness but no taut bands or trigger points, and no reproduction of pain. Hip Extension Test and Active Straight Leg Raise Test are both negative.

What are your impressions based on the history and examination? Is there any indication for diagnostic imaging, specials tests or specialist consult? Why or why not?

Diagnostic question #1:

Diagnostic question #2:

Diagnostic question #3:

Diagnosis:

The diagnosis is joint dysfunction at approximately the T5-6 segment (diagnostic question #2). There are no significant findings regarding diagnostic questions #1 and 3.

What is your initial management strategy?

The diagnosis is explained to the patient and she is told that there is much that she can do to help resolve the problem herself as well as limit the likelihood of recurrence. She is given the thoracic long axis stretch and thoracic flexion and extension self-mobilization exercises (see Chapter 8). She is also given information on anti-inflammatory nutrition. All communications are carried out in a CBT/ACT context.

She is treated twice over the following week with manipulation to approximately the T5-6 segment using an HVLA technique in the prone position. She is given additional exercises - the thoracic breathing self-mobilization exercise (see Chapter 8) and the Brugger exercise (see Chapter 7). It is recommended that she take frequent breaks when she is working at the computer (at least once per hour) and to do a few repetitions of the Brugger exercise during these breaks.

Following the second of these sessions the patient reports that her pain is less intense and the exercises seem helpful. She states that she feels that it is easier for her to reach high shelves at work and while she still has pain after prolonged computer work, this is less intense and it takes longer before the pain starts. It is recommended she continue with the exercises and return in two weeks, at which time re-examination takes place.

At re-examination the patient reports 80% improvement. She states that her pain is minimal and that reaching overhead bothers her on some days but not on others. She has been following instructions to take frequent breaks at the computer and can stand for long periods of time (such as when cooking or doing dishes) without pain. She has continued with her home exercise program.

Questionnaire data at re-examination:

STarT Back 9-Item Clinical Tool score (applied to the thoracic pain) - 8
Oswestry Low Back Pain and Disability Questionnaire (applied to the thoracic pain) - 10%
Average pain intensity over the past week - 2/10
Fear item on the STarT Back 9-Item Clinical Tool – 1/10
Catastrophizing item of the STarT Back 9-Item Clinical Tool – 0/10
Problem-Specific Depression scale – 1/10
Self-Efficacy scale – 1/10
Coping Strategies Screening Questionnaire – 12/12

The PSP and patient discuss her progress and agree that she is ready to continue on her own with her exercises. The PSP recommends she continue doing the exercises twice per day for another two weeks and, if her pain and activity interference are minimal or resolved by that point, should reduce to once per day for maintenance. The PSP recommends that if her pain is to return, she should increase the frequency of the exercises back to twice per day to see if she can resolve it herself. If, in spite of this, the pain persists after a few days, she should return to the PSP.

Case 12

History of the Present Illness:

The patient is a 25-year-old man who complains of low back pain. This began four days ago when he was at the gym and was placing a 25-pound plate on its rack. The pain is well localized to the lumbosacral junction just to the right of midline without radiation or referral. The pain is aggravated by flexion activities such as putting on shoes and socks in the morning. Sitting is generally comfortable, although if he is sitting for a long time he has trouble standing up. His most comfortable position is lying on his side in the fetal position.

He denies numbness, paresthesia or motor loss in the extremities or groin. He denies bowel or bladder difficulties, as well as any other GI or GU symptoms related to the pain. He also denies fever, chills, rigors, constitutional symptoms and unexplained weight loss.

Past Medical History:

Otherwise unremarkable. He is not currently taking any medications.

Review of Systems:

Unremarkable.

Social History:

He is single with no children. He does not smoke, drinks alcohol occasionally and goes to the gym five days per week to lift weights and use the cardio machines, although he has not done so since the onset of his pain.

Family History:

Unremarkable.

Questionnaire data:

STarT Back 9-Item Clinical Tool - 26
Oswestry Low Back Pain and Disability Questionnaire - 42%
Average pain intensity over the past week - 8/10
Fear item on the STarT Back 9-Item Clinical Tool – 2/10
Catastrophizing item of the STarT Back 9-Item Clinical Tool – 2/10
Problem-Specific Depression scale – 3/10

Self-Efficacy scale – 2/10
Coping Strategies Screening Questionnaire – 6/12

What are your impressions based on the history?

Diagnostic question #1

Diagnostic question #2

Diagnostic question #3

Physical Examination:

Reveals a well-nourished, pleasant man who appears in no acute distress. Blood pressure is 118/68 on the left. Temperature is 98.6 degrees Fahrenheit. Pulse is 68 per minute. Respirations are 12 per minute.

End range loading examination is remarkable for painful obstruction and exact reproduction of pain on extension in the prone position. The pain intensity and end rage obstruction both gradually reduce with repetition.

The patient is oriented to person, place and time. Heel, toe and tandem walking are within normal limits. Romberg's position is held with eyes closed without difficulty. Sensory examination to pinprick in the lower extremities reveals no abnormalities. Motor strength is 5/5 bilaterally in the lower extremities. Muscle stretch reflexes are 2+ and symmetric in the knees and ankles. Plantar responses are downgoing bilaterally.

What are your impressions based on the history and examination? Is there any indication for diagnostic imaging, specials tests or specialist consult? Why or why not?

Diagnostic question #1:

Diagnostic question #2:

Diagnostic question #3:

Diagnosis:

The diagnosis is acute disc derangement (diagnostic question #2) with extension as the direction of benefit for exercise.

For consideration: The examination related to diagnostic question #2 consisted only of the end range loading examination in only one direction (extension). Why were other directions not examined and why was there no examination for suspected facet pain, sacroiliac pain or radiculopathy?

As is discussed in Chapter 5 in Volume I of this series, when investigating for facet pain and for sacroiliac pain, it is necessary to first rule out disc derangement. Therefore, it is most efficient in patients with low back pain to perform the end range loading examination first. If a clear positive mechanical and symptomatic outcome is found, the diagnosis of disc derangement should be strongly suspected and a Direction of Benefit has been established. There is no need to put the patient through the potential discomfort of performing sacroiliac provocation maneuvers and the Extension-Rotation test. The most expeditious course of action would be to commence treatment according to the disc derangement diagnosis, unless there are concerns related to diagnostic question #1 that require immediate investigation.

In this case, end range loading examination in extension produced a clear positive mechanical and symptomatic outcome. Specifically, there was painful obstruction and exact reproduction of pain when testing prone extension, with lessening of both the pain and the obstruction as a result of the patient performing this movement repetitively. In addition, there was nothing in the history that would suggest the presence of radiculopathy, therefore, given the positive end range loading examination, there was no immediate need to conduct a neurodynamic examination, at least until a trial of treatment for the derangement is carried out and the response monitored.

What is your initial management strategy?

The patient is set up with a home routine of lumbar extension exercises that he is to perform 10 repetitions 4-6 times per day. He is told to limit flexion activities for the time being and to follow up in two to three days. He is also given information on anti-inflammatory nutrition. All communications are carried out in a CBT/ACT context.

The patient returns three days later and reports 70% improvement. His back pain is substantially less intense and he is engaging in most normal activities although he has not returned to the gym. He has complied well with the extension exercises and feels these have greatly helped.

Questionnaire data at re-examination:

STarT Back 9-Item Clinical Tool – 11
Oswestry Low Back Pain and Disability Questionnaire - 12%
Average pain intensity since the initial examination - 2/10
Fear item on the STarT Back 9-Item Clinical Tool – 2/10
Catastrophizing item of the STarT Back 9-Item Clinical Tool – 2/10
Problem-Specific Depression scale – 1/10
Self-Efficacy scale – 0/10
Coping Strategies Screening Questionnaire – 11/12

On end range loading examination the patient is able to nearly press up all the way but he feels a "block" toward the end of the range and this causes pain that is far less intense than when he performed this maneuver at the initial visit. When this movement is performed with practitioner overpressure, he is able to fully press up without pain. Hip Extension Test, Prone Instability Test and Active Straight Leg Raise Test are all negative.

What is the best course of action now?

The patient is instructed to continue the extension exercises two to four times per day for the next week or until the pain is completely resolved, whichever comes first. Thereafter, he should reduce the frequency to once per day, and continue that for maintenance. He is instructed how to lift while maintaining lumbar lordosis (see Chapter 9 in Volume I of this series). He is told that if he should have recurrence of similar pain he should increase the frequency of extension exercises back to four to six times per day to see if he can self-resolve the problem. If, in spite of this, the pain persists for two or more days, he should return to the PSP. Otherwise there is no need for him to schedule any follow-ups.

For consideration: The reason that this "simple" case is included here is that this will be a common scenario for the PSP. Many patients with acute low back pain, particularly if the pain results from disc derangement (which accounts for approximately 80% of cases of acute low back pain) only need to see the PSP once or a few times to resolve the problem and provide basic prevention strategies.

Patients whose acute episode is part of a chronic pattern of frequent recurrences, or whose psychological measures are elevated on initial examination and remain elevated after the acute episode resolves, may require additional stabilization exercise (in the case of frequent recurrences) or one or two follow ups to for education and guidance and to make sure they remain on track with their home exercise program (in the case of residual high psychological measures). However, most acute patients do not require more than a few sessions with the PSP.

Case 13

History of the Present Illness:

The patient is a 33-year-old woman who complains of neck pain and headaches. This began following a motor vehicle collision in which she was involved four days ago in which she was stopped at a traffic light and was struck from behind by another vehicle. She was wearing a seat belt and was unaware of the impending impact. She states that she was "in shock" immediately after the accident, and then within 20 minutes or so developed a headache that became quite severe. She was taken by ambulance to the emergency department of the local hospital where cervical radiographs were taken. She was told that these "didn't show any broken bones but my curve was messed up." She was prescribed ibuprofen and a muscle relaxant and released. The next day she awoke with severe neck pain and continued headache. She saw her primary care practitioner who referred her for PSP evaluation.

The pain is located in the upper cervical spine bilaterally extending into the occipital area. All movements of the head and neck are painful, particularly flexion. She generally feels better at rest although she still has a mild headache. She denies blurred vision, double vision, dysarthria, dysphagia, vertigo or tinnitus. She denies numbness, paresthesia or motor loss in the upper and lower extremities. She denies GI or chest symptoms related to the pain as well as fever, chills, rigors, constitutional symptoms and unexplained weight loss.

Past Medical History

Otherwise unremarkable.

Review of Systems:

Remarkable for occasional heartburn when she eats spicy foods.

Social History:

She is married with no children. She does not smoke, drinks alcohol occasionally and used to go to the gym regularly to use the cardio machines, although she has not done so since the motor vehicle collision.

Family History:

Remarkable for hypertension in both parents.

Questionnaire data:

Neck Pain Screening Tool Long Form - 42
Neck Disability Index - 66%
Average pain intensity over the past week - 7/10
Fear item on the Neck Pain Screening Tool Long Form – 6/10
Catastrophizing item of the Neck Pain Screening Tool Long Form – 7/10
Coping Strategies Screening Questionnaire - 4/12
Self-efficacy scale - 7/10
Problem-specific depression scale - 4/10

What are your impressions based on the history?

Diagnostic question #1

Diagnostic question #2

Diagnostic question #3

Physical Examination:

Reveals a well-nourished, pleasant woman who appears in no acute distress. Blood pressure is 110/70 on the left. Temperature is 98.4 degrees Fahrenheit. Pulse is 68 per minute. Respirations are 12 per minute.

End range loading examination reveals pain without abrupt obstruction in all directions. The pain does not change with repetition in any direction. The Flexion-Rotation Test is painful bilaterally. Palpation for segmental tenderness and manual joint examination reveals increased resistance to manual pressure and reproduction of the patient's neck and occipital pain at approximately the C1-2 segment. Myofascial trigger points are noted in the suboccipital muscles bilaterally, palpation of which also reproduces the patient's neck and occipital pain.

The patient is oriented to person, place and time. Heel, toe and tandem walking are within normal limits. Romberg's position is held with eyes closed without difficulty. Examination of cranial nerves II through XII is unremarkable. Pupils are round, equal and reactive to light and accommodation. Funduscopic examination is unremarkable. Sensory examination to pinprick in the upper and lower extremities is unremarkable. Motor strength is 5/5 bilaterally in the upper and lower extremities. Muscle stretch reflexes are 2+ and symmetric throughout. Plantar responses are downgoing bilaterally. Rapid alternating movements, finger-to-nose and heel-to-shin movements are carried out without dysmetria or tremor. There is no pronator drift.

DR. DONALD R. MURPHY

The radiographic report is obtained from the hospital and it reported no fractures or dislocations but it reported "decrease in the cervical lordosis, likely due to muscle spasm."

What are your impressions based on the history and examination? Is there any indication for diagnostic imaging, specials tests or specialist consult? Why or why not?

Diagnostic question #1:

Diagnostic question #2:

Diagnostic question #3:

Diagnosis:

The diagnosis is post-traumatic C1-2 joint dysfunction (diagnostic question #2).

Question for thought: Why are findings related to diagnostic question #3 other than the psychological factors not considered here?

The purpose of diagnostic question #3 is to identify important perpetuating factors. Thus, it is most relevant in the subacute or chronic patient. In the acute patient, diagnostic questions #1 and 2 are most relevant.

Question for thought: What is the significance of the radiographic finding of "decrease in the cervical lordosis, likely due to muscle spasm"?

It is common to find a statement like this in a radiographic report. However, reduction or loss of the cervical curve is likely a normal variant and should not be assumed to have any clinical significance (see Gore, et al, Christensen and Hartvigsen and Johansson, et al in the Recommended Reading list). Further, attributing this finding to "muscle spasm" is inappropriate and not supported by evidence. This is another example of an imaging finding that is of no clinical consequence but, if communicated to the patient as if it were important, risks creating unnecessary fear and catastrophizing. In this case, there is no way to determine exactly how the finding was communicated to the patient in the emergency department, but it is clear that the impression she came away with was that there was something "messed up" in her neck.

What is your initial management strategy?

The patient is taught self-mobilization exercises in cervical retraction. She is seen three times over a two week period. On each visit the C1-2 segment is treated with manipulation and she is given further self-mobilization exercises utilizing a towel, initially in rotation and then in extension (see Chapter 6). She is also given information on anti-inflammatory nutrition. All communications during these sessions are carried out in a CBT/ACT context.

At the third treatment session she is re-examined at which time she reports 50% improvement. She states that her pain is less intense and she feels the exercises are helpful. She states, "I was starting to think that I would never get better but now I am thinking that maybe it is possible. Though I am not really sure. I know you tell me that people generally recover from this type of injury but…"

She has begun to increase her activity level and returned to the gym once to ride the exercise bike. She did not try the elliptical machine. When this was discussed further she stated that "I was afraid to use my arms on the machine because it might make my neck worse." She states that while she feels better overall she still feels "vulnerable" in that she feels that if she "makes the wrong move I will worsen the injury."

Questionnaire data at re-examination:

Neck Pain Screening Tool Long Form - 31
Neck Disability Index - 42%
Average pain intensity over the past week - 4/10
Fear item on the Neck Pain Screening Tool Long Form – 6/10
Catastrophizing item of the Neck Pain Screening Tool Long Form – 7/10
Coping Strategies Screening Questionnaire - 7/12
Self-efficacy scale - 3/10
Problem-specific depression scale - 4/10

On examination, the test for gaze stability reveals difficulty maintaining focus on the target and mild dizziness during the test. On the Eye Follow Test the patient has difficulty following the target in the neck torsion position. The Cervical Stability Test is positive.

Question for thought: On initial examination cervical joint dysfunction was identified on the basis of a positive Flexion-Rotation Test, palpation for segmental tenderness and manual joint examination. Yet these procedures were not repeated at re-examination. Why would this be?

This was discussed in Case 5 in the previous chapter but bears repeating.

Before repeating pain provocation tests at re-examination, the PSP should consider carefully the value of this, as well as the potential consequences. Pain provocation maneuvers are diagnostic tests, not outcome measures. That is, the purpose of these tests is to attempt to reproduce the pain in order to gather information toward making the diagnosis. In the case presented here, the diagnosis of joint dysfunction had already been established, and the patient had experienced significant improvement following treatment directed at the joint dysfunction. Repeating the pain provocation maneuvers would serve little beneficial purpose and could possibly be detrimental.

The reason for this is that, even though the patient's pain is substantially reduced, it is likely that the cervical joint structures (or, more accurately, the nociceptive system as it relates to those structures) are still sensitive. Therefore there is a good chance that these pain provocation maneuvers will still be "positive". As it stands, the patient is feeling better and, importantly, is feeling more confident in her ability to improve further. Examining the joints and eliciting pain may put doubt in the patient's mind as to whether she really is "doing better". This could serve as a powerful message that she is not doing as well as she thought, and that she still has "damage" in her spine.

So it is important to always think carefully about whether repeating a pain provocation maneuver is important enough in providing clinical information that it is worth the risk of discouraging the patient and reducing self-efficacy.

What are your impressions now and what is the best course of action?

The pain intensity is substantially reduced but the patient has significant oculomotor dysfunction and dynamic instability and continues to exhibit high fear and catastrophizing. However she appears to be more confident in her ability to recover. This is based on her self-efficacy scale having reduced from an original 7/10 to 3/10 as well as her verbal expression of increased confidence in her recovery.

So the PSP decides to continue primary spine care without behavioral health referral at this time. Primary spine care continues with an increased emphasis on the CBT/ACT context (see Chapters 1, 8 and 11 in Volume I of this series).

A discussion takes place with regard to the patient's impressions of her progress thus far and how she feels about her present status. She states that while she is determined to "get better" she "knows" that she has significant damage to the tissues of her neck. When asked how she "knows" this she states that she has a friend who was involved in a very similar rear-end collision some time ago and experienced a "whiplash injury". This friend had been told that she had "ligamentous instability" as a result of the accident and "needed" injections, manipulation, ultrasound and electrical stimulation for nearly a year.

It is explained to the patient that there is no evidence in her case that she has severe damage to her tissues, or that she has "ligamentous instability". She is much improved and in fact her progress is right on target with the PSP's expectations. It is explained that activity is good for her and increased activity at this point should help aid in further recovery.

However, she states that, while she would love to go back to the gym, she questions whether returning to normal activities is wise because of the risk of "making the injury worse." The PSP states that it is very understandable that she would be concerned about this, given how intense the pain was at first and the manner in which it occurred. However she is reminded that both the PSP and the patient herself have been moving her neck repetitively to the end of the range of motion, and not only has that not "made the injury worse" it actually has helped with the pain. This is clear evidence that movement, under guidance, should be pursued and not avoided.

The PSP explains that, based on examination, the muscles that provide maximum protection to the neck and some of the reflexes that help coordinate neck and eye movements are not working at optimum (though it is emphasized that they are not "damaged"). It is explained that this can be corrected with simple but focused exercises.

So it is agreed that she will hold off on returning to the gym for now (though the PSP is confident that this would be perfectly safe) and will start exercises to maximize dynamic stability and oculomotor function.

She is given the cervical brace and phasic exercises (see Chapter 7) and is told to perform these twice per day. It is recommended that she return twice more over the following week to check on these exercises and to add additional exercises.

Over the following two visits she is progressed on the quadruped track for cervical stabilization and is given vestibulo-ocular/ cervico-ocular reflex and smooth pursuit exercises (see Chapter 7). At the second of these visits the patient indicates that she is comfortable returning to the gym to use the cardio machines as before. A re-examination is scheduled two weeks thereafter.

At the next re-examination the patient reports 80% improvement overall. She states that she has minimal pain only when she spends a lot of time using the computer or reading. She has complied well with her home exercise program and is back to her regular cardio workouts, 30-40 minutes per workout four days per week.

Questionnaire data at re-examination:

Neck Pain Screening Tool Long Form - 9
Neck Disability Index - 12%
Average pain intensity over the past week - 1/10
Fear item on the Neck Pain Screening Tool Long Form – 2/10
Catastrophizing item of the Neck Pain Screening Tool Long Form – 1/10
Coping Strategies Screening Questionnaire - 10/12
Self-efficacy scale - 1/10
Problem-specific depression scale - 1/10

On examination, the test for gaze stability and eye follow are normal. The Cervical Stability Test is negative.

What is the best course of action now?

The patient is told that she is recovered from the original injury and her neck muscles and eye reflexes are functioning well. There is every reason to expect that she will not experience significant sequelae. The patient asks, "Are you saying I won't have that pain again?" It is explained that neck pain is a part of life and because of this it is likely that she will have some neck pain at some time. However it is recommended that she continue with the Cervical Brace and retraction exercises to maintain mobility and keep her neck muscles working.

She is told that if she does develop neck pain, she should use the self-mobilization exercises with the towel that she had been taught. She might be able to self-resolve the problem that way but if the pain persists for more than a few days, particularly if it interferes with her ability to perform normal activities, she should return to the PSP.

Case 14

History of the Present Illness:

The patient is a 38-year-old man who complains of low back pain and right lower extremity pain. This began approximately three weeks ago when he was building a stone wall in his yard and lifted a heavy stone. He felt a "pop" in his back at the time but not much pain. He stopped working and rested. He did not feel a great deal of pain so after a period of rest he resumed lifting and carrying stones for another hour or so. Then later that day he developed low back pain that gradually became quite severe. He took over-the-counter ibuprofen and applied ice. That night he awoke with severe pain. He waited a couple of days to see if the pain would improve on its own but when it did not, he saw is primary care practitioner. The primary care practitioner ordered an MRI and prescribed 800 mg of ibuprofen, muscle relaxants and hydrocodone.

The MRI revealed a moderate-sized disc herniation at L4-5 on the right. The primary care practitioner then referred the patient to the PSP.

The patient states that since the visit with the primary care practitioner his back and leg pain have decreased somewhat in intensity but are still severe. The pain is located in the lumbosacral area with radiation down the right posterolateral thigh and leg into the lateral foot. Flexion activities and bearing weight on the right leg particularly aggravate the pain. The patient states that he is an avid runner and "I would never dream of trying to run – but I miss it!" He states that running is his passion as well as his "stress reliever." He states that there is little to no pain at rest although the pain is particularly severe when he first wakes up in the morning.

He denies numbness, paresthesia or motor loss in the extremities. He denies medial thigh or groin numbness or paresthesia. He denies bowel or bladder symptoms as well as fever, chills, rigors, constitutional symptoms or unexplained weight loss.

Past Medical History:

Remarkable for various sports injuries during adolescence with no sequelae. He is not currently taking any medications other than the ibuprofen, muscle relaxant and hydrocodone.

Review of Systems:

Remarkable for occasional headaches that he has had for years and that resolve with over-the-counter medications and occasional left knee pain that he has had for several years and that does not interfere with running.

Social History:

He is married with two children, both of whom live with him. He does not smoke, drinks alcohol occasionally and usually runs an average of 25-30 miles per week for exercise.

Family History:

Remarkable for hypertension and type 2 diabetes in his mother and prostate cancer in his father.

Questionnaire data:

StarT Back 9-item Clinical Tool - 50
Bournemouth Back Disability Questionnaire – 54
Average pain intensity over the past week - 8/10
Fear item on the STarT Back 9-Item Clinical Tool – 8/10
Catastrophizing item of the STarT Back 9-Item Clinical Tool – 5/10
Coping Strategies Screening Questionnaire - 2/12
Self-efficacy scale - 3/10
Problem-specific depression scale - 7/10.

What are your impressions based on the history?

Diagnostic question #1:

Diagnostic question #2:

Diagnostic question #3:

Physical Examination:

Reveals a well-nourished, pleasant man who appears in no acute distress. Blood pressure is 120/70 on the left. Temperature is 97.4 degrees Fahrenheit. Pulse is 56 per minute. Respirations are 12 per minute.

Straight Leg Raise with ankle dorsiflexion on the right is positive at approximately 45 degrees for exact reproduction of his leg pain. The pain is relieved by plantar flexing the ankle. Well Leg Raise is negative. End range loading examination reveals painful obstruction and reproduction of both the low back pain and right leg pain on extension. The pain peripheralizes with repetition. Specifically, as the patient performs repetitive extension maneuvers the movement restriction gradually lessens and the low back pain reduces in intensity. However the leg pain progressively increases in intensity as repetitive extension maneuvers are performed. Side gliding to either side reveals mild pain but no painfully obstructed end range.

The patient is able to walk on his toes without difficulty. Heel walking is normal on the left but there is a slight foot drop on the right. Tandem walking is normal and the patient is able to stand in Romberg's position without difficulty. Muscle stretch reflexes are 2+ and symmetric in the knees and ankles. Plantar responses are downgoing bilaterally. Sensory examination to pinprick in the lower extremities is normal with the exception of hypoesthesia over the dorsum of the right foot. Specifically, the patient reports that he "feels something" when the PSP touches the dorsum of the foot with the pin but it does not feel "sharp" as it does on the dorsum of the left foot and on the medial and lateral aspects of the right foot. On further examination, when the PSP alternately touches the dorsum of the foot with the sharp end of the pin and then the back of the pin, the patient cannot distinguish between them. Manual motor examination is 5/5 bilaterally in the lower extremities with the exception of 4+/5 weakness of the tibialis anterior on the right. Specifically, the patient is able to fully dorsiflex the right foot and when the PSP asks the patient to maintain this position and applies firm pressure to try to move the foot toward plantar flexion, the foot does not move. However, when the PSP applies very strong pressure the patient is not able to maintain full dorsiflexion.

The lower extremity peripheral pulses are intact bilaterally.

The PSP reviews the MRI images and confirms the finding of moderate-sized foraminal zone disc herniation at L4-5 on the right.

Question for thought: The End range loading examination included extension and side gliding maneuvers, but did not include flexion. Why is this?

The end rage loading examination did not include flexion maneuvers because the diagnosis is very clear and it is likely that repetitive flexion maneuvers would aggravate the condition, with very little likelihood that flexion would be determined to be the Direction of Benefit (see Chapter 5 in Volume I of this series and Chapter 3 in this volume).

What are your impressions based on the history and examination? Is there any indication for further diagnostic imaging, specials tests or specialist consult? Why or why not?

Diagnostic question #1:

Diagnostic question #2:

Diagnostic question #3:

Diagnosis:

The diagnosis is L5 radiculopathy secondary to disc herniation (diagnostic question #2).

What is your initial management strategy?

The diagnosis is explained to the patient and he is told that there is a good likelihood of success with non-surgical management. It is explained that the pressure on the nerve root from the disc herniation has caused mild weakness of the muscle that controls dorsiflexion of the foot and that, while there is good reason to expect this to improve with time, it will have to be carefully monitored. The patient is told that if progression of the weakness occurs it may be necessary to have the patient see a spine surgeon. The patient states that he would like to avoid surgery if at all possible but he will do whatever necessary to get better and return to running as soon as possible.

After this discussion the PSP and patient come to an agreement that non-surgical management will be pursued with careful monitoring of the motor loss.

The patient is treated with distraction manipulation to decompress the lumbosacral discs and is taught a co-contraction exercise (see Chapter 11 in Volume I of this series). He is also given information on anti-inflammatory nutrition. All communications are carried out in a CBT/ACT context.

He is seen four times over a three week period during which time he is progressed on low-load lumbar stabilization exercises. Motor strength of the right tibialis anterior is monitored on each visit and the patient is asked about the development of any other neurologic symptoms.

At the first two treatment sessions motor strength of the right tibialis anterior remains 4+/5. Motor strength of the right extensor hallicus longus (EHL) remains 5/5 on these sessions. On the third treatment session it is noted that the right tibialis anterior strength is 4/5 and the EHL has developed 4+/5 weakness.

Re-examination takes place on the fourth visit. The patient reports that his back and leg pain is 60% improved but he is worried because the weakness in his right foot has become more noticeable. He tried running a few times and was not limited by pain but he noticed his right foot "slapping the ground" with each step. He stopped running because of this.

Questionnaire data at re-examination:

StarT Back 9-item Clinical - 35
Bournemouth Back Disability Questionnaire – 37
Average pain intensity over the past week - 4/10
Fear item on the STarT Back 9-Item Clinical Tool – 6/10
Catastrophizing item of the STarT Back 9-Item Clinical Tool – 3/10
Coping Strategies Screening Questionnaire - 8/12
Self-efficacy scale - 3/10
Problem-specific depression scale - 8/10

On examination, Straight Leg Raise with ankle dorsiflexion on the right causes pain but the pain does not occur until approximately 60 degrees. The pain is again relieved by ankle plantar flexion. Well Leg Raise is negative. There remains hypoesthesia to pinprick over the dorsum of the right foot. Manual motor strength of the right tibialis anterior is now 3/5 and the EHL motor strength is also 3/5. Hip Extension Test is positive bilaterally for deviation of the lumbar spine. The Prone Instability Test is also positive. Active Straight Leg Raise is negative.

What is the best course of action now?

Over a two week period the patient's tibialis anterior motor loss has progressed from 4+/5 to 3/5. In addition, the patient has developed new motor loss in the EHL, which has also progressed to 3/5. The reader will recall from Chapter 12 in Volume I of this series the "3/5 rule". That is, for the PSP the general rule of thumb should be that when motor loss secondary to radiculopathy reaches the point of 3/5 or worse, surgical consult should be considered.

A shared decision making discussion takes place between the PSP and the patient regarding the patient's present status and possible options. It is explained to the patient that while there is no way to know at what point motor loss becomes permanent, progression of motor loss to the 3/5 level is generally considered an indication that referral to a spine surgeon should be considered. Particularly important in the conversation with this patient is the fact that he is passionate about running, and running is a very important part of his life. So while there are cases in which a patient's motor loss can progress to the 3/5 level yet still improve with time, one must consider the potential consequences of waiting and risking the possibility of permanency. In this patient's case, permanent motor loss in the tibialis anterior would have a dramatic effect on his quality of life. Given this, it is the PSP's advice that immediate referral to a spine surgeon be pursued. The patient is in agreement with this.

The patient is fast-tracked to a spine surgeon who agrees that surgical intervention is the best course of action. Discectomy is performed and the patient follows up with the PSP four weeks later. At that time the patient reports being pain-free. He states that the strength in the right foot has improved but not to the point at which he feels comfortable trying to run. He is performing all other activities of daily living without problem.

On examination, heel walking reveals a slight foot drop. Manual muscle testing of the right EHL reveals 4+/5 strength. No motor weakness is noted on manual testing of the right tibialis anterior. Sensation to pinprick in the left foot is intact. Hip Extension Test remains positive bilaterally for deviation of the lumbar spine. The Prone Instability Test also remains positive.

Question for thought: On examination there is a slight foot drop on heel walking, yet manual testing of the tibialis anterior reveals full strength (i.e., 5/5). Why would this be?

The tibialis anterior is a very strong muscle. Thus, subtle motor loss may not be detected on manual testing. Heel walking is a more sensitive test for subtle weakness than is manual testing.

What is the best course of action now?

The patient is started on lumbar stabilization exercises and is advised to start using the elliptical machine at the gym. During the stabilization sessions the patient is also taught how to bend forward while maintaining lumbar lordosis (see Chapter 9 in Volume I of this series). After four sessions of stabilization exercises, with emphasis on building a home exercise program, the patient is reassessed.

The patient reports that he remains pain-free and has been able to use the elliptical machine without difficulty. He feels that there is normal strength in the right foot when walking but he has not tried to run. At this time heel walking is normal and manual motor strength is 5/5 in both the EHL and tibialis anterior. Hip Extension Test and Prone Instability Test are negative. The patient is able to perform 15 repetitions of lumbar extension in the prone position without pain or difficulty.

It is recommended that the patient return to running, starting with 1-2 miles and gradually building up to his usual 5-6 miles over a period of four weeks. He is instructed to continue with his home lumbar stabilization exercises and is prescribed prone extension exercises (see Chapter 5 in Volume I of this series) 15 repetitions once per day. He is instructed to continue to maintain lordosis during flexion activities as much as possible. It is recommended he return to the PSP if he has any future problems.

Case 15

History of the Present Illness:

The patient is a 37-year-old woman who complains of low back pain and bilateral buttock and posterior thigh pain. This began approximately eight months ago when she was shopping at a local grocery store and stepped in a puddle of milk that had spilled onto the floor. She slipped and landed on her buttocks. She states that she felt immediate pain. She reported the incident to the store manager and her husband took her to the local emergency department where lumbar radiographs were unremarkable. She was given ibuprofen, cyclobenzaprine and hydrocodone/ acetaminophen and released.

She saw her primary care physician who referred her for "physical therapy". She states that the therapy consisted of hot packs, electrical stimulation and stretching exercises and that she had some pain relief immediately after the treatments but this was short-lived. After two months of "physical therapy" she returned to her primary care physician who ordered an MRI. She states that she was told the MRI showed "two disc bulges."

Her primary care physician referred her to a neurosurgeon. The appointment took place two months later. The patient states that the neurosurgeon told her that hers was not a surgical case and recommended additional "physical therapy". She states that she felt the neurosurgeon "didn't believe me and treated me like I was faking." She returned to "physical therapy" without benefit. She then sought the services of a PSP.

The pain is located in the lumbosacral area with referral into both buttocks and posterior thighs. She states that the pain is constant and "everything I try to do kills me." She states that she has had to give up going to the gym as well as biking and rollerblading. She points out that because of the lack of exercise "I've gained a lot of weight and feel like a blimp." She states "they've ruined my life." The PSP asks her who "they" are she states, "That store." The PSP asks her to elaborate on that and the patient states, "They left that mess there for me to slip on and they couldn't care less about what happened to me." She explains that after she fell some workers helped her up and she asked to see the manager. She states that the manager "became very defensive and treated me like it was my fault." She states that she then "had to deal with the store's insurance company and they treated me like there is nothing wrong with me. It got so aggravating I had to hire a lawyer."

She states that she has "constant numbness in both legs." When asked to elaborate she states that her entire lower extremity on each side is numb in a stocking distribution from the hips to the toes. She denies focal motor loss in the extremities. She denies medial thigh or groin numbness or paresthesia. She denies bowel or bladder symptoms, as well as fever, chills, rigors, constitutional symptoms or unexplained weight loss.

She is a stay-at-home mom and states, "I can barely take care of my house and my kids because of this pain." The PSP asks how she feels about this and she states, "I feel like a failure as a mother and wife." She states that fortunately her husband has been very supportive and has "picked up the slack" with regard to household activities, but she feels guilty about this.

Past Medical History:

Otherwise unremarkable. She currently does not take any medications and states that she "gave up on all the pills they had given me before because none of them helped." She sees her primary care physician regularly.

Review of Systems:

Otherwise unremarkable.

Social History:

She is married with two children age 12 and 14, both of whom live with her. She does not smoke, drinks alcohol occasionally and does not exercise regularly "because I can't."

Family History:

Unremarkable.

Questionnaire data:

StarT Back 9-item Clinical Tool - 64
Oswestry Low Back Pain and Disability Questionnaire - 82%
Average pain intensity over the past week - 10/10
Fear item on the STarT Back 9-Item Clinical Tool – 10/10
Catastrophizing item of the STarT Back 9-Item Clinical Tool – 10/10
Coping Strategies Screening Questionnaire - 0/12
Self-efficacy scale - 10/10
Problem-specific depression scale - 10/10

What are your impressions based on the history?

Diagnostic question #1

Diagnostic question #2

Diagnostic question #3

Physical Examination:

Reveals a somewhat overweight woman who appears in distress. She shifts in her chair frequently during history taking. She grimaces when getting up from the chair and walking to the examining table. She walks with a limp.

Blood pressure is 120/80 on the left. Temperature is 98.6 degrees Fahrenheit. Pulse is 76 per minute. Respirations are 20 per minute.

The patient is oriented to person, place and time. Heel, toe and tandem walking are within normal limits. Romberg's position is held with eyes closed without difficulty. Sensory examination to pinprick in the lower extremities is unremarkable. Motor strength is 5/5 bilaterally in the lower extremities although breakaway weakness is noted in all muscles. Specifically, when the patient is asked to hold a body part in position and resist pressure, she is able to give full 5/5 resistance but then after a few seconds she releases the resistance, stating "I just can't hold it any longer." This happens with each lower extremity muscle that is tested. Muscle stretch reflexes are 2+ and symmetric in the knees and ankles. Plantar responses are downgoing bilaterally. It is noted that nearly full knee extension is possible during the examination of plantar responses in the seated position with no report of pain.

End range loading examination is attempted but every direction of movement is extremely painful and the patient is not able to tolerate repetition. Straight Leg Raise is positive bilaterally for reproduction of her low back and leg pain at approximately 20 degrees. Superficial palpation causes extreme pain reactions throughout the lumbopelvic spine. Waddell's nonorganic signs are 5/5 (see Chapter 6 in Volume I of this series).

At the end of the examination the patient starts crying and states, "I used to be so active and athletic and this is what I have been reduced to because of those people."

The MRI images and report are reviewed. They are essentially unremarkable, only revealing normal age-related changes in the form of disc bulges at L3-4 and L5-S1.

What are your impressions based on the history and examination? Is there any indication for further diagnostic imaging, specials tests or specialist consult? Why or why not?

Diagnostic question #1:

Diagnostic question #2:

Diagnostic question #3:

Question for thought: Can diagnostic question #2 be answered? If not why not?

In this case there are no findings that are relevant to diagnostic question #1. Diagnostic question #2 cannot be answered because of extreme pain reactions with all movements and with superficial palpation. This does not allow for meaningful information to be derived from the end range loading exam and pain provocation tests.

The reason for this can be explained on the basis of findings relating to diagnostic question #3, specifically nociceptive system sensitization (NSS) and significant psychological perpetuating factors. Based on the questionnaire data, there is good reason to suspect that fear, catastrophizing, passive coping, low self-efficacy and depression are playing a role in the perpetuation of this patient's pain, disability and suffering experience.

However, there is another psychological perpetuating factor that appears to be playing a role here – perceived injustice. Perceived injustice is described in Chapter 2 of Volume I of this series and is elaborated on in Chapters 4 and 7 of this volume. This is a condition in which the patient perceives that his or her basic human rights have been unfairly violated, irreparable loss has occurred, people do not understand how severe the suffering is and, importantly, that this injustice is *someone else's fault*.

Question for thought: Why would the PSP suspect the presence of perceived injustice in this patient?

In Chapter 6 of Volume I of this series, when discussing the detection of important psychological perpetuating factors, it states, "it is in establishing a relationship with the patient that allows the spine practitioner to gather the most important insights." This applies to all of the important factors, but particularly to perceived injustice. Perceived injustice is frequently (though certainly not universally) an important perpetuating factor in patients whose low back or neck disorder started as a result of a "personal injury" in which another party is perceived to be "at fault". Of course, the medicolegal system requires designations such as these in order to appropriately determine compensation issues.

However when a patient has continuing anger, bitterness and desire for revenge toward another party, the pain intensity and suffering become far more intense than they would be otherwise. These emotions contribute to the development and perpetuation of NSS, which in turn further adds to the pain, disability and suffering experience. In many cases, the whole problem is compounded by the patient's (mostly negative) experience with the medicolegal aspects of their case. Then, as in the case presented here, it is further compounded by medical providers who do not understand the "big picture" of chronic pain and as a result appear (to the patient at least) to dismiss the patient's suffering, or even treat the patient as a "malingerer".

What is your initial management strategy?

The diagnosis is explained to the patient. The conversation starts with an explanation of NSS. Specifically, the patient is told that the reason the pain feels so intense is because the "pain processing system" (i.e., the nociceptive system) is on "hyperdrive". That is, the part of the central nervous system (CNS) that processes pain input is *amplifying* the pain signals. The pain signal that arises out of the back has been amplified several times before it reaches the brain. As a result, what started in the back as a whisper ends up in the brain as a scream. It is emphasized that this is very common – the patient is hardly the only person to whom this has happened. Any busy PSP sees this quite frequently.

The patient is directed to the video "Understanding Pain: What to do about it in less than five minutes" which can be found at:
https://www.youtube.com/watch?v=RWMKucuejIs [accessed 23 April 2016]

It is emphasized that "this is all good news!" After all, this means that the problem in the spine is not nearly as serious as it appears to be. Further good news is that the process is very often partially or completely reversible – but this will require a commitment on the part of the patient.

Following this, perceived injustice is discussed. The conversation goes like this:

PSP: "I can see that you are very angry about this situation."
Patient: "Of course I am! If those people at that store hadn't left that mess for me to slip on, I would not be in so much pain."

PSP: "That's understandable. It seems that you also feel like people have not shown concern for you and don't understand what you have gone through."

Patient: "That's right. The manager acted like it was all my fault. Then that insurance company person treated me like dirt. And on top of it all that specialist I saw treated me like I was a phony and that there was nothing wrong with me. If only they could feel the pain that I feel!"

PSP: "I certainly can see why you would be very upset about all this. Frankly, I am impressed with how well you have coped given all you have been through. I have a concern about this, though."

Patient: "What is that?"

PSP: "I am wondering if the anger and bitterness you feel, even though it is understandable and normal, is actually interfering with your recovery."

Patient: "What are you talking about? The fact is I fell hard and I have two disc bulges – you saw the MRI."

PSP: "Yes I did. While the bulges themselves should not concern us too much – these are normal as we get older, like gray hair - I suspect you probably did injure one of your discs when you fell. But injured tissues heal with time. When a person has ongoing pain beyond the healing time of the tissue, which is very common and something I see every day, there are usually other factors that are contributing. In your case, one of the important factors is the hyperactivity of your pain system that we talked about earlier. But we also know that anger and bitterness feeds this hyperactivity, making the pain experience more intense. I am wondering whether that might be contributing to your pain and suffering."

Patient: "Oh, don't tell me you think this is all in my head too."

PSP: "Severe back pain is not simply a matter of 'either it's all in the back or all in the head'. All pain involves the tissues that are hurting as well as our emotions, thoughts, and perceptions. A combination of factors contributes to the whole thing. Much of the problem originates in the back but our thoughts and emotions can play a strong contributing role as well. So, let me ask you a question: what happens with your pain when you get upset about that fall?"

Patient: "I do notice that whenever I think about that manager and the insurance company my back seems to tighten right up. But there is no way I am going to let them off the hook after what they have done to me."

PSP: "I don't blame you for feeling that way. My concern right now is not with them, it is with you. Specifically, helping you recover as quickly as possible. One thing that can be useful in situations like this is acknowledging the pain and relating to it differently. That is, rather than fighting the pain, and getting angry at the pain, simply noticing the pain and allowing it to be there, right here and now."

Patient: "Okay so you want me to accept the fact that I am going to be in pain the rest of my life?"

PSP: "What I am talking about has nothing to do with the rest of your life. It has to do with right now, in this moment only. Many people with chronic pain worry about it continuing into the future. That is natural. And, worrying about the pain – what do you think that does to your experience of the pain? Do you think it intensifies it or makes it better?
Patient: Oh it definitely makes it worse! But you can tell me to stop worrying, but I can't help it.
PSP: Well, I'm not telling you to stop worrying. That doesn't work. Instead, I'm wondering about helping you to focus on living in the here and now, and finding a way to accept your pain – just for today, just for now. Do you think you would be open to considering this?"
Patient: "No! I want the pain to go away!"
PSP: "Of course, I can understand that. Who wouldn't? But you've tried a number of things to make the pain go away. Have any of them worked? So assuming the pain is not going to disappear this instant, can we work on your developing the ability to accept its presence in this instant? All I am asking is whether you can be open to this possibility."
Patient: "Okay. I will consider it. I want to do whatever it takes to get better."
PSP: "Great! Me too. There is a doctor that I have utilized for help with this kind of thing whom I have found to be of great assistance. The doctor is a pain psychologist. This does not mean I think you are crazy or that 'it's all in your head'. It means that this doctor is trained to help us by teaching you skills for working with the emotional aspects of the pain, while you and I are working with the physical aspects. This can be a real asset to us in moving you along to recovery. Would you be open to this?"
Patient: "Sure, let's try it."

For consideration: There are a number of important things to note about this conversation:

- When communicating with the patient in whom perceived injustice is an important perpetuating factor, it is important to *validate* the patient's feelings about the situation. Even if it is clear that these feelings are interfering with recovery, it is essential for the PSP to *meet the patient where she is, and connect with the patient at that point.* This can only be done if the patient feels that the PSP understands her and respects how she feels.

  In the conversation presented here, this validation comes in the form of statements such as "that's understandable", "I certainly can see why you would be very upset about all this" and "frankly, I am impressed with how well you have coped given all you have been through." This validation applies to all of the psychological perpetuating factors – it is essential that the PSP makes it clear that these factors are *normal human reactions.*

- Critical with regard to validation in the presence of perceived injustice is that *it is the emotion that is validated, not the reason for the emotion*. In other words, it can be seen in this conversation that the PSP is validating the patient's anger, bitterness and emotional distress, making it clear that these things are understandable, normal and very common in people who have an experience like the one she has had.

  What is *not* being validated is the "carelessness" of the store personnel, the "thoughtlessness" of the store manager and insurance clerk and the "condescension" of the neurosurgeon. If the PSP were to come across as validating that "those bad people did bad things to you", this could potentially *exacerbate* the patient's perceived injustice.

- Note the statement by the patient, "But there is no way I am going to let them [the store manager and insurance clerk] off the hook after what they have done to me." Many patients affected by perceived injustice consider disability and suffering the only "power" of retribution they have against the perceived perpetrator of the injustice. This statement illustrates that aspect of perceived injustice.

  As discussed in Chapter 6, trying to use disability and suffering to try to get back at someone else appears to be a highly irrational way to deal with a problem. But if we were to look back honestly and mindfully over our own lives we would likely encounter many times that we have done this very same thing, to one extent or another. This is a "normal" (though usually self-defeating) human trait. It is critically important for the PSP to understand this in order to maximize patient benefit.

- Note that the PSP is not trying to get the patient to change or to convince the patient of anything. Using language such as "I am wondering whether [the anger and bitterness] might be contributing to your pain and suffering", "I'm wondering about helping you to focus on living in the here and now, and finding a way to accept your pain" and "what happens with your pain when you get upset about that fall?" allows the PSP to bring out in the patient her own ideas about the perceived injustice and the role it may be playing in her pain, disability and suffering experience, and to open herself up to taking steps to address this.

- Note that the PSP is continually speaking from a "we" orientation. Using phrasing such as "…helping you recover as quickly as possible" implies that they are working together on this and that it is the patient who is going to recover, with the PSP as the "helper". Also note, when talking about referral to the psychologist, the PSP states that the purpose is to "help *us* by teaching you skills for working with the emotional aspects of pain, while *you and I* are working with the physical aspects." They are a team working together, each with his or her specific role (as well as the psychologist in this case) in the process of moving the patient from pain, disability and suffering experience to recovery.

- Note that in the discussion of both NSS and perceived injustice the PSP repeatedly emphasizes that both these conditions happen quite often with people who are in pain – the patient is far from alone in this. This helps the patient feel more "normal". There is nothing "wrong with" the patient, she is having a problem that many other people have as well. And she is reacting to the problem in a way that, while counterproductive, is *extremely* common.

- Note that the term "perceived injustice" is never actually used in the conversation. It is not necessary to "get technical" with the patient. It is more helpful to talk in terms that are widely understood rather than in clinical terms, which can interfere with the connection between PSP and patient. In addition, recall that it was discussed in Chapters 4 and 7 that the term "experience of injustice" is often used for this construct to avoid the implication that the injustice is somehow "not real".

- Note the overall tone of the discussion regarding perceived injustice. This applies to all of the other important psychological factors that contribute to the perpetuation of spine related disorders as well. It reflects the idea that it is not a question of whether these things are "good" or "bad", "right" or "wrong", "pathological" or "non-pathological". It is simply a matter of whether they are "helpful" or "unhelpful" in any given situation. In this situation, the perceived injustice is not useful in helping the patient overcome her pain, disability and suffering experience. In fact, it serves to exacerbate and perpetuate that experience. It is for this reason that we need to help the patient make changes in her thinking and belief system, to better position herself on the road to recovery.

The patient is referred to a psychologist trained in Cognitive-Behavioral Therapy and Acceptance and Commitment Therapy to address the perceived injustice and other contributing psychological factors. In addition, the PSP and patient agree to implement a process of graded exposure for the purpose of addressing the NSS. The "green light, yellow light, red light" principle discussed Chapter 11 in Volume I of this series is followed throughout this process. The patient is also given information on anti-inflammatory nutrition.

It is decided that manipulation will be used initially for the purpose of graded exposure so that the process can begin under tightly controlled circumstances and with close involvement of the PSP in the initial stage. The PSP utilizes a muscle energy procedure (see Chapter 10 in Volume I of this series and Chapter 6 in this volume) so that the movements can be introduced slowly and gradually. The patient is told that some discomfort is likely during this process and is, in fact, necessary to desensitize the nociceptive system. However any discomfort should be mild or moderate. The patient is told that if she experiences significant pain she should let the PSP know. It is emphasized that even if severe pain were to occur, this would not reflect "worsening" of the "tissue damage", since there is no actual damage to the tissues. However severe pain is very unpleasant and is not necessary to desensitize the nociceptive system. It is for this reason that all attempts will be made to limit the elicitation of severe pain.

It is also explained that the patient will likely experience increased pain later in the day and/or the next day after manipulative treatment. Again, this is expected to be mild to moderate and is normal and necessary. This increased pain is the nociceptive system's reaction to what it "thinks" is a nociceptive stimulus, even though the stimulus is not nociceptive at all – the nociceptive system interprets the stimulus as "pain" when it is simply a "movement" stimulus that the CNS is experiencing. The purpose of the graded exposure process is, in part, to help the patient's CNS appropriately differentiate between "pain" signals and "movement" signals from the tissues.

After two sessions of this the patient is given a gentle exercise (the "cat and camel" exercise – see Chapter 10 in Volume I of this series) to provide further stimulation of the CNS as well as to promote spine mobility in the sagittal plane. After three sessions the patient is given a sacroiliac mobilization exercise (see Chapter 10 in Volume I of this series) to perform bilaterally, for the purpose of providing a new stimulus to the CNS, as well as promote spine mobility in a rotational direction.

Each session produces mild discomfort during the session and increased pain the next day. Generally, with each subsequent session the increased pain that follows is less intense than that of the previous session (although there are certain days when the pain becomes severe), an indication of desensitization of the nociceptive system. Also, the PSP notes that with each session the amplitude of the manipulative procedure can be increased, as the CNS's resistance to the movement diminishes.

At the end of six sessions the patient undergoes formal re-examination. By this time the patient has also had two sessions with the psychologist. She reports that she and the psychologist have started to review the concept of "mindfulness" – i.e., non-judgmental attention to the present moment – and she has started to practice some mindfulness exercises at home. They are also discussing the patient's values and goals, with a focus on what kinds of activities the patient has avoided because of the pain. She and the psychologist have started to set small goals for re-engaging in valued behavior. They have focused on her children.

The patient reports 30% improvement. She states that she still has severe pain but the pain is somewhat less intense and she has started to engage in activities of daily living that she had previously been avoiding. For example, she has been going for short walks with her daughter ("though I could not imagine playing catch with her or helping with her softball drills!"). She states that "sometimes I push it and pay for it the next day."

Questionnaire data at re-examination:

StarT Back 9-item Clinical Tool - 45
Oswestry Low Back Pain and Disability Questionnaire – 72%
Average pain intensity over the past week - 8/10
Fear item on the STarT Back 9-Item Clinical Tool – 6/10
Catastrophizing item of the STarT Back 9-Item Clinical Tool – 7/10
Coping Strategies Screening Questionnaire - 2/12
Self-efficacy scale - 8/10
Problem-specific depression scale - 7/10

End range loading examination can now be carried out. It is found that minimal lumbar extension in the prone position elicits a painful obstruction that exactly reproduces the patient's low back, buttock and posterior thigh pain. The PSP positions the patient in the "resting on elbows" position (see Fig. 5-6 in Volume I of this series). The patient states that this reproduces the low back, buttock and posterior thigh pain. The PSP provides manual overpressure with the patient in this position by pressing in a posterior-to-anterior (P-A) direction at the lumbosacral junction. This increases the intensity of the patient's pain, but she states that "I can handle it." The PSP asks the patient to try to "relax into the pain" and the pressure is maintained for approximately 30 seconds. The PSP stops applying the P-A pressure and the patient remains in the "resting on elbows" position. The PSP asks how the patient feels and she states that she has no pain in this position now. The PSP asks the patient to press up and she is able to extend approximately 50% greater in range, at which point there again is a painful obstruction that reproduces the low back, buttock and posterior thigh pain.

The patient is asked to perform repetitions of this press up maneuver and to observe the pain and report any changes in position or intensity. As the repetitions are continued the patient reports that the pain remains in the low back and buttocks but the posterior thigh pain lessens. With further repetitions the pain increases in intensity in the low back but the buttock pain gradually resolves. As the patient is carrying out these repetitions, the PSP notes that she is able to extend farther before reaching the point of painful obstruction. At the tenth repetition the patient only has pain in the low back.

Hip Extension Test is positive bilaterally for deviation of the lumbar spine. Prone Instability Test is also positive. Active Straight Leg Raise Test is negative.

Question for thought: What is the significance of the end range loading examination in this case?

Diagnostic question #2 can now be answered. The pain was reproduced with extension maneuvers, in which a painful obstruction was encountered. With sustained overpressure followed by repetition, the pain gradually centralized and the obstruction reduced. This indicates that the patient has disc derangement with extension as the Direction of Benefit.

Recall that on initial examination, because of the intensity of the NSS, the end range loading examination, and any examination procedure designed to seek the answer to diagnostic question #2, could not be carried out. Now that the NSS is less intense, end range loading examination was possible, and was informative.

Question for thought: Has any other important diagnostic factor been identified?

An additional perpetuating factor (diagnostic question #3) has been identified. Hip Extension Test and Prone Instability Test are both positive, suggesting the presence of dynamic instability.

What is the best course of action now?

The patient is instructed to perform lumbar extension end range loading exercises 10 repetitions four to six times per day. In addition, the graded exposure process is continued, but now it is decided that activity rather than manual therapy will be used as the mechanism for this.

The patient continues working with the psychologist. They have started to examine the question of who benefits from the patient continuing to hold on to her anger and bitterness. Her psychologist is encouraging her to notice when she is angry, to notice the angry thoughts that she has, and to see them as thoughts or feelings passing through her mind, rather than as fixed truths.

For the purpose of continuing the graded exposure process, the PSP asks the if there is an activity that the patient would very much like to return to but that she has been avoiding because of the pain. The patient states, "My psychologist said I should talk to you about this - I would love to get back to the gym but I haven't been able to do any exercise for eight months." The PSP recommends that the patient return to the gym and use whichever cardio machine the patient would most enjoy, other than the exercise bike. The PSP explains that the exercise bike will not be introduced for the time being only because sitting increases disc pressure. It is emphasized that there is no reason to think that riding the exercise bike will cause any damage or "worsen" the condition, it is just that it might slow recovery while the disc derangement is being addressed. There is every reason to think that returning to the exercise bike will be fine after the derangement is corrected. They decide that walking on the treadmill is the best exercise to start with.

The PSP explains to the patient that she should expect a similar pattern as was found with the manual therapy – there will likely be increased pain during or immediately after the exercise, or the following day. This is expected to be mild or moderate and should fade over a period of 24 to 48 hours. The patient is to use the treadmill for 20 minutes every other day. If 20 minutes does not elicit any discomfort, she is to increase to 30 minutes. If 20 minutes elicits severe pain, she should reduce the time to 10 minutes. Again, the "green light, yellow light, red light" principle is followed.

The patient is followed weekly for three weeks, with each session consisting of a discussion regarding how the end range loading exercises and the graded exposure is going, with progression of the graded exposure process (the patient sees the psychologist weekly during this time as well). Also on each session the patient is progressed on a lumbar stabilization exercise program (see Chapter 11 in Volume I of this series).

By the second of these sessions, the patient is able to perform full lumbar extension in the prone position without any pain or obstruction. At this point, she is instructed to reduce the frequency to one set per day. On the third session a formal re-examination is undertaken.

At that time the patient reports 60% improvement. Under the guidance of the PSP and psychologist she has progressed the use of the treadmill to 30 minutes per day, 4-5 days per week. She says that she would like to try light weightlifting and exercise classes but "I'm afraid to try – I don't want to set myself back." She has increased her activities of daily living, actually trying a 15-minute game of "catch" with a softball with her daughter. She states that "I paid for it the next day but I decided to try your approach – we played catch again two days later and I was sore the following day but not nearly as bad as after the first time."

She has complied well with the home stabilization exercise program and feels "thrilled to be able to do something physical." She states that she and the psychologist have decided that she is ready to apply what she has learned in the sessions on her own and she has a follow-up session scheduled in one month. She plans to continue brief moments of the "mindfulness of breath" exercise throughout the day. She finds that this calms and relaxes her, particularly when she finds that she is feeling irritable with her pain.

Questionnaire data at re-examination:

StarT Back 9-item Clinical Tool - 19
Oswestry Low Back Pain and Disability Questionnaire – 44%
Average pain intensity over the past week - 4/10
Fear item on the STarT Back 9-Item Clinical Tool – 3/10
Catastrophizing item of the STarT Back 9-Item Clinical Tool – 2/10
Coping Strategies Screening Questionnaire - 8/12
Self-efficacy scale - 3/10
Problem-specific depression scale - 4/10

End range loading examination in lumbar extension is full and pain-free. Hip Extension Test is negative. Prone Instability Test is mildly positive.

What is the best course of action now?

The PSP and patient discuss the patient's present status and it is decided that the patient will likely be able to continue her progress on her own. She will continue the graded exposure process by adding light weightlifting and continuing the gradual introduction of activities of daily living such as vacuuming and laundry. The PSP instructs the patient in maintaining neutral lordosis while performing these activities (see Chapter 9 in Volume I of this series). The patient understands the process of graded exposure and the "green light, yellow light, red light" principle. The PSP recommends that the patient follow up in four weeks although if she is having difficulty she is welcome to return sooner.

At four-week follow up the patient reports 80% improvement. She states that the pain "has its moments" but for the most part she is able to function well despite the presence or absence of pain at any given moment. When she has pain it is well localized to the lumbosacral area and there is no significant buttock or lower extremity pain.

She has been undergoing the graded exposure process and is able to vacuum a full room with minimal discomfort both during and after the activity. She is lifting weights in the gym and is almost back to her normal routine as well as her typical amount of weight ("though I never lifted heavy weights anyway"). She tried taking an exercise class and states "boy was I sore the next day." The PSP asks her to describe this soreness and she says "my leg muscles were achy and stiff and my back was hurting, but nowhere near like before." She tried the exercise class again a few days later and felt far less soreness following that class.

She has continued with her lumbar stabilization program. She states that she and the psychologist have agreed that she can carry on utilizing the skills she has developed in therapy on her own and there is no need to continue with active therapy.

Questionnaire data at re-examination:

StarT Back 9-item Clinical Tool - 12
Oswestry Low Back Pain and Disability Questionnaire – 22%
Average pain intensity over the past week - 2/10
Fear item on the STarT Back 9-Item Clinical Tool – 2/10
Catastrophizing item of the STarT Back 9-Item Clinical Tool – 2/10
Coping Strategies Screening Questionnaire - 8/12
Self-efficacy scale - 1/10
Problem-specific depression scale - 2/10

What is the best course of action now?

The PSP remarks to the patient how impressive she has been in her recovery process. It is emphasized that without her determination and persistence none of this would have been possible. The PSP indicates that there is every reason to think that the patient will be able to maintain her improvement with the home exercises and self-management strategies she has learned. It is explained to the patient that she is well on her way to being "back to normal." It is emphasized, however, that "normal" means occasionally having back pain – the vast majority of people have back pain at some time. So in her case, experiencing back pain does not mean she has "reinjured" her back or that she is "back to square one." In all likelihood, any back pain she experiences will be the typical kind of back pain that most people experience periodically.

The PSP recommends that the patient continue with one set per day of the extension exercise. However, if she should develop an episode of pain she should increase the frequency of the exercise to 4-6 times per day. She may well be able to resolve the pain herself within a couple of days. However, if she is not able to resolve the pain within a couple of days she is welcome to return to the PSP. She should also continue with the lumbar stabilization exercises. There is no need for follow up. The patient agrees that she feels confident on her own at this point.

For more information about perceived injustice, its role in the perpetuation of chronic pain and strategies to help patients overcome it, the reader is directed to the work of Michael Sullivan, PhD (see recommended reading list and **http://sullivan-painresearch.mcgill.ca/** [accessed 23 April 2016]).

Case 16

History of the Present Illness:

The patient is a 65-year-old man complaining of neck pain and left arm pain. He states that this has been gradually developing over the past eight months or so, but it has markedly worsened over the past two months. Because of this he sought the care of a PSP.

The pain is located in the left lower cervical spine with referral into the left lateral shoulder and upper arm and into the dorsal forearm. The pain is aggravated by driving and occasionally with neck movements, though he states that the pain is fairly constant. Lying supine is the most comfortable position but the pain never completely resolves.

He describes "tingling" in the dorsum of his right hand and "all my fingertips." He denies any weakness although he does note having more difficulty than usual with activities such as buttoning shirts and working a zipper. Upon further questioning he states that "my balance has been off" recently. He denies numbness, paresthesia or focal motor loss in the lower extremities. He denies GI or chest symptoms related to the pain. He denies fever, chills, rigors, constitutional symptoms and unexplained weight loss.

Past Medical History:

Remarkable for prostate cancer five years ago that was treated with radiation and for which he has had regular follow-ups, left total hip replacement three years ago and depression for which he takes buproprion. He sees his primary care physician regularly and has regular cancer screenings.

Review of Systems:

Remarkable for occasional constipation for which he takes a fiber supplement, left knee pain that he attributes to "arthritis" and occasional wheezing.

Social History:

He is married with three grown children. He smokes one pack of cigarettes a day, drinks alcohol occasionally and does not exercise regularly.

Family History:

Remarkable for heart disease in both parents and breast cancer in his mother.

Questionnaire data:

Bournemouth Neck Disability Questionnaire – 38
Average pain intensity over the past week - 7/10
Anxiety item of the Bournemouth Neck Disability Questionnaire – 3/10
Depression item on the Bournemouth Neck Disability Questionnaire – 3/10
Coping Strategies Screening Questionnaire - 3/12
Self-efficacy scale - 2/10
Problem-specific depression scale - 3/10

What are your impressions based on the history?

Diagnostic question #1

Diagnostic question #2

Diagnostic question #3

Physical Examination:

Reveals a well-nourished, pleasant man who appears in no acute distress. Blood pressure is 140/86 on the left. Temperature is 98.6 degrees Fahrenheit. Pulse is 88 per minute. Respirations are 20 per minute.

The Brachial Plexus Tension Test is positive on the left for reproduction of the patient's arm pain. Structural differentiation determines this pain to be of neural origin. Active left cervical rotation and Foraminal Compression Test both reproduce the patient's neck pain and partially reproduce the patient's arm pain. Cervical Distraction Test relieves the patient's arm pain. The Cervical Extension-Rotation Test is positive bilaterally for reproduction of the patient's neck pain. Palpation for segmental tenderness and manual joint palpation both reproduce the patient's neck pain at approximately C5-6 on the left. No significant pain is elicited at this segment on the right side or at other segments on the left side.

The patient is oriented to person, place and time. Heel and toe walking are within normal limits. The patient has some difficulty with tandem walking. The patient is unable to stand in Romberg's position with eyes closed without feeling like he is going to fall. Examination of cranial nerves II through XII is within normal limits. Pupils are equal, round and reactive to light and accommodation. Funduscopic examination is unremarkable. Sensory examination to pinprick reveals stocking distribution hypoesthesia in both feet and lower legs in addition to hypoesthesia over the left thumb and index finger. Pinprick testing of the trunk, starting in the low back and ascending, reveals a sensory level at approximately C5 or C6.

Motor strength is 5/5 bilaterally throughout. Muscle stretch reflexes are 3+ and symmetric throughout. Several beats of clonus are elicited upon rapid dorsiflexion of the ankles on both sides. Plantar responses are upgoing bilaterally. The umbilical reflexes are absent and Hoffman's and Tromner's signs are present bilaterally. The scapulohumeral reflexes are absent bilaterally. The jaw jerk reflex is normal.

What are your impressions based on the history and examination? Is there any indication for diagnostic imaging, specials tests or specialist consult? Why or why not?

Diagnostic question #1:

Diagnostic question #2:

Diagnostic question #3:

Diagnosis:

The diagnosis for the neck and arm pain is left cervical radiculopathy and joint dysfunction (diagnostic question #2). However the patient exhibits central nervous system findings on history and examination that are of concern (diagnostic question #1).

Question for thought: What are the specific historical and examination findings that are of concern with regard to diagnostic question #1?

On history, the patient reported "tingling" in the dorsum of his right hand and into his fingers. This may be attributable to the radiculopathy. However he is also experiencing difficulty with fine motor movements of the hands and with balance.

On examination, findings suggestive of an upper motor neuron lesion are present. Specifically, these are hyper-reflexia throughout, upgoing toes, ankle clonus, absent bilateral abdominal reflexes and present Hoffman's and Tromner's signs. In addition, difficulty standing in Romberg's position suggests involvement of the posterior columns of the spinal cord. Finally, the patient has sensory loss in the lower extremities and spine, with a sensory level at approximately C5 or C6.

Question for thought: Do the examination findings allow for localization of the lesion that allows for decision making regarding diagnostic imaging?

The neurologic examination localizes the lesion to the mid-cervical spine. Specifically, the hyper-reflexia in the upper and lower extremities, Hoffman's and Tromner's and sensory level, combined with the normal cranial nerve examination and normal jaw jerk reflex provides this localization. Thus, the diagnostic imaging modality of choice to identify the cause of these findings is cervical MRI.

What do you tell the patient?

The patient is told that he most likely has cervical radiculopathy along with cervical spondylotic myelopathy, which means cervical spinal stenosis that is causing compression to both his nerve root and his spinal cord. However, a cervical MRI will be needed to clarify the diagnosis.

The patient is sent for cervical MRI and the report and images are reviewed by the PSP. They reveal central and left lateral stenosis with encroachment on both nerve root and the spinal cord at the C5-6 level. There is high signal within the spinal cord at the level of compression. The transverse diameter of the cord is 5.93 mm. The cervical curve is slightly diminished but there was no focal kyphosis. The vertebrae are well aligned and no spondylolisthesis is present. There is no ossification of the posterior longitudinal ligament.

What is the best course of action?

The PSP informs the patient in lay terms that the MRI has confirmed the suspicion of both lateral stenosis causing radiculopathy and central stenosis causing myelopathy (cervical spondylotic myelopathy – see Chapter 2). It is explained that one of his conditions - cervical joint dysfunction combined with radiculopathy related to lateral canal stenosis - is one that can ordinarily be managed at the primary spine care level. However, the myelopathy can only be addressed with surgery. The patient asks if the myelopathy "will get worse if I don't have surgery" and the PSP discusses that this is highly variable but that studies have shown that many patients remain stable while others progress. There are some known risk factors for worsening (excessive range of motion, focal kyphosis or spondylolisthesis at the stenotic segment – see Oshima, et al in Recommended Reading list) but the patient does not have most these. However he does have one important risk factor, that is, the small (5.93mm) transverse diameter of the spinal cord (see Kadanka, et al in Recommended Reading list). It is also discussed that many people with conditions such as his do well with surgery (see Neo, et al in Recommended Reading list).

The PSP recommends that the patient make an appointment with a spine surgeon to discuss his surgical options as well as the risks versus benefits of surgery.

The PSP discusses with the patient that in the meantime, nonsurgical management of the joint dysfunction and radiculopathy can be undertaken to try to reduce the neck and arm pain. The PSP explains that the treatment would consist of gentle and graded mobilization of the left C5-6 joint and of the involved nerve root. This would be done via manual procedures that the PSP would apply along with exercises that the patient would self-apply on his own. The primary risk would be the possibility of worsening of the myelopathy however, the likelihood of this is very small given the fact that low-velocity, low amplitude maneuvers would be applied. In addition, the patient would already have the appointment with the spine surgeon. The PSP explains that there is a good likelihood that the treatment would improve the neck and arm pain but it would not be expected to improve the myelopathy. The PSP further explains that there is a good chance of increased neck and arm pain after the first session, but this would likely be mild or moderate (though severe pain occurs in approximately 10% of patients) and would likely resolve within 24-48 hours. The patient and PSP make a shared decision to undergo a trial of non-surgical management of the radiculopathy.

The treatment consists of manipulation at approximately the C5-6 segment using a supine anterior-to-posterior muscle energy technique and manual neural tensioning maneuvers in the median bias position. Flossing maneuvers are not used in order to minimize movement of the spinal cord. The patient is given a series of neural tensioning maneuvers to perform at home. The patient is seen four times over a two week period.

At re-examination the patient reports 50% improvement in his neck and arm pain. After the first session of manipulation and neural mobilization he experienced moderately increased neck and arm pain that returned to baseline over the following two days and steadily improved after that. He states that the difficulty with fine motor movements of the hands and difficulty with balance have remained unchanged. He has complied well with his home exercises and feels these have been beneficial.

Questionnaire data at re-examination:

Bournemouth Neck Disability Questionnaire - 22
Average pain intensity over the past week - 4/10
Anxiety item of the Bournemouth Neck Disability Questionnaire - 3/10
Depression item on the Bournemouth Neck Disability Questionnaire - 3/10
Coping Strategies Screening Questionnaire - 6/12
Self-efficacy scale - 5/10
Problem-specific depression scale - 3/10

Examination reveals normal heel and toe walking. The patient continues to have some difficulty with tandem walking and standing in Romberg's position with eyes closed but this is no worse than it was at initial exam. Motor strength remains 5/5 bilaterally throughout. Muscle stretch reflexes remain 3+ and symmetric throughout. Plantar responses are upgoing bilaterally.

Question for thought: Why was the Brachial Plexus Tension Test, Foraminal Compression Test, palpation for segmental tenderness and manual joint examination not repeated at re-examination?

For the answer, refer to cases 5 and 13.

The patient had met with the surgeon who recommended an operation that would consist of anterior cervical discectomy with fusion. He states that the surgeon expressed confidence that the operation will stop further progression of the disease and that he might regain some of his hand function as well as some of his balance. The patient had a long discussion with his wife and has decided to go forward with the surgery.

The PSP recommends that the patient continue with the home neural mobilization exercises until the time of surgery. It is agreed that the patient will follow with the surgeon as needed following surgery and will only return to the PSP if he has continued or recurrence of neck and/or arm pain.

Case 17

History of the Present Illness:

The patient is a 39-year-old man who complains of low back pain and left lower extremity pain. This began one week ago when he was cleaning his bathtub. He states that he spent approximately 15 minutes on his knees leaning forward and scrubbing the bathtub. When he got up he experienced "searing pain in my back and down my leg." He states that he fell right to the floor and could not get up because of the pain. His wife called 911 and he was taken to the emergency department of the local hospital. He states that "they shot me up with pain medication" and he had an MRI. He states that he spent "most of the night" in the emergency department before he was finally able to leave with the help of his wife. He was prescribed hydrocodone/ acetaminophen and saw his primary care practitioner three days later (he states that he had been unable to leave the house until then). His primary care practitioner changed his prescription to naproxen and referred him to the PSP.

The pain is located in the lumbosacral area with referral down the left buttock and posterolateral thigh and leg, extending to the ankle. He states that the pain is less severe than it was a first but that he "can still hardly move." He states that any movement can provoke his pain and "if I cough or sneeze it is excruciating." He states that he generally does not have pain when he is lying on either side but that it "takes quite a while before I can get comfortable."

He has "a little numbness" in the dorsum of his left foot. He denies focal motor loss in the lower extremities. He denies numbness or paresthesia in his medial thigh or groin as well as bowel and bladder difficulties. He denies fever, chills, rigors, constitutional symptoms or unexplained weight loss.

Past Medical History:

Otherwise unremarkable. He is not currently taking any medications, other than the naproxen. He sees his primary care practitioner regularly.

Review of Systems:

Unremarkable.

Social History:

He is married with one child who lives with him. He does not smoke and drinks alcohol occasionally. He works as a salesman in an appliance store and has not worked since the onset of his pain. Four weeks ago he had gotten back to a fitness regimen after some 15 years of a sedentary lifestyle. The regimen consisted of 30 minutes of cardio machines five times per week and weight training four times per week. He was "really starting to feel great" and is anxious to get back to this as soon as possible.

Family History:

Unremarkable.

Questionnaire data:

StarT Back 9-item Clinical Tool - 54
Oswestry Low Back Pain and Disability Questionnaire - 80%
Average pain intensity over the past week - 9/10
Fear item on the STarT Back 9-Item Clinical Tool - 10/10
Catastrophizing item of the STarT Back 9-Item Clinical Tool - 8/10
Coping Strategies Screening Questionnaire - 0/12
Self-efficacy scale - 8/10
Problem-specific depression scale - 7/10.

What are your impressions based on the history?

Diagnostic question #1

Diagnostic question #2

Diagnostic question #3

Physical Examination:

Reveals a well-nourished, pleasant man who appears in acute pain. During history taking he sits leaning off to his right and occasionally stands in order to avoid remaining in one position for too long. Blood pressure is 128/76 on the left. Temperature is 98.6 degrees Fahrenheit. Pulse is 80 per minute. Respirations are 20 per minute.

Straight Leg Raise with ankle dorsiflexion is positive on the left at approximately 20 degrees for reproduction of his left leg pain. The pain is immediately abolished with ankle plantar flexion. Well Leg Raise is positive for reproduction of his left leg pain at approximately 60 degrees. End rage loading examination is deferred.

The patient is oriented to person, place and time. Heel, toe and tandem walking are within normal limits, although they provoke pain. Romberg's position is held with eyes closed without difficulty. Sensory examination to pinprick in the lower extremities is unremarkable with the exception of hypoesthesia over the dorsum of the left foot. Motor strength is 5/5 bilaterally in the lower extremities. Muscle stretch reflexes are 2+ and symmetric in the knees and ankles. Plantar responses are downgoing bilaterally.

The MRI report is reviewed and the images are read online. There is a large lateral recess zone disc protrusion at L4-5 on the left contacting the descending L5 nerve root.

What are your impressions based on the history, examination and diagnostic imaging findings?

Diagnostic question #1

Diagnostic question #2

Diagnostic question #3

Diagnosis:

The diagnosis is acute L5 radiculopathy secondary to disc herniation (diagnostic question #2). There are no significant findings of concern with regard to diagnostic question #1. Diagnostic question #3 is not immediately relevant because this is an acute condition, however based on the questionnaire data there significant fear, catastrophizing, problematic coping, low self-efficacy and depression. These will need to be monitored carefully.

For consideration: Why was the end range loading examination deferred?

It was clear based on history and neurodynamic examination that the patient had severe acute radiculopathy secondary to disc herniation. It is very likely that the end range loading examination would exacerbate the nerve root pain without revealing any useful information regarding a Direction of Benefit. However, it is expected that at some point, after the acute nerve root pain reduces in intensity, end range loading examination will be possible, and useful.

What is your initial management strategy?

The diagnosis and management options are discussed with the patient. The PSP explains that there are some cases in which surgery is necessary for a condition like this but the majority of cases can be managed non-surgically. It will be important to introduce exercise as early as possible but this is difficult at present due to the severity of the acute pain. The patient states "I can't continue like this – how long will I be in this much pain?" The PSP explains that this can be quite variable but time is on his side – the intense pain decreases naturally on its own. One option is to wait for this to occur naturally. However, another option that may reduce the pain more quickly is an epidural steroid injection (ESI). This intervention is explained in detail to the patient (see Chapter 11 in Volume I of this series).

The patient states that he would like to reduce the pain as quickly as possible so he can start resuming activity again ("I can't afford to stay out of work any longer!"). The patient is fast-tracked to see an interventional pain specialist for consideration of an ESI. The patient is scheduled to follow up with the PSP 3-5 days after the injection.

The interventional pain specialist agrees that an ESI is clinically indicated and provides the injection. The patient follows up with the PSP four days later and reports 70% improvement in his leg pain. He still has considerable low back pain. He rates the intensity of his leg pain 4/10 and his back pain 7/10.

End rage loading examination is carried out and prone extension is somewhat painful but there is no obstruction. Right side gliding reveals painful obstruction that reproduces the patient's low back pain and part of the patient's lower extremity pain. Specifically, during movement into right side gliding a painful obstruction is noted and the patient reports pain in the left side of the low back extending into the left buttock and posterior thigh, remaining above the knee. There is no change in the pain or the obstruction after 10 repetitions. The PSP explores sustained positioning by moving the patient to the obstructed end range and maintaining this position for 30 seconds. The PSP asks the patient to observe the pain and report any changes during the sustained positioning. The patient reports that the pain lessens in intensity as the position is maintained although there is no change in location. The PSP moves the patient out of the position and asks the patient if he has any pain in neutral standing. The patient reports that he does not. The patient is then again placed in the right side gliding position and moved to the point of obstruction. The PSP notes that the point of obstruction occurs later in the range of motion than it did before. That is, the range of motion in right side gliding prior to the point at which the painful obstruction is met has increased. The PSP asks how this position feels and the patient reports pain in the low back and buttock, but not in the posterior thigh. Also, the patient reports that the pain is less intense than it was upon initial positioning. The patient is again held at that position for 30 seconds. During this time the patient reports that the pain gradually abolishes. The patient is then moved farther into side gliding until another point of obstruction is encountered. The patient reports only low back pain with no buttock or posterior thigh pain in this position.

Question for thought: What is the significance of the findings on the end range loading examination?

It is determined that the nerve root pain is much reduced after the ESI and the disc pain centralized with end range loading examination in right side gliding. This indicates that right side gliding is the Direction of Benefit for exercise. The PSP and patient discuss the next steps.

It is decided that because it appears that the patient is ready to start active exercise (specifically, end range loading in right side gliding) the best course of action is to start right side gliding exercises four to six times per day. The PSP also performs distraction manipulation to decompress the L4-5 disc (see Cox in Recommended Reading list). It is decided that the ESI has been effective enough in reducing the nerve root pain to allow for exercise to be instituted. Therefore, the PSP decides that no further injections are indicated at the present time. The patient is given information on anti-inflammatory nutrition. All communications are carried out in a CBT/ACT context.

The patient states that he loves his job and would like to try to get back to the store as soon as possible, though he does not want to "set myself back." The PSP and patient agree that he should return to work but he should limit flexion and prolonged sitting as much as possible.

The patient is followed four times over the next two weeks at which point re-examination take place. At this time the patient reports 90% improvement. He states that he has occasional mild pain in his low back but no leg pain. He has continued the side gliding exercises and states that these have been quite helpful. He states that his back is "stiff" in the morning and he gets out of bed very slowly. His back "loosens up" soon after doing a set of the side gliding exercise. He is engaging in most normal activities although he states that he is limiting any flexion activities "because I feel like I will tweak it if I bend too much." He has not tried going back to the gym. He reports no new symptoms.

Questionnaire data at re-examination:

StarT Back 9-item Clinical Tool - 16
Oswestry Low Back Pain and Disability Questionnaire - 26%
Average pain intensity over the past week - 2/10
Fear item on the STarT Back 9-Item Clinical Tool - 3/10
Catastrophizing item of the STarT Back 9-Item Clinical Tool - 2/10
Coping Strategies Screening Questionnaire - 10/12
Self-efficacy scale - 1/10
Problem-specific depression scale - 3/10

On examination, right side gliding is mildly painful at end range but there is minimal obstruction. Heel and toe walking are within normal limits. Sensory examination to pinprick in the lower extremities is unremarkable. Motor strength is 5/5 bilaterally in the lower extremities. Muscle stretch reflexes are 2+ and symmetric in the knees and ankles. Hip Extension Test is positive on the right for deviation of the lumbar spine. Prone Instability Test is positive. Active Straight Leg Raise Test is negative.

What is the best course of action at this point?

Both the nerve root pain and the disc pain have resolved. The patient does have signs suggestive of dynamic instability, which is relevant to diagnostic question #3 (i.e., positive Hip Extension Test and Active Straight Leg Raise Test).

It is explained to the patient that the disc and nerve root pain have resolved and he is ready to transition to a stabilization exercise program. The patient asks "has the herniated part of the disc gotten sucked back in?" The PSP explains that the herniation is still there but in all likelihood will "dry up" over the coming weeks or months. The important thing at this point is to train the muscles to protect the disc as much as possible while this is taking place and to minimize disc pressure during everyday activities. The patient asks "you say the herniated piece of disc will dry up. Don't I need that piece of the disc? Will the disc be less healthy after that piece dries up?" The PSP explains that the nucleus of the disc dries up as a normal process of aging and this, in and of itself, does not make the disc vulnerable – this drying up would have happened anyway.

The patient is taught how to bend forward while maintaining a normal lordosis (see Chapter 9 in Volume I of this series). He is also set up with a basic home stabilization exercise program (see Chapter 11 in Volume I of this series). This takes place over the course of three sessions. He is told that if he should experience recurrence of pain he should utilize the right side gliding exercise four times per day and there is a good likelihood that he will be able to self-resolve the pain. The patient is scheduled to follow up in one month. He should return sooner if he has recurrence of pain that he is not able to self-resolve.

Question for thought: On the initial visit, questionnaire data suggested significant psychological factors. Is that still a concern at this point?

On reexamination the questionnaire findings with regard to fear, catastrophizing, coping, self-efficacy and depression are much improved. In the majority of cases these factors improve with effective primary spine care that is carried out in a CBT/ACT context. Therefore, they usually do not need to be addressed directly. But they always need to be monitored in order to identify the minority of patients whose psychological perpetuating factors do not improve with primary spine care (see Case 15).

The patient returns in one month, reporting that he is virtually pain free, although he has had a few mornings in which he has awakened with mild to moderate pain and stiffness that he was able to immediately self-resolve with the side gliding exercise. He has continued with his home stabilization exercise program however he states that he as "slacked off" at times because of his work schedule.

Questionnaire data at re-examination:

StarT Back 9-item Clinical Tool - 3
Oswestry Low Back Pain and Disability Questionnaire - 8%

Average pain intensity over the past week - 1/10
Fear item on the STarT Back 9-Item Clinical Tool - 0/10
Catastrophizing item of the STarT Back 9-Item Clinical Tool - 0/10
Coping Strategies Screening Questionnaire - 12/12
Self-efficacy scale - 1/10
Problem-specific depression scale - 0/10

On examination, right side gliding reveals no painful obstruction. Lumbar extension in the prone position reveals a mild painful obstruction at end range. Hip Extension Test remains positive on the right for deviation of the lumbar spine. Prone Instability Test is negative.

What is the best course of action now?

The patient is set up with a basic "prevention" program, designed to minimize the likelihood of recurrence. This includes one set of 15 repetitions of lumbar extension exercises per day, continued basic stabilization program (the patient is told that four times per week is adequate) and following the principles of maintaining lumbar lordosis with forward bending whenever possible. The PSP reiterates that if he should develop low back pain despite this program (or if he has "decided to be human and slack off the program") he should try the right slide gliding exercises to see if he can self-resolve the problem. If the pain should persist for a few days despite these exercises, the patient should return to the PSP.

The PSP explains that there is no way to guarantee with 100% certainty that he will not have back pain in the future – in fact, since back pain is a normal part of life, it is likely that he will have back pain at some point. However, there is no reason to expect, barring severe trauma, that he will ever be hampered by chronic, nagging back pain, as long as he follows these basic instructions.

Question for thought: If the PSP and patient had decided not to pursue the ESI, would this likely have changed the clinical course and the final outcome?

ESI is designed to bring about quick relief in patients with an inflammatory radiculopathy. There are some cases in which the benefit is long term, but typically it is short term. Also, it is designed to reduce the pain arising from the inflamed nerve root; it is not intended for any other pain source. The reason that the shared decision making process in this case led to referral for consideration for ESI is that both the PSP and patient decided that commencement of active treatments and return to normal activity as quickly as possible were a high priority in this case. Also, it was determined that the nerve root pain was the most disabling aspect of the clinical picture. It was decided that ESI would be a good way to bring about rapid reduction in the nerve root pain, which would lead to rapid return to active (self-)treatment strategies and normal activities.

Note that the ESI reduced the severe radiating leg pain (that portion of the pain that was arising from the nerve root) but not the disc pain (which ended up centralizing with end range loading examination). It is likely that, without the ESI, the institution of end range loading maneuvers to correct the disc derangement (in this case, right side gliding maneuvers) would have been delayed. Thus, the ESI was very beneficial in helping bring about rapid improvement. However, there is every reason to think that the end result of this case would have been the same with or without the ESI; the nerve root inflammation would likely have resolved with the passage of time. Thus, the ESI sped up the process of recovery, but it did not impact the final outcome.

Question for thought: On the final session, when the PSP was setting the patient up with a "prevention program", why did the PSP make it a point to suggest that the patient might "decide to be human and slack off on the program"?

It is important to impress upon the patient that the key to success in limiting the frequency and impact of recurrences is to be consistent with basic exercises (prone extension, stabilization) and spine-sparing habits (maintaining lordosis with forward bending activities) as well as self-management of recurrences if they do arise (end range loading exercises, self-mobilization maneuvers). However, it is also important for the PSP to take guilt out of the picture by giving the patient an "out". The fact is that many patients will "slack off" their exercises and self-management strategies. Some patients, when this happens and they experience a recurrence of pain, will be too ashamed to return to the PSP because they feel guilty about not having followed the PSP's instructions. They might instead seek out a different practitioner who would have no reason to be "mad at them" for slacking off. This is certainly not desirable for the PSP nor beneficial to the patient.

Case 18

History of the Present Illness:

The patient is a 29-year-old woman complaining of low back pain. She works as a certified nursing assistant and eight months ago was assisting a patient in transferring from a chair to a bed when she felt sudden pain. She states that she tried to finish her shift but pain prevented her from doing so. She reported the incident to her supervisor and went home. The next day she awoke with severe pain and attended a walk-in center. She was prescribed naproxen, cyclobenzaprine and tramadol and was referred to the occupational medicine physician of a local orthopedic group. She states that this physician referred her for "physical therapy", which consisted of stretching exercises and manual mobilization. She states that she had some relief immediately after the sessions but there was no lasting benefit. After three months she stopped physical therapy on her own and returned to the occupational medicine physician who referred her for an MRI.

The patient states that the MRI "showed that I have a disc problem" and that the occupational medicine physician told her that she needed injections. The patient underwent a series of three ESIs without benefit. The occupational medicine physician referred her to an orthopedic spine surgeon who told her that hers was not a surgical case. The patient confides that she felt that both the occupational medicine physician and the orthopedic surgeon made her feel like she was "faking it." She states that she feels the physical therapists were kind to her and "tried to help but they couldn't." She saw her primary care practitioner who referred her for primary spine care. She has not worked in any capacity since the original incident.

The pain is located in the right lumbosacral area without radiation or referral. She states that "everything I do aggravates the pain" although upon questioning she indicates that she can walk without pain. She has no pain when standing from a sitting position and she has no pain when sitting. She has trouble finding a comfortable position when lying down although she states that eventually she is able to "relax into it" when she is in bed. She denies numbness, paresthesia or motor loss in the lower extremities. She denies GI or GU symptoms related to the pain. She denies fever, chills, rigors, constitutional symptoms and unexplained weight loss.

Her job entails caring for elderly residents of a nursing home. This includes bathing residents and helping them transfer from bed to chair and getting up out of a chair.

Past Medical History:

Otherwise unremarkable. She is not currently taking any medications. She sees her primary care practitioner regularly.

Review of Systems:

Remarkable for occasional heartburn when she eats spicy foods, and depression due to her prolonged disability.

Social History:

She is single with an eight-year-old son who lives with her. When she was working her mother cared for her son. She smokes one-half pack of cigarettes per day ("but never in front of my son"), does not drink alcohol and takes daily walks for exercise.

Family History:

Remarkable for hypertension and type 2 diabetes in her mother and older sister and heart disease in her father.

Questionnaire data:

StarT Back 9-item Clinical Tool - 48
Oswestry Low Back Pain and Disability Questionnaire - 80%
Average pain intensity over the past week - 8/10
Fear item on the STarT Back 9-Item Clinical Tool - 9/10
Catastrophizing item of the STarT Back 9-Item Clinical Tool - 9/10
Coping Strategies Screening Questionnaire - 2/12
Self-efficacy scale - 8/10
Problem-specific depression scale - 8/10

What are your impressions based on the history?

Diagnostic question #1

Diagnostic question #2

Diagnostic question #3

Physical Examination:

Reveals a well-nourished, pleasant woman who appears in no acute distress. End range loading exam reveals painful obstruction on extension that reproduces the patient's pain. The pain progressively increases in intensity with repetition and overpressure. Side gliding to either side and flexion are unremarkable. Sacroiliac provocation maneuvers are unremarkable. The Extension-Rotation Test is positive to the right for reproduction of the patient's low back pain. The Hip Extension Test is positive bilaterally for deviation of the lumbar spine. Active Straight Leg Raise Test is positive. Prone Instability Test is negative.

The patient is oriented to person, place and time. Heel, toe and tandem walking are within normal limits although they provoke pain. Romberg's position is held with eyes closed without difficulty. Sensory examination to pinprick in the lower extremities is unremarkable. Motor strength is 5/5 bilaterally in the lower extremities. Muscle stretch reflexes are 2+ and symmetric in the knees and ankles. Plantar responses are downgoing bilaterally.

The MRI images and report are obtained. They reveal a small central disc herniation at L5-S1.

What are your impressions based on the history and examination? Is there any indication for diagnostic imaging, specials tests or specialist consult? Why or why not? Specifically, what is the significance of the MRI finding?

Diagnostic question #1:

Diagnostic question #2:

Diagnostic question #3:

Diagnosis:

The diagnosis is lumbosacral facet joint dysfunction (diagnostic question #2) with dynamic instability and significant psychological factors (diagnostic question #3). Of great concern as a perpetuating factor is the eight months of continuous disability. There are no significant findings of concern with regard to diagnostic question #1.

The MRI finding of small central disc herniation at L5-S1 is incidental and of no clinical significance. Despite what she reportedly was told by the occupational medicine physician, the patient does not have "a disc problem".

The PSP opines that the patient is not totally disabled and that she is capable working at a Light Physical Demand Level (PDL) with a lifting limit of 20 pounds and no patient transfers.

Question for thought: What is the significance of the PSP opining on disability and Physical Demand Level (PDL)?

In all patients, particularly those with work related spine problems, managing disability is as important as managing the other aspects of the problem. In other words, it is important not only to address the specific diagnostic factors identified through the CRISP® protocols, but also to guide the patient in returning to normal activities.

In addition, the PSP can expect others involved in the case, such as Workers' Compensation case managers, work conditioning/ work hardening facilities, attorneys and judges, to ask for opinions regarding what work related activities the patient is capable of. Determining work capabilities is not an exact science, however a reasonable estimation of occupational capabilities is possible in the majority of patients. Also, the estimation of disability status is not entirely separate from patient care; they are inter-related. In other words, opining about work capabilities needs to be part of the conversation with the patient as well as with others involved in the case.

It is common for patients to underestimate what they are capable of. This partly arises from the understandable fear for many patients of "re-injury" if they were to engage in activities they feel they are not "ready for". This fear is often particularly marked in the patient whose pain started at work, since returning to normal activity means returning to the very environment at which the problem initiated. This is why it is essential for the PSP to function as "leader" in guiding the patient along the path from "disability" to "ability". Part of this involves establishing a baseline functional level at which the patient is capable, to serve as the foundation of recovery and return to a normal life.

Important in determining disability level is the understanding that extremely few patients with spine related disorders are "totally disabled". "Totally disabled" means that the individual is incapable of performing any kind of work for any amount of time. People who are bedridden can be considered totally disabled. If the patient is able to attend a doctor's office or therapy center, it is highly questionable that the person is totally disabled. There are some exceptions to this, certainly, but in the majority of cases, individuals who can attend a health care facility can also attend work.

Now, it may be that the patient's employer does not have a position available that can accommodate their current limitations. However, that is between the patient and the employer – it is the job of the PSP to determine what level of work activity the person is *capable of*, independent of whether there is a job available that matches that capability.

So the vast majority of patients the PSP sees will either have "no disability" - (i.e. capable of performing normal work duties) or "partial disability" - i.e., capable of certain work duties but not all work duties that are required by the patient's job.

The Physical Demand Level estimated for each patient should be based on the categories provided by the Dictionary of Occupational Titles. These categories are summarized here but details can be found at **http://www.occupationalinfo.org/appendxc_1.html #STRENGTH** [accessed 23 April 2016].

Sedentary:
- Exerting up to 10 pounds occasionally
- And/or exerting a negligible amount frequently
- Primarily sitting
- Occasional walking and standing

Light:
- Exerting up to 20 pounds occasionally
- And/or exerting up to 10 pounds frequently
- Significant walking and standing with negligible weight

Medium:
- Exerting 20-50 pounds occasionally
- And/or exerting up to 10-25 pounds frequently
- And/or exerting up to 10 pounds constantly

Heavy:
- Exerting 50-100 pounds occasionally
- And/or 25-50 pounds frequently
- And/or 10-20 pounds constantly

Very heavy
- Exerting greater than 100 pounds occasionally
- And/or greater than 50 pounds frequently
- And/or greater than 20 pounds constantly

Sometimes hybrid designations are used if an individual's PDL falls between two categories, e.g., Light-Medium, Medium-Heavy, etc.

What is your initial management strategy?

The diagnosis is explained to the patient and she is told that she has a good likelihood for recovery but this will require a concerted team effort on the part of the patient and the PSP. It is explained that recovery will require determination and consistency on the part of the patient and the patient is assured that the PSP, perhaps with the help of others who are utilized along the way, will guide her along the path to recovery.

It is explained that one of the most important aspects of "therapy" will be return to some form of work as soon as possible. Work is healthy and therapeutic and the sooner return to work occurs the more rapid and robust her recovery will be.

The PSP asks the patient how she feels about her job. She states, "It's OK; it's not a great job but they generally treat me well. And it gets me out of the house – I am tired of sitting around all day. I get my son off to school in the morning, then I sit around and watch television. It's boring. And I love my son, but it is good to have another aspect to my life other than being a mother."

The patient states that, "I have been told that I shouldn't try to go back to work until I am 100%, otherwise I might injure myself even worse. Then I will really have serious problems." The PSP replies, "This is very understandable, and it seems logical. Which doctors told you this?" The patient answers "Oh it wasn't any doctors, it was friends who have had similar problems." The PSP says, "I can understand this concern. Do you follow other medical advice from these same friends?" The patient says, "Well not really but this is my body and my life and I am concerned about my future." The PSP says, "Of course you are. So am I. The idea of not returning to work until you are 100% is a very common misconception."

The PSP further explains that "a large number of studies have looked at the reasons people who develop back pain at work fail to recover and study after study has shown that it is not the people who return to work before they are 100% who end up 'really having serious problems'. It is the people who *don't return to work soon enough* who are at risk. I would not want you to be at risk of developing serious problems, so I am going to recommend that return to work activities, in a gradual fashion if necessary, should be an important aspect of our efforts together. But we can talk more specifically about that when the time comes."

The PSP asks the patient, "Are you willing to work with me in doing whatever it takes to get better?" The patient says she is, but seems to be somewhat reluctant. It is difficult for the PSP to determine whether this reluctance is a reflection of lack of confidence (self-efficacy), lack of motivation, fear, or a combination of the three. But then the patient says, close to sobbing, "I just want to get my life back!" The PSP asks, "What does getting your life back mean to you?" She says, "Being able to do the things I used to do – take care of my son without burdening other people, do my job, have some fun." The PSP then asks, "What if we set that as our goal – for you to get your life back?" The patient responds, "I'm all for it." But, again, she does not seem very convincing.

The initial treatment consists of self-mobilization maneuvers targeted at the right lumbosacral facet joints, as well as manipulation targeting these joints. After the initial few sessions, stabilization exercises are instituted. The patient is also given the pelvic tilt exercise and then transitioned to the "Good Morning" exercise in order to prepare to teach her how to maintain a neutral lumbar lordosis while performing activities that require flexion (see Chapter 9 in Volume I of this series). The patient is given information on anti-inflammatory nutrition. All communications are carried out in a CBT/ACT context.

The PSP puts a call in to the case manager who is assigned to the patient's Workers' Compensation case to find out if there are any light-duty positions available at her place of employment and finds out that there are not. The PSP counsels the patient on increasing her home activities, starting with some light house work that she had previously been avoiding. She is also provided with smoking cessation information.

On the sixth session re-examination takes place. At this time the patient reports 30% improvement. She states that her pain intensity has lessened overall and that she "feels great after the treatments" but her pain returns shortly after. She is able to lessen the pain with the self-mobilization exercises but "it's not as good as when you do it." She states that she has been doing the initial-level stabilization exercises but states that "those are boring so I don't always do them." The PSP asks how often the patient is doing the stabilization exercises (the recommendation was twice per day) and she states that she gets in at least one set per day, but sometimes she forgets to do the second.

The patient states that she has started to do some additional housework, even carrying the laundry basket down to the laundry room ("I hate to see my 60-year-old mother doing it!"). This gives her some pain but she was surprised that she was able to do it at all.

Questionnaire data at re-examination:

StarT Back 9-item Clinical Tool - 46
Oswestry Low Back Pain and Disability Questionnaire - 60%
Average pain intensity over the past week - 6/10
Fear item on the STarT Back 9-Item Clinical Tool - 8/10
Catastrophizing item of the STarT Back 9-Item Clinical Tool - 7/10
Coping Strategies Screening Questionnaire - 4/12
Self-efficacy scale - 6/10
Problem-specific depression scale - 7/10

On examination, Hip Extension Test remains positive bilaterally for deviation of the lumbar spine. Active Straight Leg Raise Test remains positive. Prone Instability Test remains negative.

What is the best course of action now?

The patient has experienced clear improvement in pain and has begun to increase her functional abilities. The improvement in pain intensity can be considered minimally clinically meaningful (two points on the Numeric Rating Scale) and the improvement in Oswestry score falls just short of the threshold for clinically meaningful change (25% change *versus* the accepted threshold of 30% to be considered clinically meaningful). She has begun to increase her activities, but is still far from the point at which transition back to work on a full-duty basis is realistic.

The patient remains out of work, there being no light-duty work available and she is not ready to return to her full-duty position. She has residual signs of dynamic instability. It has now been nearly nine months since she last worked and she is showing signs of increased functional ability and self-efficacy, in addition to decreased pain intensity. However she still has significant pain and disability as well as psychological distress.

The PSP decides that it is best to transition her to a Work Hardening program. The strategy is for her to continue with the stabilization exercises and to start work simulation activities in the Work Hardening program. In addition, she will meet with the behavioral health specialists to help with the psychological barriers to recovery.

This is discussed with the patient and she is reluctant about stopping manipulation because "that gives me so much relief." She is also nervous about work simulation activities for fear of "re-injuring myself."

The PSP tells the patient that this is certainly understandable given all she has been through. It is also made clear to the patient that she does not *have to* do work hardening. The patient asks, "What is the alternative?" To which the PSP responds "What do you think?"

The patient does not have an immediate answer, so the PSP asks her what the two of them had discussed on the initial session was her primary goal in their work together. "To get my life back!" is the patient's reply. The PSP then asks, "what about 'relief', was that the primary goal?" "Well the relief certainly is great. But the *primary* goal? No, pain relief was secondary." The PSP then asks, "So what do you think your alternatives are?" The patient responds "staying the way I am or trying to get better?" To which the PSP responds, "From the first time we met, I knew you were smart!"

The PSP explains that the purpose of manipulation is to decrease the intensity of the pain arising from the joint so that transition to more active approaches, such as exercise and, in her case, work simulation, can be instituted. So manipulation is a "means" in helping her to her primary goal, not an "end", in and of itself.

For consideration: Many patients might not realize this until they are challenged to really think about it. For most, the primary goal of recovery is not "relief" *per se* but improvement in the ability to engage in meaningful life activities, both personal and work related. They might think, on the surface, that they want "relief" or "to make the pain go away" but in fact, when it comes down to it, what they *really* want is to be able to live a life that is consistent with their values, without interference by pain. However, if we never bring out in patients what is *really* important to them, they might not ever realize this and might fall into the trap that "relief" is the answer to their problems. As was discussed in Chapter 8 of Volume I of this series, this can actually lead patients *away* from recovery because focusing on "making the pain go away" actually increases pain perception (see Notebaert, et al in Recommended Reading list). It gives the pain power that it would not otherwise possess.

The PSP reminds the patient that she will be able to continue her self-mobilization maneuvers, which are designed to further the process of reducing joint pain that had been begun by manipulation. The effect of the self-mobilization maneuvers might not be as dramatic as that of manipulation but are more enduring, since the patient can do these daily.

The PSP also discusses with the patient that it is normal to be nervous about returning to work-related activities after experiencing a severe and protracted episode of back pain. However, the patient is assured that the physical and occupational therapists at the Work Hardening facility are experts in identifying her current level of ability and gradually progressing her to increasingly higher-level activities. With that, however, it is explained that she should expect to be challenged somewhat, even in performing activities that she is not sure she is quite ready for. She is assured that this will always occur under close expert guidance. This is the best way to bring about steady improvement and, ultimately, recovery.

The PSP asks the patient, given what they have discussed, which she thinks is more useful in her attaining her primary goal, continued manipulation or facing the challenge of work hardening. The patient asks, "But what if I have a flare up of pain while I am there?" The PSP asks, "What do you think you should do if that happens?" She answers "I wouldn't know what to do!" The PSP asks, "What has been helpful with the pain so far?" After thinking for a moment, she replies "The treatment you provided me." To which the PSP responds, "Do you think it would be more accurate to say 'the treatment we engaged in together'?" The patient chuckles and nods in agreement. She states that she is willing to give work hardening a try.

The patient is directed to return to the PSP in three weeks. But she is welcomed to return sooner if she has a flare-up of pain that she is not able to manage herself with self-treatment strategies she has been given.

For consideration: Did you notice the PSP's use of Motivational Interviewing with this patient? See Chapter 9 in Volume I of this series and the book by Rollnick, Miller and Butler in the Recommended Reading list.

At three-week follow up the patient reports 70% improvement. She states that she has progressed well in Work Hardening and has begun doing simulated patient transfers with a 40 kg dummy. She has also been doing strength training. She has met with the psychologist three times to learn relaxation techniques as well as to challenge her beliefs about back pain and about her capabilities.

The initial report that the PSP received from the Work Hardening facility had indicated that Functional Capacity Evaluation (FCE) had determined the patient to be functioning at a Light PDL. The Work Hardening facility had determined, based on discussion with the patient's employer as well as a written job description, that the patient's required PDL for return to work is Medium-Heavy. The most recent FCE, performed the day before her follow-up visit to the PSP, determined that she is now functioning at a Medium PDL.

Questionnaire data at re-examination:

StarT Back 9-item Clinical Tool - 30
Oswestry Low Back Pain and Disability Questionnaire - 20%
Average pain intensity over the past week - 4/10
Fear item on the STarT Back 9-Item Clinical Tool - 4/10
Catastrophizing item of the STarT Back 9-Item Clinical Tool - 3/10
Coping Strategies Screening Questionnaire - 7/12
Self-efficacy scale - 2/10
Problem-specific depression scale - 3/10

On examination, Hip Extension Test, Prone Instability Test and Active Straight Leg Raise Test are all negative.

What is the best course of action now?

The patient has progressed well in Work Hardening and has almost reached the required PDL for return to work. What is more, her fear, catastrophizing and self-efficacy have markedly improved. The PSP comments on what a great job she is doing and discusses that she is close to being able to finally get back to her usual work. The patient expresses some trepidation about this although she is happy with the progress she has made.

The PSP explains that being nervous about going back to usual work duties after this long, and given all the difficulties she has been through, is perfectly normal. She is reminded that her situation is completely different than it was just a couple of months ago – her condition has improved, she has become stronger and better able to perform work-related activities and she is more confident in her ability to recover. The PSP asks the patient to "remind me one more time so I don't forget – what was our goal at the very beginning of all this?" The patient responds with an enthusiastic, "To get my life back!"

The patient continues Work Hardening and returns to the PSP in three weeks. At that point she reports 80% improvement. She states that she has further increased the amount of weight she is lifting at the Work Hardening facility and has been doing simulated patient transfers with a 70 kg dummy without pain. She states that she feels ready to return to full-duty work although she is "pretty nervous that I might tweak it."

The most recent FCE from the Work Hardening facility indicates that the patient is functioning at a Medium-Heavy PDL. Specifically, the report states that she is "exerting 75 pounds occasionally and 30 pounds frequently" and that she is "able to tolerate repetitive bending with good body mechanics."

Questionnaire data at re-examination:

StarT Back 9-item Clinical Tool - 8
Oswestry Low Back Pain and Disability Questionnaire - 6%
Average pain intensity over the past week - 2/10
Fear item on the STarT Back 9-Item Clinical Tool - 1/10
Catastrophizing item of the STarT Back 9-Item Clinical Tool - 1/10
Coping Strategies Screening Questionnaire - 10/12
Self-efficacy scale - 1/10
Problem-specific depression scale - 1/10

On examination, Hip Extension Test, Prone Instability Test and Active Straight Leg Raise Test all remain negative.

The PSP and patient discuss that she is fully recovered and ready to return to work on a full-duty basis. The PSP explains that it is very likely that she will have some back pain at first when she returns to her usual work activities. It is explained that in the vast majority of cases this reflects "pain memory" rather than re-injury. The "pain memory" typically fades gradually over a period of days or, occasionally, weeks. If the patient has severe pain, or pain that persists beyond the initial two weeks she should return to the PSP.

The PSP recommends that she continue her home lumbar stabilization exercises once per day and instructs her in performing lumbar extension exercises once per day for 10-15 repetitions. She should continue utilizing the body mechanics techniques she learned in Work Hardening.

The PSP recommends that the patient schedule a one-month follow to make sure she remains on track and to trouble shoot any problems that may arise. The patient agrees that this is a good idea.

At one-month follow up the patient reports that, as expected, the first week of work "was tough". When asked to describe this she states, "I was really sore at the end of each workday, but the soreness became slightly less with each passing day. There was one day when I had to do a number of patient transfers and I was hurting all day. But I used my self-mobilization exercises and by the next day I was OK. Gradually the soreness at the end of the day stopped and now I am doing fine". She states that she has continued with her home exercises and has been applying her body mechanics techniques ("I really feel the difference when I occasionally forget").

The PSP congratulates the patient on a job well done, emphasizing that without her determination, openness and consistency, the positive outcome would not have been possible. There is no need for the patient to schedule any more appointments but she is welcomed to return if she should have any future problems.

Recommended Reading:

Balaji VR, Chin KF, Tucker S, Wilson LF, Casey AT. Recovery of severe motor deficit secondary to herniated lumbar disc prolapse: is surgical intervention important? A systematic review. Eur Spine J. 2014 Sep;23(9):1968-77.

Blumenfeld H. Neuroanatomy Through Clinical Cases. 2nd ed. Sunderland, MA: Sinaouer Associates, 2010.

Bogduk N. Evidence-informed management of chronic low back pain with facet injections and radiofrequency neurotomy. Spine J. 2008 Jan-Feb;8(1):56-64.

Christensen ST, Hartvigsen J. Spinal curves and health: a systematic critical review of the epidemiological literature dealing with associations between sagittal spinal curves and health. J Manipulative Physiol Ther. 2008 Nov-Dec;31(9):690-714.

Cox, JM. Low Back Pain: Mechanism, Diagnosis, and Treatment, 7th edition, 2011, Philadelphia: Lippincott, Williams & Wilkins. http://www.coxtechnic.com/ [accessed 19 October 2015]

Gore DR, Sepic SB, Gardner GM. Roentgenographic findings of the cervical spine in asymptomatic people. Spine (Phila Pa 1976). 1986;11:521–4.

Gore DR. Roentgenographic findings in the cervical spine in asymptomatic persons a ten-year follow-up. Spine (Phila Pa 1976). 2001;26(22).

Gudavalli M, Cambron J, McGregor M, Jedlicka J, Keenum M, Ghanayem A, Patwardhan A. A randomized clinical trial and subgroup analysis to compare flexion-distraction with active exercise for chronic low back pain. Eur Spine 2005;15(7):1070-1082.

Johansson MP, Baann Liane MS, Bendix T, Kasch H, Kongsted A. Does cervical kyphosis relate to symptoms following whiplash injury? Man Ther 2011;16(4):378-83.

Kadanka Z, Bednarik J, Vohanka S, Vlach O, Stejskal L, Chaloupka R, et al. Conservative treatment versus surgery in spondylotic cervical myelopathy: a prospective randomised study. Eur Spine J. 2000 Dec;9(6):538-44.

Kadanka Z, Mares M, Bednarik J, Smrcka V, Krbec M, Chaloupka R, et al. Predictive factors for mild forms of spondylotic cervical myelopathy treated conservatively or surgically. Eur J Neurol. 2005 Jan;12(1):16-24.

Neo M, Fujibayashi S, Takemoto M, Nakamura T. Clinical results of and patient satisfaction with cervical laminoplasty for considerable cord compression with only slight myelopathy. Eur Spine J. 2012 Feb;21(2):340-6.

Notebaert L, Crombez G, Vogt J, De Houwer J, Van Damme S, Theeuwes J. Attempts to control pain prioritize attention towards signals of pain: an experimental study. Pain 2011;152(5):1068-73

Oshima Y, Seichi A, Takeshita K, Chikuda H, Ono T, Baba S, et al. Natural course and prognostic factors in patients with mild cervical spondylotic myelopathy with increased signal intensity on T2-weighted magnetic resonance diagnostic imaging. Spine. 2012 Oct 15;37(22):1909-13.

Overdevest GM, Vleggeert-Lankamp CL, Jacobs WC, Brand R, Koes BW, Peul WC, et al. Recovery of motor deficit accompanying sciatica--subgroup analysis of a randomized controlled trial. Spine J. 2014 Sep 1;14(9):1817-24.

Rollnick S, Miller WR, Butler CC. Motivational Interviewing in Health Care: Helping Patients Change Behavior. New York; The Guilford Press, 2008.

Salvi FJ, Jones JC, Weigert BJ. The assessment of cervical myelopathy. Spine J 2006;6(6 Suppl):S182-9.

Spijker-Huiges A, Vermeulen K, Winters JC, van Wijhe M, van der Meer K. Epidural steroids for lumbosacral radicular syndrome compared to usual care: quality of life and cost utility in general practice. Arch Phys Med Rehabil. 2015 Mar;96(3):381-7.

Sullivan MJ, Adams H, Martel MO, Scott W, Wideman T. Catastrophizing and perceived injustice: risk factors for the transition to chronicity after whiplash injury. Spine (Phila Pa 1976) 2011;36(25 Suppl):S244-9.

Sullivan MJ, Scott W, Trost Z. Perceived injustice: a risk factor for problematic pain outcomes. Clin J Pain. 2012;28(6):484-8.

Sullivan MJL, Davidson N, Garfinkel B, Siriapaipant, N, Scott W. Perceived Injustice is Associated with Heightened Pain Behavior and Disability in Individuals with Whiplash Injuries. Psychol Inj Law. 2009;2(3-4):238-47.

Tortolani PJ, Carbone JJ, Quartararo LG. Greater trochanteric pain syndrome in patients referred to orthopedic spine specialists. Spine J. 2002 Jul-Aug;2(4):251-4.

Webster BS, Bauer AZ, Choi Y, Cifuentes M, Pransky GS. Iatrogenic consequences of early magnetic resonance diagnostic imaging in acute, work-related, disabling low back pain. Spine (Phila Pa 1976) 2013;38(22):1939-46.

Webster BS, Cifuentes M. Relationship of early magnetic resonance diagnostic imaging for work-related acute low back pain with disability and medical utilization outcomes. J Occup Environ Med. 2010 Sep;52(9):900-7.

Williams BS, Cohen SP. Greater trochanteric pain syndrome: a review of anatomy, diagnosis and treatment. Anesth Analg 2009 May;108(5):1662-70.

CPSIA information can be obtained
at www.ICGtesting.com
Printed in the USA
LVHW021725030822
725003LV00005B/188